The Principles and Practice of Nutritional Support

Stephen J.D. O'Keefe

The Principles and Practice of Nutritional Support

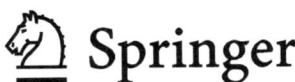 Springer

Stephen J.D. O'Keefe, M.B.B.S. (London), M.D. (London),
  M.Sc., Human Nutrition (London), M.R.C.S. (England),
  F.R.C.P. (England)
Director of Nutrition and Intestinal Health
Division of Gastroenterology
Department of Medicine
University of Pittsburgh
Pittsburgh, PA, USA

ISBN 978-1-4939-1778-5   ISBN 978-1-4939-1779-2 (eBook)
DOI 10.1007/978-1-4939-1779-2
Springer New York Heidelberg Dordrecht London

Library of Congress Control Number: 2014952901

Printed on acid-free paper

Springer is part of Springer Science+Business Media (www.springer.com)

This book is dedicated to my family and other animals

*Liz, Alex, Sebastian, Fergus the German shepherd,
Mhlope the Golden Retriever, and Zambezi the
Siamese cat, who could never understand why
I sometimes chose to write inside rather than
join them running in the fields.*

Foreword

Published in 1959, Dr. Francis D. Moore's textbook on *Metabolic Care of the Surgical Patient* was the only volume on the subject by a single author. It used case studies to cover the years from 1941 to 1952 and was followed by a textbook based on his publications and lectures during that time.

Much has changed since then. In a seminal 1968 article, Stanley Dudrick, M.D., and colleagues showed that total parenteral nutrition (TPN) accelerated healing and improved prognoses in patients with poorly functional gastrointestinal tracts and catabolic disease processes. Their research, first in 6 beagle puppies and then in a clinical trial in 30 patients with chronic gastrointestinal disease, established TPN as a valuable way to address malnutrition in hospitalized patients (1).

The second advance came in 1974, when Bistrian et al. (2) found that approximately 50% of surgical patients in an urban hospital had protein-calorie malnutrition. This high prevalence spurred the development of dedicated nutrition support services to prevent malnutrition in critically ill patients. At that time, the stress response to injury and infection in those with baseline malnutrition was of particular concern (3).

In the following decade, the focus shifted to overfeeding and the risk of hyperglycemia. Cases of mild malnutrition now outnumbered those of severe malnutrition, yet treatment remained the same: 44 kcal/kg and over 550 kcal from lipids, with the rest from dextrose (4). This formula increased infections and only significantly reduced noninfective sequelae in the 5% of patients with severe malnutrition. However, it put the remaining 95% at risk for hyperglycemia, infections, and subsequent complications that led to increased morbidity and mortality (5).

The American College of Chest Physicians consensus statement (6) defined an adequate dose of TPN as 20–25 kcal/kg and 1.5 g of protein/kg per day. In a landmark study by Van den Berghe et al. (7), early and adequate TPN combined with aggressive glucose control achieved normoglycemia and decreased hospital mortality by 33% in surgical ICU patients. That report also validated data from a high-quality meta-analysis (8) that compared enteral and PN in ICU patients. It showed that early and adequate feeding significantly decreased mortality and so did tight glucose control, with the use of exogenous insulin to hold glucose levels at less than 150 mg/dl for at least the first 3 days in the ICU (9).

In critically ill patients, administration of tight glucose control should be managed by highly trained RNs and certified medical assistants; nutrition support services should be led by physician-directed teams to provide the highest quality of care. The mode, timing, and adequacy of nutritional support affect glycemic control and outcomes. The delivery of correctly formulated and safely delivered nutritional and metabolic support is a matter of life and death in surgical and critical care units (10). Yet nutrition support practices vary widely and would benefit from well-designed and executed randomized controlled trials that can help define optimal procedures for nutritional support.

Dr. O'Keefe's research is in the field of nutritional gastroenterology. Most of his investigations are translational, evaluating the physiological and pathophysiological responses to dietary intake and interventional feeding. He entered the field via the London School of Hygiene and Tropical Medicine, London, where he mastered the use of isotopic measurements of body nitrogen dynamics in surgery.

He served his fellowship in internal medicine and nutrition at the Center for the Study of Nutrition Medicine at the Deaconess Hospital, Harvard Medical School, Boston, Massachusetts, and the MIT Department of Nutrition and Food Science, Cambridge, Massachusetts. He is now a Professor of Medicine and Medical Director of the Small Intestinal Rehabilitation and Transplant Center at the University of Pittsburgh Division of Gastroenterology, Hepatology, and Nutrition in Pittsburgh, Pennsylvania.

In his textbook, Dr. O'Keefe has followed in the footsteps of Dr. Moore, combining his publications and academic presentations over 40 years to describe the science of the metabolic response to acute illness and injury and the use of interventional nutritional support to improve patient outcomes and survival.

The volume starts with a discussion of cellular function to provide the foundation for understanding the basic metabolic and nutritional needs of single cells to maintain life. It progresses from there to the second half of the book, which focuses on nutrition support. The following chapters offer a framework for best practice based on randomized controlled trials or experimental studies combined with years of clinical experience.

The text emphasizes the importance of well-organized nutritional support teams, and drives home the message that the field is dynamic, with advances that require specialized knowledge to maximize patient outcomes. It covers nutritional support under varying conditions, such as home parenteral and enteral feeding, and diseases that affect digestion, absorption, and assimilation of nutrients. It ends with chapters on obesity and postbariatric surgery and nutritional support of the elderly. Dr. O'Keefe's wife, Elizabeth, an academic geriatric physician, is responsible for this superb contribution to the field.

The roles of food reward and cognition are dramatically changed by certain bariatric procedures. The use of new technologies, such as functional magnetic resonance imaging (fMRI), has enhanced our insight into these changes in ways that might lead to safer surgeries (e.g., sleeve gastrectomy) as well as new directions for medications that will reset the optimal homeostatic body weight (11, 12).

Dr. O'Keefe's textbook will serve as an effective resource for diverse health-care professionals, from medical school students to nurses, surgeons, and physicians. It will educate those just entering the field and provide an updated reference for those with years of experience in the use of nutrition support to preserve and sustain life in critically ill patients.

George L. Blackburn, M.D., Ph.D.

References

1. Dudrick SJ, Wilmore DW, Vars HM, Rhoads JE. Long-term total parenteral nutrition with growth, development, and positive nitrogen balance. Surgery. 1968;64:134–42.
2. Bistrian BR, Blackburn GL, Hallowell E, Heddle R. Protein status of general surgical patients. JAMA. 1974;230:858–60.
3. Bistrian BR. Recent advances in parenteral and enteral nutrition: a personal perspective. JPEN J Parenter Enteral Nutr. 1990;14:329–34.
4. Buzby GP, Knox LS, Crosby LO, et al. Study protocol: a randomized clinical trial of total parenteral nutrition in malnourished surgical patients. Am J Clin Nutr. 188;47(2 suppl):366–81.
5. The Veterans Affairs Total Parenteral Nutrition Cooperative Study Group. Perioperative total parenteral nutrition in surgical patients. N Engl J Med. 1991;325:525–32.
6. Cerra FB, Benitez MR, Blackburn GL, et al. Applied nutrition in ICU patients. A consensus statement of the American College of Chest Physicians. Chest. 1997;111:769–78.
7. van den Berghe G, Wouters P, Weekers F, et al. Intensive insulin therapy in critically ill patients. N Engl J Med. 2001;345:1359–67.
8. Simpson F, Doig GS. Parenteral vs. enteral nutrition in the critically ill patient: a meta-analysis of trials using the intention to treat principle. Intensive Care Med. 2005;31:12–23.
9. Malhotra A. Intensive insulin in intensive care. N Engl J Med. 2006;354:516–8.
10. Blackburn GL, Wollner S, Bistrian BR. Nutrition support in the intensive care unit. Arch Surg. 2010;145:533–8.
11. Shin AC, Berthoud HR. Obesity surgery: happy with less or eternally hungry? Trends Endocrinol Metab. 2013;24:101–8.
12. Madsbad S, Dirksen C, Holst JJ. Mechanisms of changes in glucose metabolism and body-weight after bariatric surgery. Lancet Diabetes Endocrinol. 2014;2:152–64.

Author's Preface

The wonderful thing about food is that everybody – physicians, nurses, pharmacists, dietitians and patients and their families – believes in the importance of nutrition in the maintenance of good health. The problem arises when sickness intervenes and the patient, or person, cannot eat. Until relatively recently, we simply waited for the illness to resolve, for appetite to return, and for normal eating to resume and catch up what was lost during the period of inanition. However, the dramatic advances in the development of nutritional support techniques in the 70s changed all of this. In particular, the use of intravenous feeding, or parenteral nutrition (PN), meant, for the first time, that there was no situation where feeding could not be maintained during sickness.

Unfortunately, the faith in the healing powers of feeding often led to the over enthusiastic use, supported by demands from the family, of interventional feeding in the previously well-nourished. The recognition that all forms of interventional feeding, in particular parenteral feeding, were accompanied by significant complications that could outweigh the benefits of nutritional maintenance, have forced us to more closely examine starvation physiology and the metabolic response to stress and acute illness. Crucial to the debate, was the recognition that body stores of most essential nutrients exist, and that hormonal mechanisms regulate their controlled release during acute illness, obviating the need for short-term nutritional support. Indeed, the recent publication of two large randomized controlled studies support the view that full feeding in the first week of illness offers no benefit to the average, non-malnourished ICU patient, and that the best approach may be to simply maintain renal function and metabolic stability with simple IV solutions, and gut function with slow enteral feeding whilst body stores last.

This book was written to address issues such as these. First, we discuss cellular function to provide the foundation for our understanding of the basic metabolic and nutritional needs of single cells to maintain life. Next, we apply this knowledge to how more complex organisms create a survival advantage by differentiating cells with specific functions, for example protein and fat storage, so that continuous feeding is no longer essential for viability. This, in turn, is applied to our understanding of normal human physiology, digestive function, and the interdependence between food and the gut. We then examine the influence of stress and acute illness on these processes to better understand where interventional nutritional support can best be used to improve patient outcome and survival.

The second half of the book is dedicated to the Practice on Nutritional Support, providing a framework for best practice based, wherever possible, on the results of robust randomized controlled clinical trials, and in their absence, the results of experimental studies combined with years of clinical experience. The importance of the development of a "nutritional support team" is emphasized, acknowledging the fact that few physicians have specialized training in NS and that the field is dynamic and progressive, with advances that are difficult for the average physician to keep up with. Most of the discussion involves the principles and practice of NS techniques and where they should most appropriately be used. Notably, much discussion is spent on the relative attributes of enteral versus parenteral feeding, not that one is better than another, but rather what their specific indications are.

Recognizant of the fact that many patients are left with feeding problems after recovery from acute illness that can be managed at home, thus cutting costs and improving quality of life, the third section of the book delves into the expanding field of home nutritional therapy, where we work together with home care companies to carefully manage this special group of patients dependent on home parenteral (HPN) and home enteral nutrition (HEN).

In general the book provides principles for the management of all forms of acute illness. However, in the last section, I single out special acute disease states, namely the short bowel syndrome, acute pancreatitis, renal and hepatic failure and obesity, which either account for most of our service requests and clinical effort, or which intrinsically alter usual nutritional requirements, necessitating specialized feeding. The book is appropriately concluded by a chapter (contributed by my wife, an academic geriatrician) on nutrition and the aged, with important discussion on the ethics of forced feeding in the terminal stages of life.

Despite the extra effort needed, I decided to make this a single author, rather than a multiple-author, textbook, as the nutritional support of patients with different diseases follows similar principles, unlike their medical or surgical management. Thus, the assembly of multiple experts to contribute specific chapters on nutrition in specific diseases, for example "nutritional support of pancreatitis" (as I am often asked to provide), inevitably results in considerable overlap with the other authors' contributions, with loss of focus on how we can best use nutritional support to improve patient outcome.

Pittsburgh, PA, USA   Stephen J.D. O'Keefe

Contents

Part I
The Principles

Chapter 1
Cell Biology

Cell Structure and Function

Intrinsic to survival, all systems and organisms exist within microclimates that are contained by barriers that allow the system components to interact and function. The world itself is protected by an outer shell, the atmosphere, the atom by a canopy of electrons, and the cell by its membranes. The cell could be regarded as the unit of life. Its survival in a hostile environment is assured by the remarkable amphipathic properties of its phospholipid membranes. Key to membrane structure is its physicochemical composition of fatty acids, which have at one end a hydrophobic tail and on the other a hydrophilic head. If randomly mixed, phospholipids self-assemble into sheets arranged with the hydrophilic heads on one side and hydrophobic tails on the other, forming rafts that can coat aqueous surfaces as a monomeric film. However, because the ends are unstable, they unite spontaneously forming bilayers or vesicles with the hydrophobic surfaces inside and the hydrophilic outside, allowing interaction with the aqueous environment. Glycosylated proteins also have amphipathic properties that enable them to integrate with the fatty acid sheets. Although outnumbered 50–1 in membrane surfaces, the relative masses of the proteins are greater resulting in a 50/50 weight-to-weight composition. It is the presence of these proteins that allow membrane systems to become dynamic in transport and metabolism allowing the cell not only to maintain its structure but also to sense and communicate with the external environment through receptors. Other proteins are active in energy transfer through the generation and oxidation of ATP. Specialized proteins also form the pumps that utilize the ATP to pull soluble nutrients from the external to the internal environment. Finally, proteins provide the flexible, adaptable structure of the membrane itself [1].

The contents of the cell are further divided into organelles by internal membranes that segregate countless cellular functions. Most cells contain a similar composition of organelles or compartments with the cytosol taking up 54% of the cell, the mitochondria 22%, and the nucleus only 6% of the volume (Fig. 1.1).

© Springer Science+Business Media New York 2015
S.J.D. O'Keefe, *The Principles and Practice of Nutritional Support*,
DOI 10.1007/978-1-4939-1779-2_1

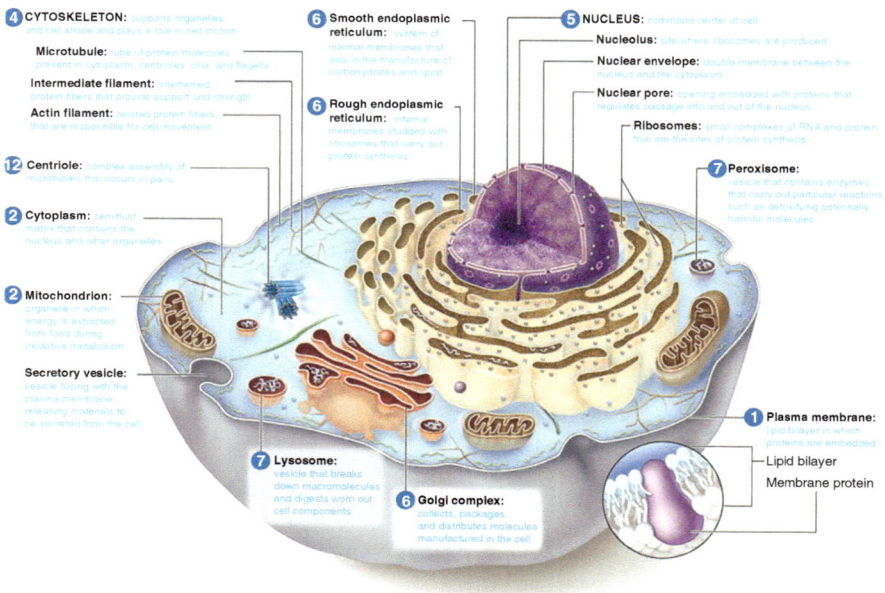

Fig. 1.1 Illustration of the anatomy of the cell (reproduced with permission from [2], Molecular Biology of the Cell. Ed Alberts B et al. 5th edition. Garland Science, Taylor and Francis Group, LLC 2008, New York)

All of these organelles are separated by semipermeable membranes, which consist of lipid protein bilayers. The composition of the cell varies, but its water content remains remarkably constant at 72%, with proteins contributing 18%, DNA 1%, RNA 6%, and phospholipids 2–3% of the mass. Animal and plant cells are very similar in composition, both containing a nucleus responsible for cell division and replication, but differ fundamentally in their possession of either the mitochondria or chloroplasts. The fact that both the mitochondria and chloroplasts have their own DNA–RNA protein synthetic capacities independent of nuclear DNA suggests that they might have been derived from independent organisms that became fused symbiotically to form primitive protocells when oxygen and carbon dioxide first appeared in the atmosphere about 1.5 billion years ago. This dramatically increased the functional independence of both plant and animal cells, as it allowed the plant cell to capture and synthesize atmospheric CO_2 into sugar and animal cells to produce energy both anaerobically (yields 10 mol ATP from 1 mol glucose) and now aerobically (generates an extra 20 mol ATP/mol glucose) in the mitochondria. In consequence, sugar was oxidized fully back to CO_2, which was released back into the atmosphere, completing a cyclical process and leaving the cell with 30 mol ATP to drive its machinery. It is likely that plant cells predated animal cells as they alone are capable of generating complex, stable, and transportable energy substrates from atmospheric gas. Perhaps the key to evolutionary life, therefore, was the ability of

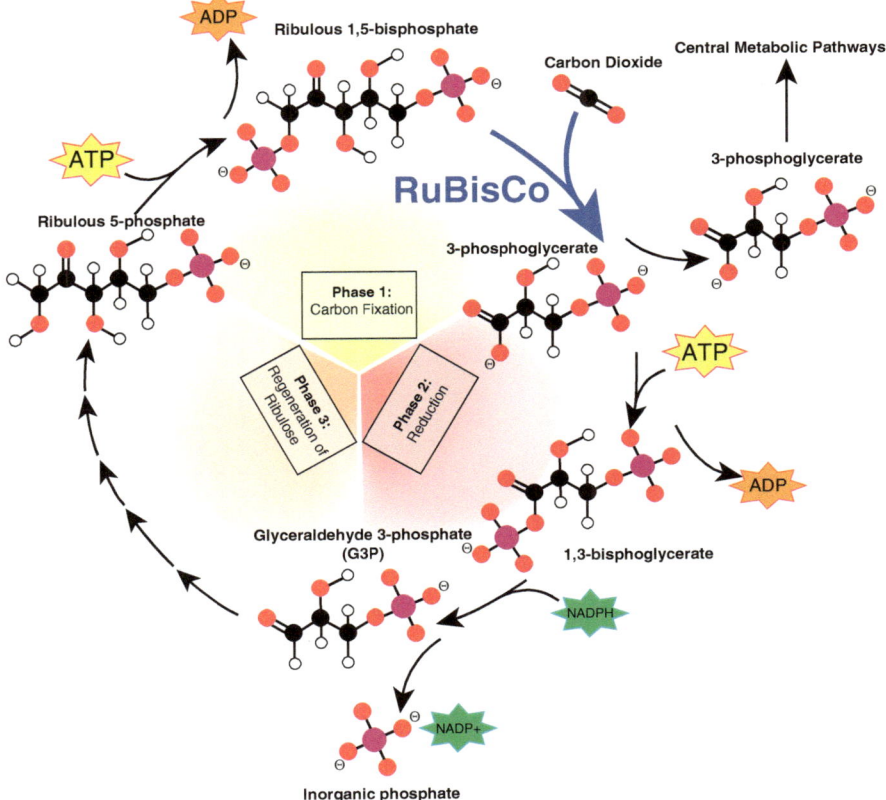

Fig. 1.2 The Calvin cycle: fundamental to life is the ability of plants to fix atmospheric carbon dioxide for the synthesis of carbohydrate, the essential fuel for all living cells. In many ways, it functions as the reverse of the Krebs cycle, which liberates CO_2 and energy

the chloroplast-specific enzyme *ribulose bisphosphate carboxylase* to trap and convert atmospheric carbon dioxide gas into sugar. The complete enzyme, ribulose-1,5-bisphosphate carboxylase oxygenase (RuBisCO), contained in plants fixes atmospheric carbon dioxide in the synthesis of energy-rich molecules, such as glucose, in a process termed the Calvin cycle (Fig. 1.2), which is the reverse of the Krebs cycle (Fig. 1.3). RuBisCO is probably the most abundant protein in nature.

Proteins form not only the structure but also the machinery of the cells to maintain life and reproduction. In essence, each cell is a tiny factory performing millions of reactions every second. The ability of the nucleus to synthesize myriads of different proteins is remarkable. How simple structures, such as repeats of only four different types of nucleotides, can unite to form a double helix of DNA which, in turn, becomes copied to form mRNA, which then fuses with ribosomes to trigger tRNA subunits to charge specific amino acids to combine to form a specific protein, is one of the wonders of life. The rate at which these reactions occur is determined by

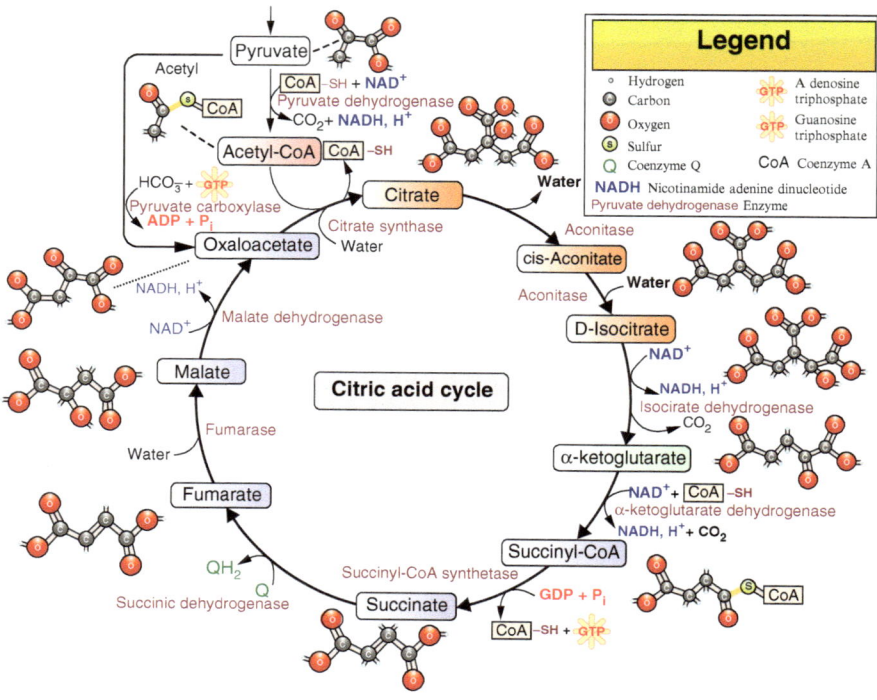

Fig. 1.3 The Krebs cycle: the way we release most of the energy from the foods we eat

other specific proteins, termed enzymes, which act as catalysts and shift the reaction at a remarkable rate. Enzymes have been shown to speed up cellular reactions 10^6 times such that diffusion forces alone limit the rate of reactions. It has been estimated that proteins can move along a DNA strand at a rate of 1,000 nucleotides per second. Although our knowledge of how cells work is expanding at an exponential rate following the unraveling of the human genome, we are still far from understanding how all these processes act in symphony and do not self-destruct. All molecules within the cell are in continual motion through translational, vibrational, and rotational movements, and it is estimated that there are about 500,000 random collisions per second. However, everything holds fast by the amalgamation of strong and weak forces provided by ionic, covalent, hydrogen bonding, and van der Waals attraction and repulsion actions.

This does mean, however, that there is no single reaction within the cell that is truly independent of another and helps explain why noncellular studies of the function and regulation of cellular pathways might bear little relationship to what happens in life. Figure 1.4 gives a glimpse of this, showing how much more complex the Krebs cycle and Embden–Meyerhof pathway are than we learned in medical school. Each dot represents a molecular substrate, which may be used in many

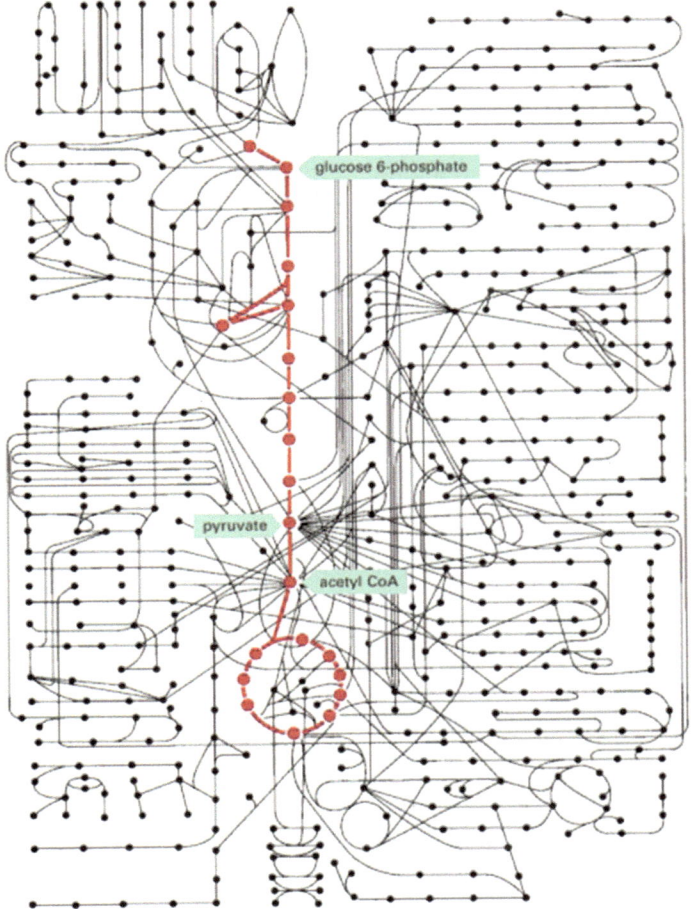

Fig. 1.4 An illustration of the complexity of metabolism with a vast array of interconnecting pathways feeding into the glycolysis pathway and Krebs cycle. It indicates that loss of one enzyme can be circumvented but also that loss of function in one segment can influence the function of another (reproduced with permission from [2])

different pathways. For example, pyruvate is currently recognized to be a substrate for at least six different enzymes, which all produce different products.

Order is maintained by the net product of these forces, which directs cellular traffic in the same way that a stream continues to flow downstream despite all the impediments in its way. This helps us understand the fact that the loss of function of a specific enzyme due, for example, to a genetic polymorphism rarely results in death as there are many interconnecting pathways which flow around the impediment. Consequently, such obstructions only result in a *loss of efficiency* of function. On the other hand, it can also benefit the cell if the specific protein can simultaneously take part in multiple different processes resulting in conservation of action. For example, it has been estimated that each protein enzyme domain may interact simultaneously with 5–20 different partners.

The Krebs cycle well illustrates the critical interactions between macronutrients and micronutrients (Fig. 1.3). First, it offers a common pathway whereby amino acids, carbohydrates, and fats are broken down to synthesize acetyl coenzyme A, which enters the cycle to generate energy, carbon dioxide, and water, i.e., the reverse of the Calvin cycle. In doing so, vitamins such as thiamine, pantothenic acid, nicotinamide, and riboflavin as essential cofactors in energy transfer and trace elements such as magnesium, manganese, zinc, copper, molybdenum, and iron are intricate components of the enzyme catalyzing the reactions.

I offer the above superficial view of the composition and workings of the cell to remind the reader of the exquisite sophistication of the process of life that we are trying to support with interventional feeding during sickness. Providing nutrition is not akin to pouring gasoline into a hungry engine to maintain speed. Nutrients provide not only the fuel for human cells but also the engine, the chassis, and the body of the car. *Consequently, the feed must contain a balanced mixture of all these components and not an excess of specific nutrients that might support fuel or structural needs.* This is a fundamental principle that I will keep coming back to during the course of this book. *All too often in nutritional support, overenthusiasm and commercialism team up to develop nutritional supplements that are essential for health, but cannot support health on their own, and if given in excess not only result in a waste of money and resources but also commonly pose a danger to health due to toxicity.* Furthermore, the timing and quantity of support will vary depending upon the endogenous stores which are released in a tightly controlled manner, and overprovision may produce deleterious effects, as in flooding the engine. It must also be remembered that the body consists not of one type of cell but of a society of cells with different functions that compliment one another increasing their ability to survive in times of stress and deprivation. The following section will expand on this theme.

Chapter 2
Physiology of Human Nutrition: Starvation and Obesity

Life is a dynamic state in which plants and animals are being formed and broken down continuously with reutilization of some constituents and replacement of others, termed "nutrients," from the environment. It therefore follows that life can be modified by nutrient availability within and outside the cell. Thus, nutrition is essential for the maintenance of the organisms' health and ability to withstand disease.

In the simplest forms of life, for example, single cell organisms, the organisms will only survive if placed in a constant nutritive environment. In contrast, animals, such as humans, consist of 10^{13} cells that survive as a community with each cell having specialized functions on which the others depend. Consequently, no cell can exist on its own, and removal of cells with specialized function can result in failure of the whole animal to survive. Recent investigations have shown that even this is an oversimplification, as within our body, there exists a live, metabolic "organ" that contains 100 times as many cells as we have, namely, the microbiota. The intimate proximity and interdependence of host cells and microbes has led to the recognition that we are actually "superorganisms" which enables us to survive in an otherwise hostile environment [3].

Perhaps the most fundamental development within our body was the ability of some cells to become *storage organs*, thus enabling the organism to become independent of a nutritive environment for variable periods of time. This allowed animals to move from one hunting area to the next and permitted survival in times of famine or immobilization because of injury. In humans, the depth of stores of different nutrients varies considerably such that survival without water is measured in days, whereas survival without fat-soluble vitamins is measured in months. Furthermore, the rate of consumption of stores varies. For example, the rate of metabolism gradually decreases during starvation. Resting energy expenditure diminishes, and the rate of nitrogen loss in the urine decreases from 10–14 to only 2–3 g per day [4, 5]. The reduced energy expenditure is related to the diminished active cell mass, while the reduced nitrogen excretion represents a loss of labile protein, reduced protein turnover, and the redistribution of amino acid stores from

© Springer Science+Business Media New York 2015
S.J.D. O'Keefe, *The Principles and Practice of Nutritional Support*,
DOI 10.1007/978-1-4939-1779-2_2

the skeletal muscle to vital visceral organs [6]. This process is termed *adaptation* as it maintains the function of essential organs, such as the brain, liver, and heart, while curbing physical work and activity.

These processes have made it almost impossible for international health authorities, such as the FAO and WHO, to agree on what the ideal nutritional requirements for health within a community are. The essence of the question is "for *optimal* function, is it better for humans to be lean or overweight?" Clearly, the overweight have expanded stores and therefore will survive acute starvation better than the lean. Indeed, there is some evidence that the moderately obese have a survival advantage in critical illness (Chapter 16) [7]. On the other hand, studies in mammalian models have shown that leanness is associated with a longer life span [8]. In the 1960s, the WHO recommended protein intakes of 0.8 g/kg/day for adults. Subsequent studies questioned whether this level was too high – bearing in mind the fact that nitrogen losses in the urine only measure 0.3 g/kg/day in adapted starvation as discussed above. After a series of further conferences, the requirement level was reduced to 0.6 g/kg/day. This change, namely, 25%, had enormous consequences (termed *the protein fiasco*) [9] in the developing world as it led to the emphasis on a general increase in total *food* consumption rather than the prioritization of the development of *high-protein* foods. In many ways, this instigated a paradigm shift in agricultural policy away from efforts to increase the production of specialized high-protein crops, such as soybeans, to the increased production of the time-honored staple foods of the community, e.g., wheat, potatoes, or corn.

Another problem is the question of *sufficiency*. Many errors have been made by the misinterpretation of the essentiality of specific food items. An excellent example is vitamin nutrition. In general terms, vitamins are complex molecules that are difficult to synthesize. Through evolution, predators have given up their ability to make these substances, as they are freely available in their prey. The classic studies that demonstrated the essentiality of specific vitamins in the diet for the maintenance of health, for example, the development of scurvy in around the world sailors who had no access to fresh foods [10], led to the belief that a diet *enriched* in such substances would be even *more* healthy. Other examples of this in the world today are far too many to cover but suffice it to say that food supplementation is a thriving business in the USA and accounts for a turnover of over two billion dollars per year. Although some cautioned that too much of a good thing might be bad, others argued that the excesses would simply be excreted from the body. However, certain fat-soluble vitamins and trace elements are difficult to excrete, and over-supplementation can lead to toxic accumulation [11]. For example, oral vitamin A supplementation can easily exceed removal rates leading to vitamin A toxicity and hepatic fibrosis [12]. Concern has recently been expressed about the safety of unphysiologically high intakes of water-soluble vitamins, which were previously thought to be safe because they are rapidly excreted in the urine. For example, high folate consumption may increase the rate of neoplastic progression [13]. We must be reminded, *more is not necessarily better*. We shall see that this is particularly pertinent to IV feeding, where physiological safeguards against excessive intakes into the body are bypassed and life-threatening acute metabolic derangements can suddenly appear.

Nothing could be nearer the truth than the state of health and nutrition in western countries such as the USA today where 1/3 of the population are now obese [14, 15]. Because we are designed to survive feast and famine, we store excess food during times of feast so that we can survive periods of famine. Because of the greater access to food throughout life, our present society is in a continual state of feast and so the flux of stored nutrients does not occur. A dominant characteristic of all functions of digestive and absorptive function is its *reserve capacity*, which allows survival after injury or loss. For example, we can lose up to 90% of our intestine and pancreatic function before death will occur due to malabsorption. This enables us to survive seemingly catastrophic injury that results in permanent anatomical losses. However, the downside of this is that given an intact GI tract and excess food, we can absorb considerably more than we need and thus become obese. The costs to health care are enormous, with the development of diseases associated with the metabolic syndrome, such as diabetes, hypertension, and cancer. It may be considered surprising that intense research is being invested into curtailing the physiological processes that result in obesity, when these processes are simply a product of the 3.5 billion years of human evolution that has allowed us to survive as a species. No doubt, in the not too distant future, famine will return and the excesses will be consumed. The answer should be simple: *educate the population to eat sufficiently*. Unfortunately, the solution is complex, as changing established eating patterns is extremely difficult, and is not helped by the mass of highly effective food-related advertising on television which encourages the consumption of appetizing, easily available, and cheap fast foods.

In summary, we know that the cellular mechanisms of the body are dependent on a constant supply of nutrients either from the environment or from body stores to sustain life, and we know that illness can disrupt the utilization and rate of consumption of these nutrients. This book will provide guidelines on how best we can maintain essential supplies for our patients during sickness to support the intrinsic mechanisms of repair that have allowed us to evolve into the dominant species of the world we know.

Organ Function and Survival in Starvation: The Critical Importance of Body Stores

It is fundamental that we understand the fact that the human body has evolved through millions of years to survive trauma and illness without eating and *without* nutritional support. An injured animal cannot hunt for food and therefore cannot eat, but it survives because it mobilizes its body stores for repair and recovery. Although we commonly think of body stores as those of the macronutrients fat, carbohydrate, and protein, they consist of a complex mixture of *all* nutrients—just like the composition of food. However, our capacity to store different nutrients varies considerably, and their rates of utilization also vary, particularly in sickness.

Most critical is our limited ability to store water and electrolytes. Much was learned about metabolic needs in starvation from the studies of Gamble on survival on the life-raft ration (1946 [16]). He was able to show that water was most limiting, followed by potassium. All metabolic processes are directly dependent on a constant 73% aqueous environment, and although fluid losses are minimized by hormonal–renal mechanisms if oral intake is deficient, a contraction in the intravascular volume will progressively reduce renal cortical perfusion, reducing urine flow. A decrease in urinary output below 500 ml/day will result in irreversible renal failure if prolonged. Potassium becomes a problem before sodium as its loss in urine is constant and independent of hormonal (aldosterone) regulation. Other minerals such as calcium, magnesium, and phosphorus are stored in the bone and are released at a rate to maintain normal blood levels for months. Loss of these minerals from the body is also minimized by the conservational actions of vitamin D on the kidneys. The depth of stores of the macronutrients, protein, carbohydrate, and fat is considerable, and provided that hydration is maintained, survival continues for several weeks, as illustrated by the IRA hunger strikers [17] where death only commenced after they lost over 40% of their normal weight. If fluid, electrolytes, and vitamins are given, survival can continue in otherwise healthy previously well-nourished individuals for as long as 8 weeks until fat deposits are expended. Death occurs rapidly after this point, as endogenous protein is the only remaining source of fuel and the demand would be 500 g/day, equivalent to a loss of 2 kg of lean tissue a day.

In clinical nutrition, this state is never reached, and the demand for nutritional support is usually early during critical illness in patients who commonly were well nutritioned, and commonly obese, before the onset of illness. In this situation, stores of nearly all nutrients other than water and electrolytes are adequate to support survival for weeks. Much attention has, however, been placed on the need for protein, or amino acid, support, bearing in mind the known importance of an adequate supply of amino acids for tissue repair and immunological function. While there are recognized stores for fat (adipose tissue) and carbohydrate (glycogen), there aren't strictly for protein, as all body proteins have functional roles. However, not all these functions are critical to survival, the best example being skeletal muscle, which increases with exercise and reduces with bed rest with no discernable influence on "vital" organ function, for example, the heart, the brain, and the viscera. Another interesting fact is that the more protein that is fed in the diet, the greater the incremental gain in body protein. Furthermore, there appears to be no survival benefit for this gain. In fact studies in rats have shown that survival during long-term starvation is greater in rats that were previously fed with low-protein diets [18]. Studies in human volunteers show that if subjects are fed a high-protein diet and then given a normal protein diet, they go into a period of negative nitrogen balance, while if they were previously fed a low-protein diet, they went into positive nitrogen balance on the same diet [19, 20]. This has made it difficult or even impossible to define "ideal" protein requirements. Indeed, McGilvery concluded that "...*there is no nutritional basis for an absolute requirement of any particular food!*" [20]. Studies in acute starvation have led to the proposal of the existence of "labile protein" stores, representing 3–5% of total body protein. The subject is reviewed in detail by Munro in

Fig. 2.1 Through the process of evolution, complex organisms have developed the capacity to store excess nutrients to maintain life during starvation to increase survival

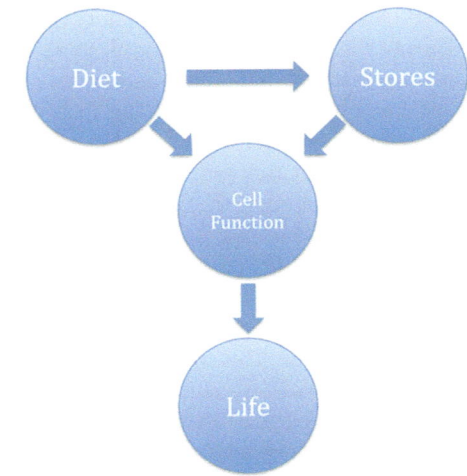

Fig. 2.2 Illustration of the changes in protein–nitrogen metabolism following fasting in humans. Initial losses are high, representing the consumption of "labile protein" for gluconeogenesis, but drop exponentially to basal rates ~2 g/day coincident with fat mobilization and oxidation to protein-sparing ketones

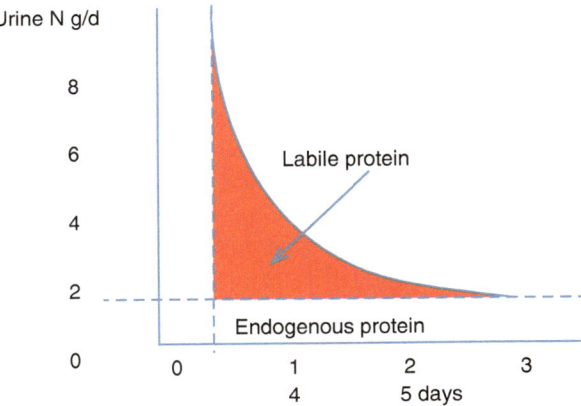

his book *Mammalian Protein Metabolism* [6], summarizing the classic observations of Voit from the 1800s [19], showing that the initial high losses of nitrogen drop exponentially during the first 3–6 days of starvation to a basal level of only 2.2 g/day, representing a loss of only 13.5 g protein per day (Fig. 2.2). Based on measurements in rats [22], it has been postulated that the high initial losses are accounted for by loss of "labile proteins" from fast turning over proteins contained chiefly in the liver (chiefly enzymes), intestine (proliferative cells), and pancreas (pancreatic enzymes). Basal losses after this point are considered to be derived from "endogenous" proteins, particularly those in skeletal muscle, which will support survival for several weeks of further starvation.

Protein metabolism is intimately tied up with carbohydrate and fat metabolism. During this acute stage, blood glucose levels are maintained by the breakdown of glycogen stores in the liver and muscle, together with gluconeogenesis in the liver and kidney in order to maintain neurological function. After 3 days, glycogen is spent, and the need for gluconeogenesis is progressively diminished by the increased mobilization of free fatty acids from adipose tissue and the production of ketones from fat oxidation by the liver governed by the key hepatic enzyme, acylase. Ketones can substitute for 75% of the glucose needs of the brain. Once this basal state has been achieved, it is possible to maintain nitrogen balance, and "endogenous" body proteins, with as little as 22 g of dietary protein per day. The addition of 100 g glucose to the diet reduces this need even more as it reduces the residual need for gluconeogenesis. This forms the basis for the common use of 5% dextrose IV solutions in hospitalized patients. However, protein turnover is never 100% efficient, and, in the nonstressed state, 10–20% enter oxidative pathways with the release of nitrogen, which is predominantly incorporated into urea by the key hepatic enzyme carbamoyl phosphate synthetase and excreted in the urine. Protein turnover is essential to life as it allows amino acids stored as body proteins to be redistributed to the area of most need: in critical illness, this enables survival and organ repair as labile protein supplies, predominantly from skeletal muscle, are mobilized to vital organs within the splanchnic bed. Energy expenditure, like protein, also decreases exponentially during prolonged starvation, but conservation of energy is less critical *as there is approximately 75,000 kcal stored as fat, a quantity that would provide energy needs for approximately 6 weeks.*

From this, it can be seen that nitrogen balance can be maintained by a wide range of dietary protein intakes, a fact that has made it extraordinarily difficult to define "optimal dietary protein intake" levels. In the west, we are accustomed to eating approximately 100 g of protein per day; in less developed countries, usual intakes are commonly only 40 g per day [9]. Which is better, no one knows. Studies have shown that underfed animals survive longer than well-fed animals [23]. There are intrinsic adaptation factors that allow us to survive on lower-protein and energy diets, but it has been suggested that such diets impair work capacity and productivity. However, other studies have suggested that obesity also impairs cognitive function and performance [24]. What is clear is that acute change in nutrition is of greater consequence than chronic change, as adaptation takes time to develop.

The functional consequence of the loss of labile stores is still debated. Loss from the pancreas and liver is chiefly from the cytosol as the number of cells remain unchanged, whereas loss from the intestine is associated with atrophy and hypoplasia. Most of the protein lost from the liver represents the diminution in enzyme production resulting from decreased need for metabolic activity associated with food assimilation. However, there is some evidence that early loss of protein from the liver impairs enzyme function, exemplified by the observed reduction in the ability to clear sulfobromophthalein [25] and the heightened toxicity of anesthetic agents [26]. Protein loss from the intestine is also related to the reduction in intestinal work with starvation, both with regard to enzymatic digestion and absorption, which is of little concern. The greater concern is related to the stagnation of the

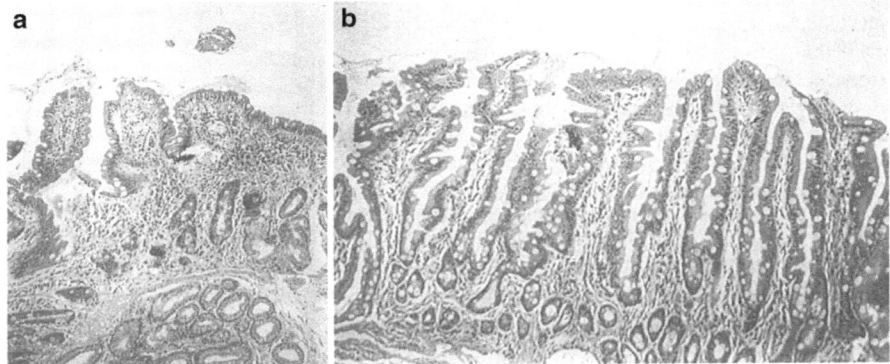

Fig. 2.3 Duodenal biopsies from patient No. 8 (Crohn's colitis). (**a**) Prior to nutritional support histological examination revealed partial villous atrophy, with no evidence of parasites or increase in inflammatory cells in the lamina propria. (**b**) Following the period of intensive enteral nutritional support, normal villous structure is now evident

intestine, the potential for bacterial overgrowth and dysbiosis, and possible toxin diffusion due to reduced tight junction proteins and leaky membranes. These observations have been used to support the use of early nutritional support in the critically ill, but we need to be cautious, particularly with regard to the overenthusiastic use of parenteral feeding, not to stress the liver with high infusions of amino acids which will demand increased hepatic enzyme synthesis and elevate protein catabolic rates which are associated with *worse* outcomes [27].

Thus, in conclusion, *the composition of nutritional support should be geared to the depth of body stores*. First, as stores of fluid and electrolytes are shallowest, initial support must contain sufficient fluids and electrolytes to maintain renal function and normal blood levels. Next, the urgency for provision of vitamin and mineral support is less, as there are significant body stores of vitamins and minerals that need to be provided, and finally, protein and energy must be supplied to prevent organ dysfunction. There is no clear evidence to support the need for early protein or amino acid infusions to prevent labile protein losses in the previously well-nourished patient. On the other hand, it will be critically important to assess the depth of protein stores and monitor the rate of loss of protein from the skeletal muscle, as depletion in this compartment will inevitably lead to impairment of vital organ function.

What we need to know is how much of any stored nutrient can we lose before vital organ function becomes impaired? Unfortunately, the tools to measure this have not been available, and, at best, we can only make educated guesses. With regard to protein stores, we attempted to answer this by measuring protein turnover rates by isotope amino acid labeling techniques in patients with BMIs <17 kg/m^2 [28]. All these patients were physically weak and bedbound. Focusing on vital organ function, we found clear evidence of mucosal atrophy and reduced mucosal turnover [28] (Fig. 2.3). Furthermore, pancreatic enzyme synthesis and secretion was impaired. Fat and carbohydrate digestion was mildly impaired, but enteral feeding was generally well tolerated if started slowly and resulted in rapid restitution of both the mucosa and digestive enzyme secretion.

We did, however, also perform these measurements in one extremely malnourished patient who had lost 60% of his body weight (a level of depletion associated with death in the IRA hunger strikers), with a BMI of only 9 kg/m² [29]. Initial attempts at oral refeeding resulted in exacerbated diarrhea and dehydration indicating intestinal failure. He needed TPN for a short period to supply the building blocks for metabolism and protein synthesis and thus to break the vicious cycle of food-induced malabsorption and diarrhea. Recovery thereafter was rapid, with excellent enteral tolerance, progressive increase in pancreatic function (Fig. 2.5) and a doubling of body weight within 3 months (Fig. 2.4).

Similar evidence of malnutrition-associated intestinal failure and pancreatic atrophy was witnessed in survivors of Nazi concentration camps, with reports of early deaths occurring in survivors who were refed orally too rapidly. The **refeeding syndrome** is all too commonly encountered in clinical practice and can be equally fatal unless managed appropriately. It is akin to flooding the engine with too much fuel but is even more complex than that because food provides not only the energy for the car but also essential components for the spark plugs (proteins, trace elements, and vitamins for enzyme function), the engine (proteins, vitamins, minerals

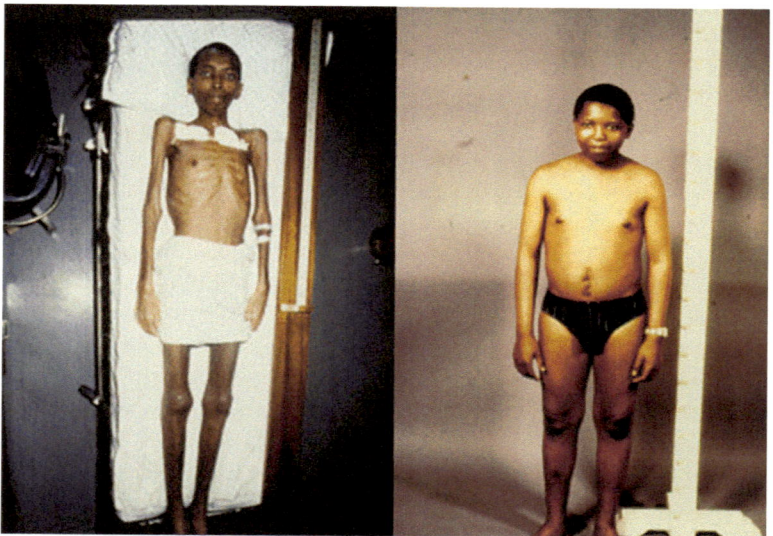

Fig. 2.4 A 20-year-old marasmic (weight depletion 62%, fat depletion 79%) patient with a 5-month history of severe diarrhea 10–15/day, unresponsive to antibiotics and antidiarrheals, associated with a weight loss of 20–30 kg. Diagnosed with α-heavy chain disease (immunoproliferative small intestinal disease (IPSID)) treated with oral tetracycline and nutritional support alone. Initial enteral feeding failed as it exacerbated diarrhea, necessitating short-term (10 days) PN, with recovery of pancreatic secretion (see Fig. 2.5) and conversion to full enteral feeding

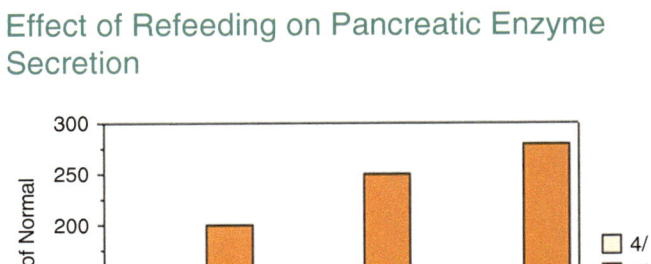

Fig. 2.5 Pancreatic secretion in the patient above expressed as % control during refeeding at start, 2 months, and 9 months after full recovery

for DNA, RNA, and mitochondrial function), the chassis (structural proteins and minerals), and the grease for the wheels (fluids and electrolytes), as discussed in the opening chapter. The goal in refeeding should always be to introduce a *balanced mixture* of all essential nutrients *slowly*, allowing the machinery to recover first, before filling the tanks. There is also substantial experimental and clinical evidence that while IV feeding does allow patients with permanent intestinal failure to survive, it is not a substitute for enteral feeding as it bypasses processes which are essential for the efficient utilization and distribution of nutrients, increasing the risks of severe complications that worsen outcome. *Thus, the urge to aggressively feed critically ill patients with TPN early in the acute event has to be tempered by knowledge of how to support the recovery process properly.*

Based on our data, we have evidence that patients with a BMI between 11 and 17 kg/m² have impairment of gut function but not enough to be considered "intestinal failure" necessitating IV feeding. Furthermore, we know that villous growth is dependent chiefly on luminal nutrients. Consequently, enteral feeding should initially be used, given as a slow continuous infusion to maximally stimulate mucosal recovery and to allow sufficient quantities of balanced nutrients to enter the portal blood stream to stimulate hepatic recovery, which in turn will orchestrate the recovery of all other internal organs. We do know, however, that patients with extreme marasmus with BMIs <10 kg/m² (see case study above) will have critical levels of protein deficiency with insufficient free amino acids to support the synthesis of digestive enzymes and the function of mucosal absorptive cells, leading to problems with nutrient digestion and absorption, which when taken together with increased mucosal permeability will result in explosive diarrhea with overzealous enteral feeding. The subsequent losses of endogenous fluid are likely to precipitate life-threatening fluid and electrolyte instabilities. Here, a short period of judicious IV support, first to correct fluid and electrolyte deficiencies and next to provide the full complement of essential nutrients, exemplified by amino acids to provide the building blocks for structural and functional repair, will break the vicious cycle, leading to the return of gut function and subsequent tolerance to enteral or oral feeding.

Chapter 3
Physiology of Digestion and Absorption: The Functional Interdependence Between Food and the Gut

Physiology

The process of digestion commences with the sight and smell of food, which triggers the "cephalic phase" mediated by the vagus nerve, which primes the system with increased contractions and the commencement of secretion of digestive juices from the salivary gland, the stomach, the pancreas, and the liver [30] (Fig. 3.1). These responses are amplified in a stepwise manner by the consumption and mastication of food, swallowing, and contact of the ingesta with the gastric mucosa, which culminates in the "gastric" phase. Mucosal contact in the stomach releases gastrin and pepsin, which, together with salivary amylase, initiate the digestive process. The grinding action of the stomach breaks the food down to a fine emulsion. Once particulate matter is reduced to <2 mm in diameter, the emulsion is slowly ejected into the duodenum, where a final boost of pancreatic secretion is generated by the combined hormonal and neurologic stimulants, CCK and acetyl choline, leading to the final, and most active, "intestinal" phase. The consequence of these events is the intimate and graded breakdown and mixing of food, fluid (massive quantities 5–7 l per day), digestive enzymes, and biliary secretions to expose maximum surface areas of food particles for efficient enzyme action in lysis and hydrolysis. It is also important to note that the protein synthetic potential of the exocrine pancreas is one of the highest in the body, which explains why protein deficiency will impair digestive capacity [28, 29].

It must be remembered that food is highly contaminated with environmental bacteria, which are tolerated by the gut, but deadly if they gain access to the bloodstream. One of the chief roles of the intestine is to sterilize nutrients so that they can be safely absorbed into the portal venous system. Gastric acid commences the sterilization process, followed by the antibacterial actions of pancreobiliary secretions together with their key roles in emulsifying and digesting the food particles and bacterial structures. The digesta is then filtered across the brush border of the intestinal mucosa, and any residual bacteria are phagocytosed or lyzed by the profuse

© Springer Science+Business Media New York 2015
S.J.D. O'Keefe, *The Principles and Practice of Nutritional Support*,
DOI 10.1007/978-1-4939-1779-2_3

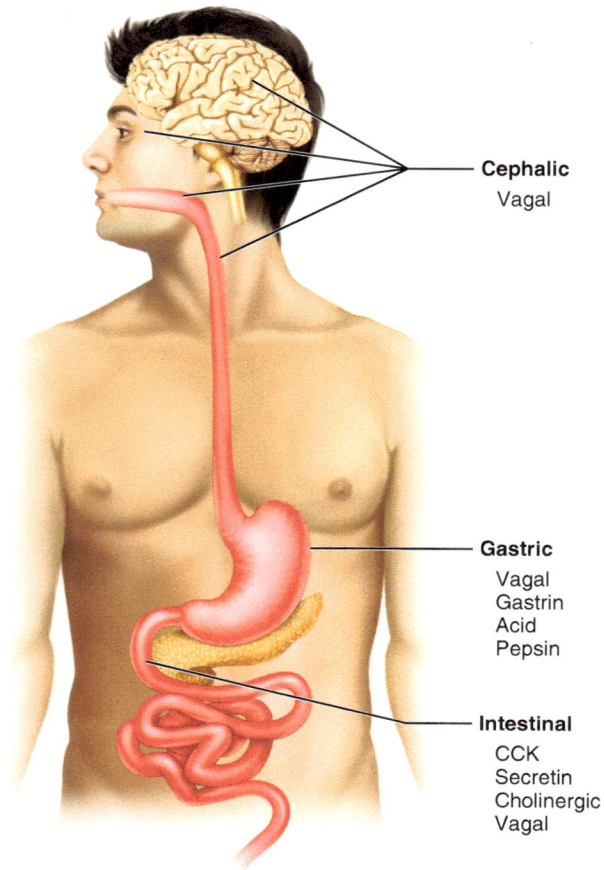

Fig. 3.1 The physiology of pancreatic secretion. The three phases of pancreatic stimulation

gut-associated lymphoid tissue (GALT). The role of GALT cannot be overemphasized in this regard. It is the largest lymphoid organ within the body and is responsible not only for ensuring sterility of absorbed fluids and nutrients but also in immune recognition and tolerance, which allow us to survive the onslaught of thousands of foreign antigens consumed in our diet each day. *It is important to remember that the luminal interaction between food, microbes, and the mucosa represents the chief site of interaction between us and the environment.* The sterilized nutrient solution then passes into the portal venous system, and is sensed by the pancreas, which, together with the liver, orchestrates the transport, uptake, and assimilation of absorbed nutrients into vital organs or body stores. This process stems the otherwise large fluxes in the concentration of nutrients during feasting and fasting within the systemic blood circulation.

Another important key principle to recognize is that most of the absorption of nutrients occurs in the duodenum and proximal jejunum, and the reason we have such a long small intestine is to reabsorb the 5–7 l of secretions needed for efficient digestion. To facilitate secretion and to maintain isotonicity between luminal and body fluids, proximal gut mucosa is permeable to body fluids, and it is only when the chime reaches the ileum that a concentration gradient can be established by the combination of tight intercellular junctions and active transport of water and electrolytes. This will be addressed again later under the section on the management of the short bowel syndrome (Chapter 11), where dehydration threatens life before malnutrition, due to loss of absorptive surface area.

Nutrition and the Gut

The development of techniques of total parenteral nutrition indirectly taught us a great deal about the importance of luminal nutrition in maintaining digestive and mucosal function. This will be discussed in greater detail under the complications of parenteral feeding in Chapter 9. While TPN was able to maintain nutritional balance and life, its long-term use was shown to suppress all aspects of gut function, and stasis causes problems, just like a car that is left out in the yard for too long— the tires go flat. While the suppression of digestive and absorptive capacity was not a problem, disuse of the gut has a major effect on our resident luminal microbiota, leading to dysbiosis, inflammatory, and infective complications. First, the absence of eating results in suppression of gastric acid secretion, the first line of defense against bacterial invasion. Second, the absence of luminal food results in reduced motility and suppressed pancreobiliary secretions. Pancreobiliary secretions are also bacteriostatic. This combination prevents the normal "housekeeping" of the gut, resulting in stasis and the ability of colonic microbiota to migrate caudally, culminating in increased colonization of the small intestine, causing the condition termed "small bowel bacterial overgrowth." This condition interferes with the normal process of digestion and absorption, and induces an inflammatory response, both at the local level of the mucosal and distally in the systemic circulation via endotoxemia. Stasis within the biliary system leads to intra- and extrahepatic cholestasis and subsequent liver dysfunction. The absence of luminal nutrients exacerbates the problem, as luminal nutrients are essential for normal mucosal growth and function. Luminal food or enteral nutrition stimulates mucosal blood flow and the release of growth factors, which maintain barrier function and gut immunity. PN cannot compensate for this and both conditions of starvation and PN result in progressive villous atrophy, suppression of sIgA production, plus alterations in innate immunity to a pro-inflammatory state, resulting in decreased mucosal defense and increased permeability to bacteria and their toxins [32].

Downstream, colonic mucosal function also becomes impaired by the lack of topical nutrients, but this time the problem is mediated through the microbiota. The absence of dietary residues, e.g., fiber, starves the microbiota, suppressing fermentation and the production of short-chain fatty acids, such as butyrate, which are essential for colonic mucosal health and function [33]. The lack of food for the microbiota also leads to a contraction in their population numbers and diversity, increasing the risk of overgrowth with pathogens, culminating in a state of "dysbiosis" [34]. The net result of all these changes is the establishment of an acute-on-chronic inflammatory state within the small bowel and colonic mucosa, setting the stage for pathogen overgrowth, enteritis, colitis, bacteremia, and eventual septicemia. From this, it is easy to see how prolonged bowel rest will result in a vicious cycle of events: mucosal atrophy, increased permeability, reduced gut (innate) immunity, cholestasis, and bacterial overgrowth—which sounds very much like an abscess waiting to rupture!

Nutritional Needs of the Small Intestine

Topical nutrients are the most important trophic stimuli for the small intestinal mucosa, and bowel rest results in progressive atrophy of all segments of the bowel, especially the surface epithelium. Interestingly, the amino acid glutamine is the preferred fuel for enterocytes, not glucose [35]. Furthermore, amino acids derived from the digestion of food are used in preference to and more efficiently for the synthesis of mucosal proteins (Fig. 3.2) [31], and we have shown that 30% of dietary protein is used on "first pass" by the gut and splanchnic mucosa [31]. In the pig model, it has been shown that protein balance can be maintained in the small intestine if as

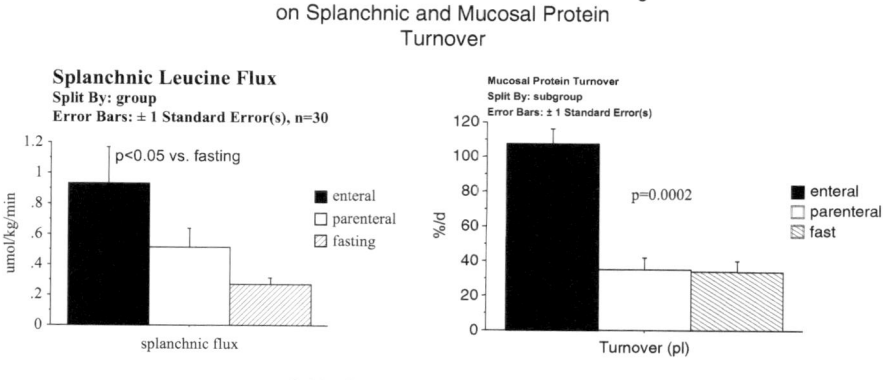

O'Keefe et al. Am J Physiol 2005

Fig. 3.2 Studies in normal healthy volunteers infused with stable isotope-labeled amino acids fasting, enteral, and parenteral feeding (same quantities of nutrients) illustrating higher levels of splanchnic amino acid turnover and higher rates of mucosal protein turnover during enteral feeding

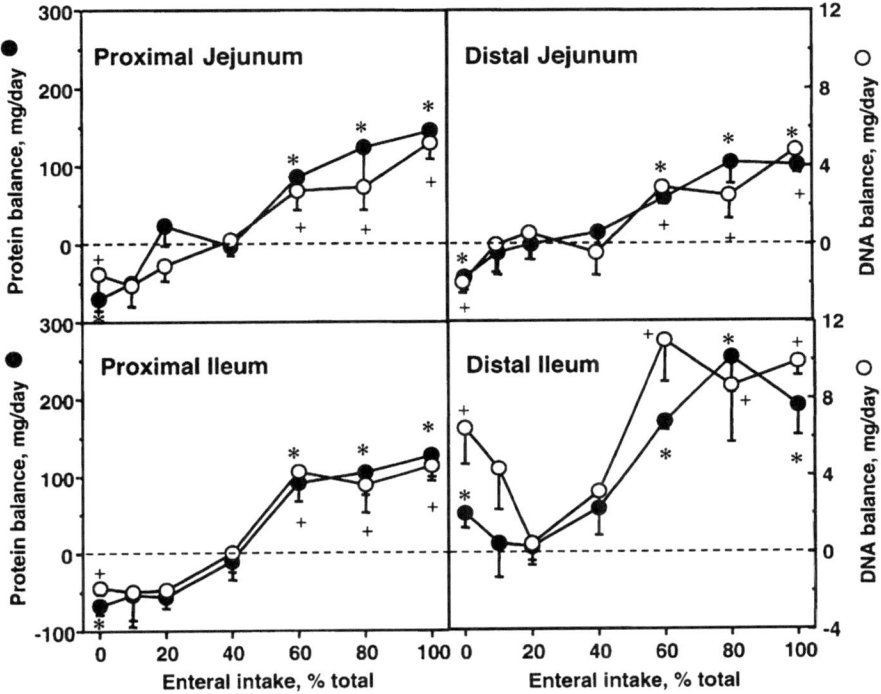

Fig. 3.3 The effect of progressive enteral feeding (0–100% of their nutrient intake) on protein balance in the small intestine in pigs. *Stoll et al. AJP 2000*

little as 20% of normal dietary requirements are provided enterally (Fig. 3.3) [36, 37], supporting the wisdom of "trickle" or "trophic" enteral feeding (not at 10 cc/h, but at 20–30 cc/h) in critically ill patients. In addition, there is good experimental evidence for compartmentation between splanchnic and systemic amino acid circulations [38], such that the ability of IV administered amino acids to support mucosal—and hepatic (e.g., albumin)—protein synthesis is considerably less than enterally administered amino acids [31, 39].

A complex, normal, balanced diet, not surprisingly from evolutionary point-of-view, best supports the health of the gut. The fact that the prolonged use of TPN results in mucosal atrophy in experimental animals, and that the atrophy can be *partially* prevented by glutamine supplementation, has led to extensive research on the essentiality of glutamine in the regulation of mucosal turnover, the preservation gut-immune function, and mucosal integrity [40]. However, it must be remembered that glutamine is an *inessential* amino acid synthesized from copious supplies of glycolysis and Kreb's cycle intermediates (Chap. 1, Fig. 1.3), and that there is prolific inter-conversion between glutamine, citrulline and arginine. Consequently, once again, the best nutritional support for the gut is going to be food. *It is fundamental to understand that no one amino acid is superior to another, just like no "nutrient" is superior to another*—unless, of course, an inborn error of metabolism is present. The belief that amino acid requirements change in critical illness has led to the development of "specialized" amino acid formulae, which will be discussed further on, but it is important to note that in the majority of experiment studies under which these were based showed that simple "rat-chow" (or a normal complex diet) was the most effective in maintaining mucosal integrity and gut function. For example, in a recent study, Li et al. randomized 30 rat pups to gastrostomy feeding with either whole milk, or 25% milk with or without glutamine supplemented up to the level obtained in whole milk. After 7 days, weight gain, villus growth, and tight junction protein production were highest in the whole milk diet. In the 25% milk diet, the addition of glutamine did not affect any of these parameters (Fig. 3.4) [41].

Diets have also been marketed that are "elemental" so that they can be immediately used by the mucosa or be absorbed without the need for digestion. However, digestion is normally so efficient that if a polymeric diet is infused at a slow continuous rate, the body forms its own elemental formula within the duode-

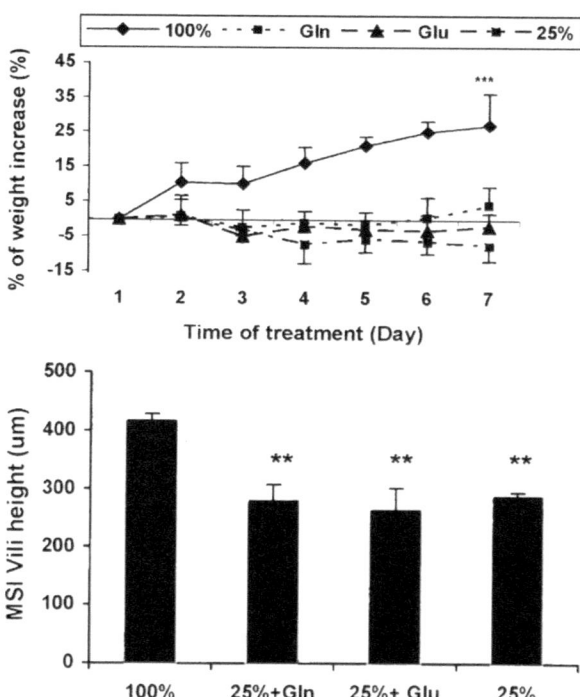

Fig. 3.4 Effects of glutamine (Gln) versus glutamate (Glu) on pup growth. The rat pups were nourished using rat milk substitute with 100% protein or 25% protein. Two protein-deprived (25% protein) groups were provided with Gln or Glu. Line graphs represent the rate of pup body weight with the time expressed as a percentage increase from the beginning of the study (***: $P<0.001$ vs. protein deprived groups). Mid-small intestinal villus morphology was determined by measuring villus height (**a**), Villus area (**b**), and crypt depth (**c**) using a light microscope (*$P<0.05$; **$P<0.01$, vs. 100% protein group). Weight gain and intestinal morphology were consistently higher in rats given the complete non-glutamine-supplemented formula [41]

num and proximal jejunum, obviating the need for the more expensive elemental diet. Furthermore, we will argue that gut stimulation is beneficial and elemental diets are less stimulatory [30]. Clearly, the situation is different if pancreatic insufficiency exists, but it must be remembered that you need to lose >90% of exocrine secretion before malabsorption occurs [42]. Pancreatic stimulation may also be detrimental in patients with acute pancreatitis, as food stimulates the synthesis of trypsinogen, and trypsinogen pre-activation within the pancreas is the cause of the disease [43].

Nutritional Needs of the Colon

In years past, the colon was considered a simple organ whose primary function was to reabsorb secretions for the conservation of water and electrolytes. However, recent investigations, based on non-culture gene sequencing techniques of conserved regions of 16S-rRNA, have exposed *a complex organ with metabolic functions that rival the liver, which affect not only the health of the colon but also the whole body* [3, 44].

The investigations have revealed that the gut microbiota outnumber the total number of cells in the body by one order of magnitude and that they contain 100 times as much DNA. This has led to the proposition that we are *superorganisms,* where mutualism between "external" microbes and human "internal" cells allows us both to function and survive together. Studies from germ-free rats have proven that our gut immune system cannot develop and remain functional without our normal microbiota, and that germ-free rodents fail to thrive and develop acute colitis [45]. The microbiota composition is balanced by intimate cross-talk not only between the different microbial species but also between microbe and host, maintaining the production of essential mucosal nutrients and preventing the overgrowth of potential pathogens. Thus, our resistance to injurious environmental antigens is closely bound to a healthy microbiota. Most importantly, the microbiota synthesizes essential nutrients, such as short-chain fatty acids (SCFA) and vitamins, notably folate, B-12, biotin, and vitamin K, which maintain mucosal and body health [46]. The short-chain fatty acid, butyrate, is what glutamine is to the small intestine, the preferred food for the colonic epithelium. It also has profound anti-inflammatory and anti-proliferative effects, which account for the reduced risk of colon cancer in populations consuming high complex carbohydrate diets with high rates of fermentation [44]. Advances in high-throughput technology have led to an explosion in the fascinating new world of "omics," with closer definition of the microbiome (bacteria, viruses, fungi), the metagenome (the synthetic genetic potential of the microbiome), the transcriptome (the genetic expression (RNA transcripts) of the microbiome), and the metabolome (metabolic products of the microbiome and human genome). The extraordinary complexity of the interactions between the host and the microbiome in the colon is well illustrated by Fig. 3.5, which shows the integration of metabolic pathways of carbohydrate, fat, protein, and bile acid metabolism, based on the enzymes of bacterial groups identified by phylogenic microarray analysis, host metabolic enzymes, and fecal and urinary metabolites by ^{1}H NMR [47]. Recent

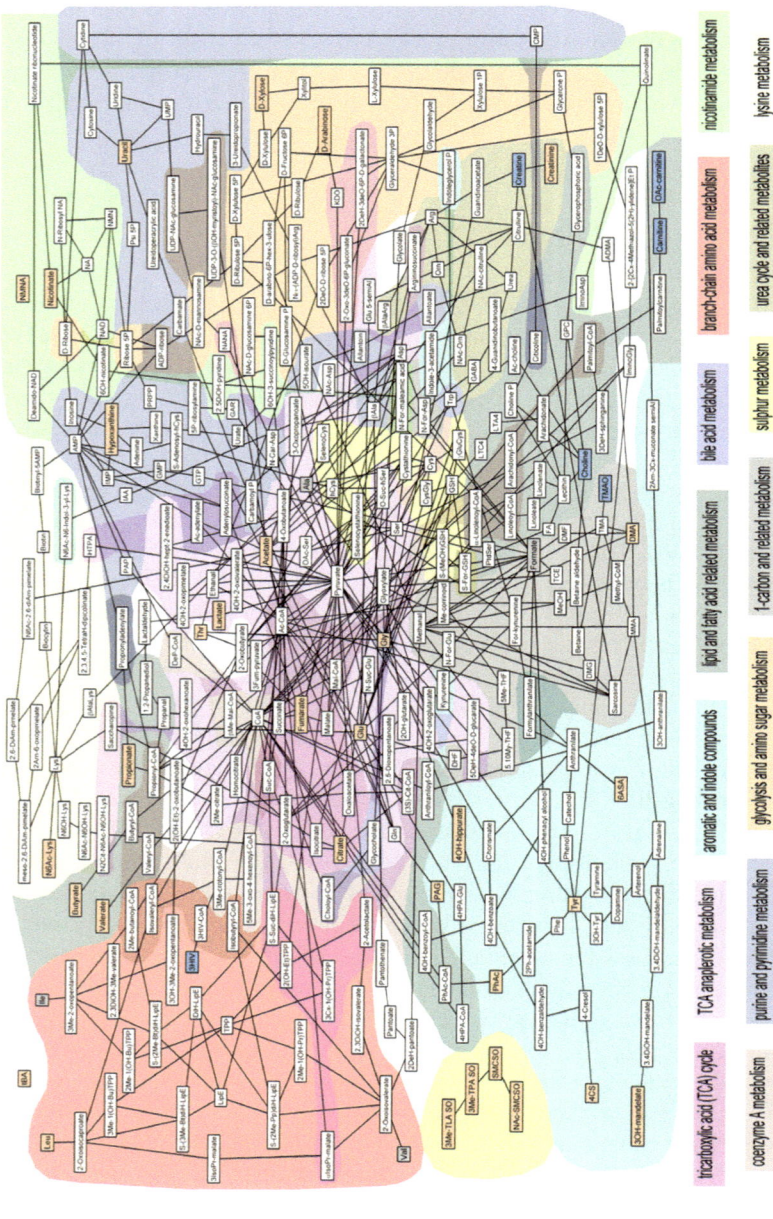

Fig. 3.5 Global network of changes observed in fecal water and urine between different dietary comparisons, created using the MetaboNetworks software. The network shows links between metabolites if the reaction entry in KEGG indicates a main reactant pair and the reaction is either mediated by an enzyme linked to human genes, enzyme linked to genes from identified microbial groups using the HITChip phylogenic microarray analysis, or it is part of a spontaneous process. The background shading indicates different interconnected pathways

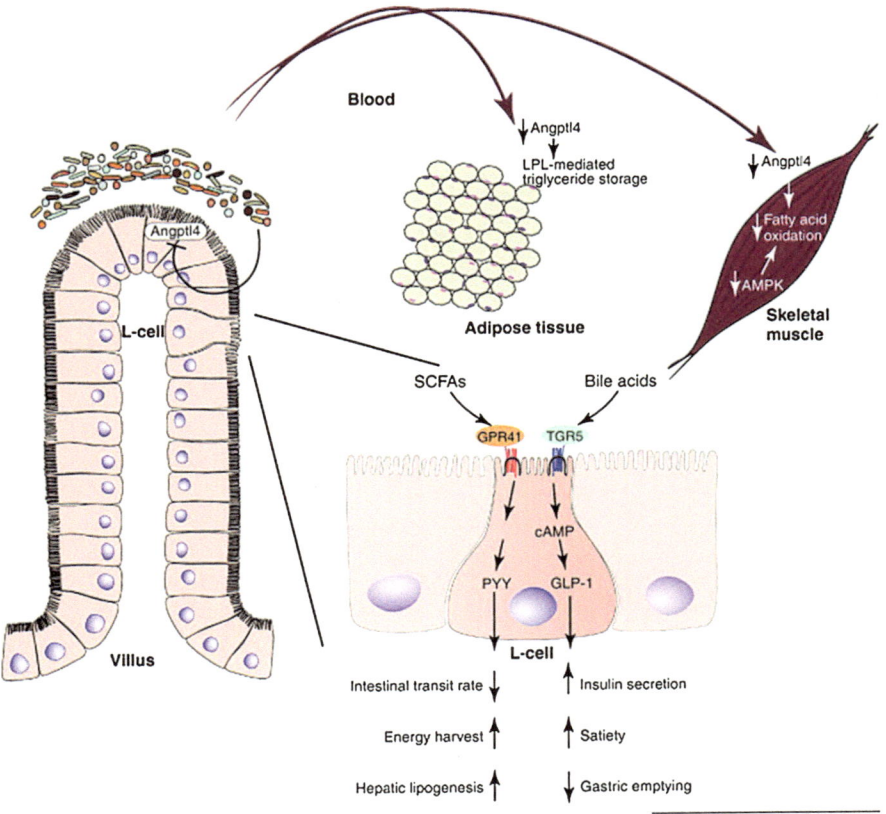

Fig. 3.6 Gut microbiota regulation of host metabolism. The gut microbiota suppresses enterocyte expression of Angptl4; this alleviates LPL inhibition and promotes LPL-mediated triglyceride storage in adipose tissue. In addition, reduced Angptl4 levels together with diminished activation of AMPK reduce fatty acid oxidation in skeletal muscle. The gut microbiota has also direct effects on enteroendocrine L-cells: microbially generated short-chain fatty acids (SCFAs) bind to the G-protein-coupled receptor (GPCR) Gpr41 which stimulates secretion of the gut hormone PYY. Secretion of PYY leads to reduced intestinal transit, increased energy harvest, and stimulates hepatic lipogenesis. The gut microbiota generates secondary bile acids that are the major ligands for the GPCR TGR5. Stimulation of TGR5 enhances GLP-1 secretion, and this promotes increased insulin secretion, satiety, and reduced gastric emptying [48]

experimental studies suggest that the microbiota also influences body homeostasis and energy balance via a complex network of actions mediated by microbial metabolites (e.g., SCFAs and secondary bile acids), gut innate immunity, and the gut neuroendocrine system [48]. Key features include the ability of the microbiota to suppress enterocyte expression of Angpt14, which promotes lipoprotein lipase-mediated triglyceride storage in adipose tissue. In addition, SCFAs bind to G-protein-coupled receptors on neuroendocrine L-cells in the ileum to release PYY, which in turn increases energy harvest and lipogenesis (Fig. 3.6).

Chapter 4
Pathophysiology: Nutrition in Illness

Metabolic Response to Starvation
With or Without Acute Illness

It is important to understand the effects of starvation on metabolism and gut function in order to understand what goes on in acute and chronic illness, as illness is commonly associated with anorexia and the inability to eat normally. However, acute illness disrupts the processes of adaptation to starvation described above, and results in an escalation, rather than conservation, of the rate of consumption of body stores. Figure 4.1 illustrates the differences between nitrogen metabolism in starvation and starvation associated with acute illness. Unlike in simple starvation, nitrogen loss from the body continues at an elevated rate, demanding the breakdown of more substantial body protein stores, chiefly in muscle, once labile stores are exhausted to substitute for the diet.

Feeding on top of this response results in further elevation of nitrogen losses because of the change in counter-regulatory hormones that promote mobilization and suppress whole-body synthesis: this is simple substrate-driven kinetics. Evidence that this is hormonally mediated was gained from studies which showed that IV infusions of glucose and insulin suppressed nitrogen, or "catabolic" losses [49]. However, our own investigations showed that the suppression of catabolism was not necessarily a good thing, as the resulting suppression of amino acid flux resulted in suppressed hepatic protein (albumin) synthesis [50] (Fig. 4.2). The simultaneous infusion of amino acids restored flux and albumin synthesis, while at the same time suppressing whole-body protein breakdown, indicating that conventional IV feeding can substitute for body stores in maintaining metabolism during acute illness. But, what is the value of doing this in someone with adequate body stores? All we are achieving is the preservation of body stores and the inducement of potential TPN complications. Measurements of the mechanisms underlying this change have allowed us to design interventional feeding techniques that best *support* organ function, thus allowing repair to commence, paving the way to recovery.

© Springer Science+Business Media New York 2015
S.J.D. O'Keefe, *The Principles and Practice of Nutritional Support*,
DOI 10.1007/978-1-4939-1779-2_4

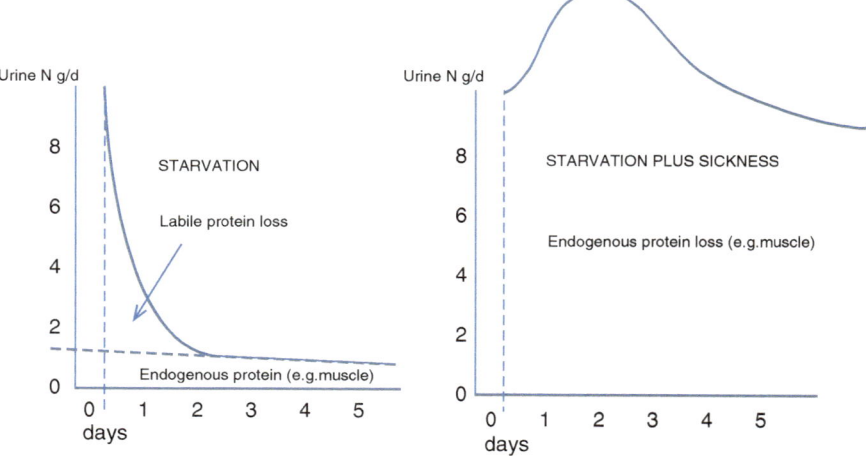

Fig. 4.1 Illustration of the differences starvation has on urine nitrogen loss, whether the person was previously well (*left*) or sick (*right*)

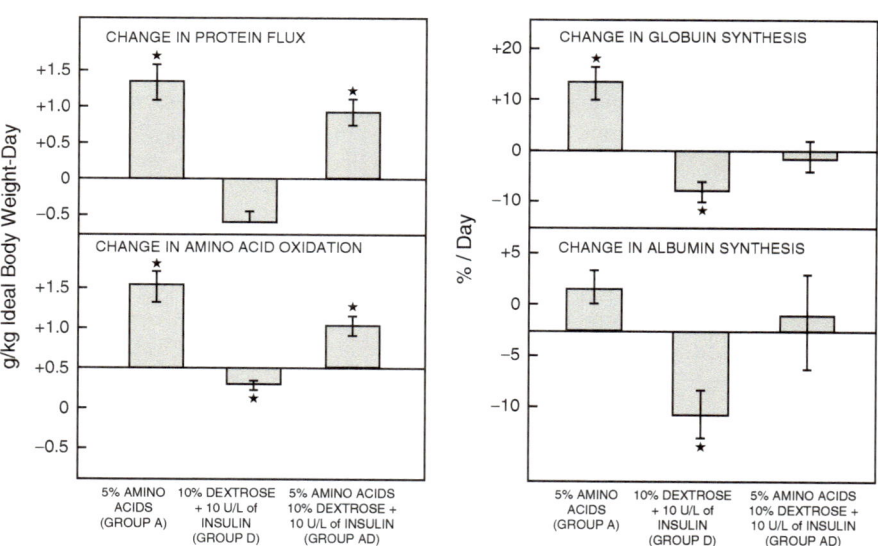

Fig. 4.2 Illustration of the differential effects of IV feeding with amino acids alone (1.5 g/kg/day), dextrose (10 kcal/kg/day) with sufficient insulin to suppress hyperglycemia, and a combination of the two in patients recovering from major surgery. Whole-body protein flux and oxidation, together with albumin and globulin synthesis, were measured by primed continuous 8-h IV infusions of ^{14}C-labeled leucine. Results showed that although dextrose was most effective in suppressing protein oxidation, it also suppressed amino acid flux and its incorporation into hepatic export proteins, namely albumin and globulin

However, it must be emphasized that although food is therapy for starvation, it is not for disease. Consequently, patient management should focus on specific treatment of the underlying condition (e.g., antibiotics for infective disease, surgery for mechanical obstructions) together with equipping the body with the tools (nutrients) to optimize conditions for tissue/organ repair: *this is the role of nutritional support.*

The Metabolic Response to Acute Illness

Protein Catabolism

Following the classic studies of Cuthbertson in the 1930s on patients with hip fractures that showed "nitrogen wasting" in the urine [51], *protein catabolism* was recognized as a characteristic feature of acute stress, whether it be due to trauma or acute illness. Using isotope-labeled amino acid infusions in Waterlow's unit in London, we were able to trace the changes in metabolism responsible for catabolism in patients recovering from abdominal surgery who were not fed, showing that the balance of protein turnover was disturbed, with a suppression of whole-body protein synthesis and relative increase in protein breakdown, allowing an efflux of "stored" amino acids, predominantly from muscle, into the circulation (Fig. 4.3) [52].

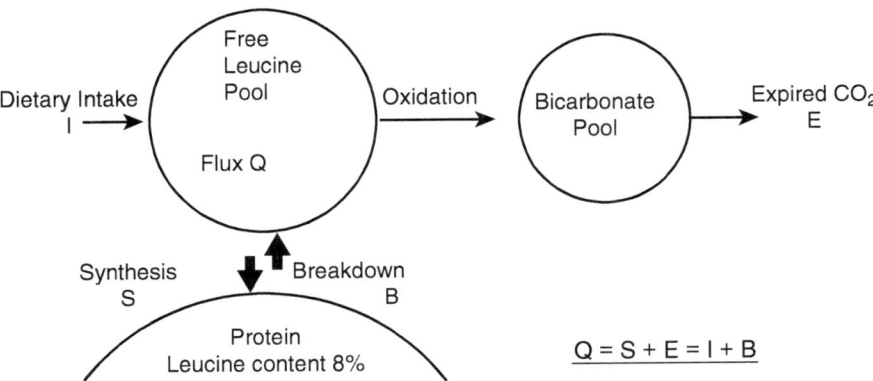

$$Q = S + E = I + B$$

Fig. 4.3 The 8-h intravenous infusion of ^{14}C-labeled leucine allowed measurement of the rates of flux of amino acids through the body (plasma) pool (Q) at steady state, and simultaneous measurement of the rate of excretion of label as $^{14}CO_2$ allowed calculation of amino acid oxidation rates (E). As the dietary intake of amino acids (I) was known, the quantity of amino acids released from body protein (B=catabolism) and taken up into body protein synthesis (S) could be calculated from the simple equation $Q=S+E=I+B$. *O'Keefe et al. Lancet 1974*

   This was an appropriate response as it generated a strong flow of substrate amino acids from stores to organs most in need, chiefly the viscera. Further studies showed that more severe forms of critical illness, such as acute tetanus, predominantly increased the rate of protein breakdown, resulting in remarkably high plasma flux rates of amino acids and high hepatic oxidation rates, exhibiting a general state of body protein "catabolism" [53]. Subsequent studies, discussed above, showed that the IV infusion of amino acids reduced the rate of catabolism of body proteins and maintained the synthesis of visceral proteins, while the infusion of glucose and insulin without amino acids also reduced protein catabolism, but also suppressed the mobilization of amino acids and their utilization for visceral protein synthesis, for example hepatic albumin synthesis [50] (Fig. 4.2).

   The change in balance between protein synthesis and breakdown is hormonally mediated, but initiation of the response is probably governed by immune responses to tissue injury, and increased generation and release of pro-inflammatory cytokines such as IL-1, IL-6, and TNFα. For example, insulin tips the balance in favor of anabolism by promoting the uptake of amino acids into protein synthesis, while corticosteroids, catecholamines, and glucagon accelerate the rate of protein catabolism and, at the same time, counteract the anabolic actions of insulin (insulin resistance) and growth hormone. The increased flux of amino acids also increases substrate for hepatic transaminase pathways and oxidation, resulting in accelerated gluconeogenesis with the liberation of nitrogenous metabolites, which are removed by the liver and incorporated into urea synthesis, accounting for the increased "catabolic losses" of nitrogen in the urine. Insulin resistance also prevents the storage of glucose and fat leading to increased plasma fluxes of all metabolic substrates, and stress-associated hyperglycemia (see below).

   These fundamental alterations are responsible for differences in metabolism between stress and starvation, and *account for the difficulty in improving nutritional status by forced feeding in critically ill patients*. We argue that the goal should be to *support* the normal response, which is the mobilization of body stores, and to only intervene when body stores become limiting. A pivotal illustration of this is Munro's original observation that the catabolic response to femur fracture in rats was directly related to its previous nutritional state, and that malnourished rats exhibited minimal catabolic responses, and yet their survival was lower [54] (Fig. 4.4).

   While most of the studies have focused on changes in protein metabolism induced by stress, it is important to understand that overall metabolism is altered, with similar increases in the mobilization of energy stores, particularly with mobilization of fat stores. However, the urgency for support of fat and energy mobilization is considerably lower as the depth of fat stores is much higher, particularly in Western populations where up to 40% are obese. The needs for glucose are also increased, but gluconeogenesis is increased from protein catabolism and care needs to be taken to avoid excessive infusions for fear of inducing hyperglycemia, a condition that is associated with higher complication rates and mortality, whatever the disease process [55].

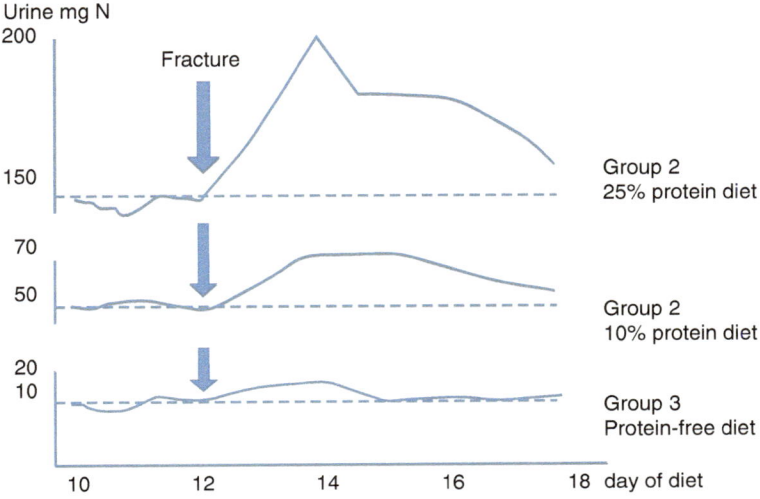

Fig. 4.4 The catabolic response to hip fracture in rats, demonstrating that losses are higher if rats are given higher protein intakes before trauma. Despite lower catabolic rates in malnourished rats, survival was also lower [54]

Hyperglycemia

The acute stress response in critical illness is characterized by increased gluconeogenesis from protein and rapid glycogenolysis, resulting in increased glucose turnover [56]. Basal blood glucose concentrations increase, and hyperglycemia will develop in prediabetics given oral or IV, particularly IV, glucose infusions (often the obese) because, unlike the situation in healthy subjects, gluconeogenesis is not suppressed by glucose infusion. It is well recognized that glucose infusions suppress protein catabolism, a process termed "protein sparing" [57]. This popularized the use of high glucose (>40 kcal/kg/day) containing parenteral nutrition solutions in the 1970s and 1980s, but the benefits on protein conservation were outweighed by the complications of the resultant hyperglycemia. Concern about the risks of hyperglycemia, including immunoparesis, dysmotility, increased infections, and liver dysfunction due to increased hepatic fat synthesis (i.e., "*pate de foie*" syndrome), and the recognition from the results of measurements of energy expenditure in the ICU that resting metabolic expenditure was rarely over 25 kcal/kg/day, led to the rise in popularity of "hypocaloric feeding" in the 1990s in the critical stages of illness [58]. It was, however, subsequently shown that outcomes could be improved if the hyperglycemia induced by full feeding was controlled by high rates of insulin infusion [59] (Fig. 4.5).

What these studies did not tell us was whether "full feeding" and insulin infusions were better than no feeding. The recent publication of two large-scale studies

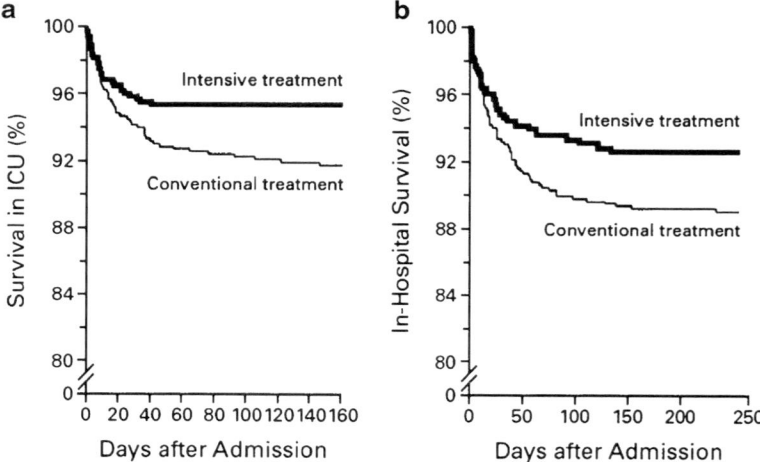

Fig. 4.5 Preventing hyperglycemia (maintenance of blood glucose at a level between 80 and 110 mg per deciliter) in patients in the ICU receiving a mixture of parenteral and enteral feeding with "intensive insulin treatment" improves survival (van den Berghe et al. N Engl J Med 2001; Ref. [55])

in fact suggests that full feeding in the first week is associated with more complications (see Chapter 5), endorsing our view that forced feeding to conserve stores in the previously well nourished is unphysiological and possibly harmful.

Chapter 5
Nutritional Support

The Evolution of Nutritional Support

The discipline of nutrition support was born when Dudrick and colleagues demonstrated that parenteral feeding on its own could support normal mammalian growth and function [60]. Their classic studies of TPN feeding in Beagle pups opened up the "TPN Era" of the 1970s and 1980s. The subsequent development and commercial production of safe IV nutrient solutions meant, for the first time, that any sick patient who was unable to eat could be fed, artificially. As a consequence, there was a boom in nutritional intervention, and the American Society of Enteral and Parenteral Nutrition (ASPEN) was born, soon followed by the European (ESPEN), Australian (AuSPEN), and South African (SASPEN) societies among others, to foster the nutritional care of hospitalized patients. Dramatic improvements in the survival of patients with incapacitating abdominal catastrophes, who previously would have died due to the exhaustion of body stores (e.g., massive intestinal resection/loss), led to the *overenthusiastic application of TPN*, such that nearly every patient in the ICU who was unable to eat after 3–5 days was placed on TPN. Caloric infusion rates were usually excessive (>3,000 kcal/day), and the term "hyperalimentation" was coined. Unfortunately, experience was soon to show that the combinations of TPN, bowel rest, and excessive nutrient infusions were associated with their own set of serious septic and metabolic complications, which often worsened outcome. The premature or inappropriate use of TPN usually led to a worsening of outcome because of the failure to appreciate the following:

(a) The body stores are sufficient to support life in a well-nourished patient for weeks
(b) TPN has septic and metabolic complications because we were not designed to receive food into our veins
(c) Disuse of the gut leads to disturbance of the microbiota and bacterial overgrowth that leads to a risk of sepsis from endogenous organisms and heightens systemic inflammatory responses

© Springer Science+Business Media New York 2015
S.J.D. O'Keefe, *The Principles and Practice of Nutritional Support*,
DOI 10.1007/978-1-4939-1779-2_5

(d) Parenteral nutrients are ineffective in maintaining overall gut mucosal health and liver function

For example, a number of studies demonstrated that patients actually did better with "standard care" (no nutrition, just IV fluids and electrolytes) compared to TPN. An excellent illustration of this was the study of Sax et al. where patients with mild acute pancreatitis were randomized to TPN or simple IV fluids [61]. The group given TPN had more septic complications (from the IV catheter) and ended up spending more time in hospital (Table 5.1). This could have been anticipated because endogenous stores were sufficient so IV infusions were superfluous, as was the need for invasive procedures such as central catheter placement. Today, we would not advise any form of nutritional intervention in this group of patients with mild acute pancreatitis, as they would likely be eating normally by day 4 [62, 63]. Another key study was the VA TPN Cooperative Study which investigated the hypothesis that "perioperative TPN would reduce the 30-day rate of major complications in patients undergoing non-emergency laparotomy or thoracotomy for conditions from which they were likely to die from within 90-days" [64]. Irrespective of whether they had functional guts or could eat normal food, they were randomized to no perioperative TPN or TPN for 7–15 days before surgery. In addition, the TPN group was allowed to eat, consuming on average 3,000 kcal/day. The TPN was continued for at least 3 days after surgery. The intended number of patients was not enrolled as the study was stopped after interim analysis showed no benefit after the enrollment of 395 patients. In fact, mortality was numerically higher (26% vs. 25%) in the TPN group and there were significantly more infectious complications (14 vs. 6%, $p=0.01$). Subgroup analysis suggested that there might be some benefit from this approach if the patient was initially malnourished, as noninfectious complications were significantly lower—but on the other hand, infectious complications were more commonly encountered in the malnourished. Again, today, we would not give TPN to any patient after thoracotomy or laparotomy unless they were shown to have intestinal failure.

Table 5.1 Using TPN in well nourished patients worsens outcome

TPN can worsen outcome in acute pancreatitis
• *Controlled* study: TPN vs. IV fluids; Sax et al. Am J Surg (1987):
– 54 patients with mild disease (average Ranson's score 1)
– TPN group did worse
• Catheter sepsis 11 vs. 2%, $p<0.01$
• Length of hospital stay 16 vs. 10 days
• TPN arm more expensive
Perioperative TPN can worsen outcome in surgical patients
• Controlled trial: TPN for 7 days before and 3 days after surgery vs. no TPN
• VA TPN Cooperative Study: N Engl J Med (1991)
• 395 patients
– Infectious complications higher in TPN group, 14% vs. 6%, $p=0.01$
– Mortality 26% in TPN group, 25% control
– TPN arm more expensive

Enteral vs. Parenteral Feeding

In patients with underlying GI disease or disturbance, improved understanding of the physiology of the upper GI tract has enabled us to restore intestinal function with interventional feeding tube placement [63]. This has allowed us to provide enteral feeding in even the sickest of ICU patients who previously were considered to have "intestinal failure" (because of the presence of ileus, dysmotility, or subacute or upper GI obstruction) and in need of parenteral feeding. This led to the "Enteral Nutrition Era" in the 1990s, which continues to the current time. The lag in appreciation that interventional feeding tube placement could avoid the need for TPN in most ICU patients, plus the relative ease of use of TPN, led to the persistence of the preferred use of TPN in many centers during the 1980s, until the conduct and publication of several prospective controlled clinical trials, and their eventual meta-analysis (Fig. 5.1), showed that TPN should never be used if there is a functional gut.

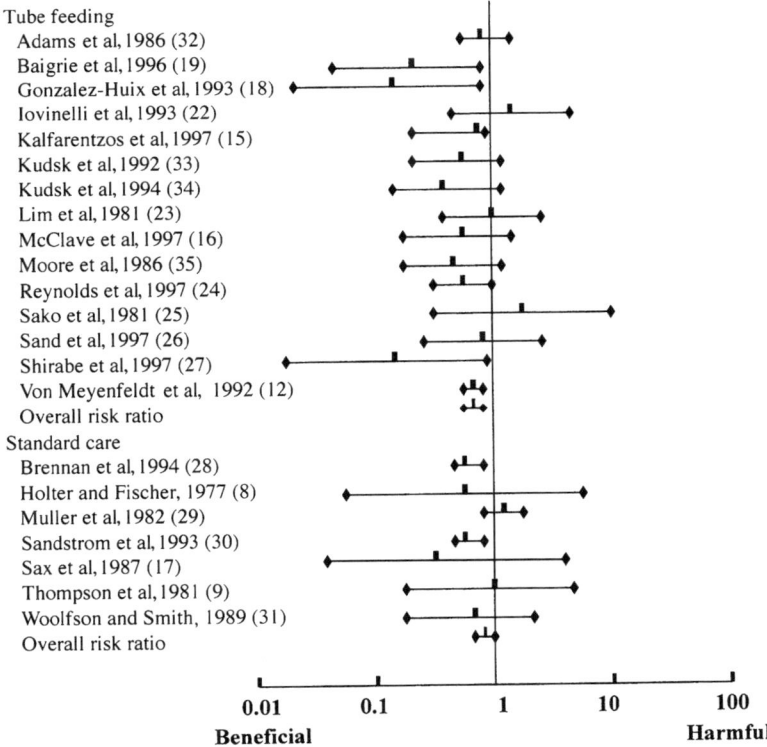

Fig. 5.1 Meta-analysis: enteral nutrition and no nutrition vs. TPN: Risk factors and associated 95% CIs for the effect of enteral nutrition (tube feeding or standard care) compared with that of parenteral nutrition on infection [67]. Nearly all studies showed that the groups randomized to EN fared better (Note: we now know that there are different indications for EN and PN, and randomizing them to one or the other today would be unacceptable! See Table 5.2)

One of the early studies conducted by Kudsk et al. randomized 98 patients with abdominal trauma to enteral or parenteral nutrition within 24 h of admission [66]. The results showed clearly that enteral feeding was superior particularly with regard to the incidence of pneumonia (11.8% vs. 31%), abdominal abscess (1.9% vs. 13.3%), and catheter sepsis (1.9% vs. 13.3%). Further, they noted that these differences were most pronounced in patients with the most severe degrees of illness. Moore and Moore reported similar findings in trauma victims following laparotomy procedures [65]. Patients were randomized to early enteral feeding via a needle jejunostomy placed at the time of surgery or to TPN after postsurgical day 5. The results again showed the superiority of enteral feeding with better nitrogen balance and a lower incidence of major infections (8% vs. 29%). The results of 27 evaluable randomized controlled trials were combined in the meta-analysis reported by Braunschweig et al. [67]. The analysis included 1,828 patients and included comparisons between both enteral and parenteral feeding and parenteral feeding and "standard" care (i.e., no nutrition, IV fluids, and electrolytes). The analysis detected a significantly lower risk of infections with both standard care and tube feeding compared to TPN. The only situation where TPN was shown to be superior to standard care was in a sub-analysis of malnourished patients, which is what we would have anticipated from our discussions in the last chapter. The results of this analysis are illustrated in Fig. 5.1.

The results of a recent large scale 'pragmatic', randomized trial of enteral vs. parenteral feeding involving 2400 adults with an unplanned admission to one of 33 English intensive care units should not be allowed to confuse this issue [68]. In this study, nutritional support was initiated within 36 hours of admission and used exclusively for 5 days. The primary outcome was all-cause mortality at 30 days, the secondary outcomes included the duration of organ support, treated infectious and noninfectious complications and length of stay in the ICU and hospital. From what we have discussed above, it should come as no surprise that they found no significant difference in 30-day mortality associated with the route of delivery of early nutritional support. I say this because virtually none of the patients were malnourished (< 5%) and 5 days of interventional feeding could only have caused complications. Because a non-fed control group was not included, we cannot claim that either form of feeding was beneficial or detrimental. Finally, as concluded earlier, *EN and PN should not be used interchangeably*; they both have their own specific indications. Thus, the majority of patients included in this study should not have been given PN as the chief inclusion criterion was "patients who *could be fed through either the parenteral or the enteral route*", indicating that they all had functional guts.

The consequence of the above meta analysis was a massive increase in the demand for feeding tube placement and the increasing involvement of gastroenterologists, radiologists, and surgeons to place specialized feeding tubes for enteral feeding in ICU patients with upper GI disturbances. This can be readily appreciated by a visit to any of our ICUs, where most patients will be seen to be sporting nasoenteric feeding tubes! Only a small minority of patients needing nutritional support, namely those with severe malnutrition (i.e., BMI <15 kg/m^2), where protein

Table 5.2 TPN and enteral feeding both have their own specific indications and should not be applied interchangeably

- If the gut is functional, *enteral feeding* should be used
- If the gut cannot be used for extended periods of time, *TPN* should be used
- If the patient is marasmic (e.g., on physical examination or BMI <15) and where enteral feeding results in diarrhea/malabsorption, short-term supplemental *TPN plus enteral (or oral) feeding* ("bridge TPN") is needed to break the vicious cycle

depletion impairs digestive and visceral organ function [28, 29] and those with true intestinal failure, are given TPN (Table 5.2).

Why Is Enteral Feeding Superior?

It is fundamental to understand that enteral feeding is physiological whereas intravenous feeding (TPN) is not. Our ability to tolerate nutrients infused into the right side of the heart with TPN is considerably less than our ability to tolerate nutrients fed via the gut as there are protective mechanisms within the gut, but not within the central veins, to (a) prevent microorganisms entering the body with food, to (b) prevent overfeeding, and to (c) prevent excessive fluctuations in bloodstream nutrients during feeding and fasting.

Explanation for the Complications of Parenteral Nutrition

In Chapter 3, we reviewed the physiology of normal feeding via the gut. In contrast, intravenous feeding bypasses the highly orchestrated processes of digestion, absorption, and distribution of absorbed nutrients to specific organs, and, at the same time, breaks the septic barrier with infusions directly into a central vein and right side of the heart (Fig. 5.2). The catheter not only can introduce infection into the systemic circulation but also can injure the intima of the vein, setting up a nidus for thrombosis and subsequent venous occlusion. By bypassing the regulatory effects of the pancreas and the liver, IV infusions result in excessive fluxes in nutrient levels during times of TPN infusions, for example, at night. Consequently, the long-term problems of TPN include recurrent bacteremia and septicemia, hyperglycemia, hyperaminoacidemia, hypertriglyceridemia, central vein thrombosis, and perhaps the most serious of all, impaired liver function because of depleted hepatic nutrition from the portal bloodstream, which may progress to liver failure and death. There is strong experimental evidence that nutrients infused by vein are not utilized as efficiently by the liver as portal nutrients derived from enteral feeding because of compartmentation [38]. In a study of healthy volunteers, we infused exactly the same quantity of amino acids and glucose (1.5 g of protein and 40 kcal energy/kg ideal body wt/day) into the gut and then into a vein and showed that the plasma amino acid and glycemic responses were always greater with IV infusion [30] (Fig. 5.3).

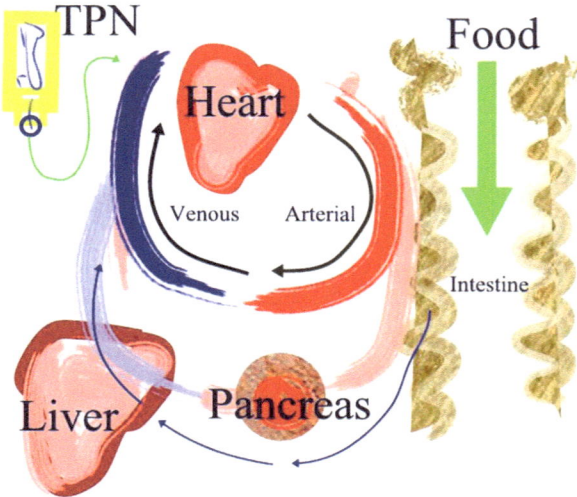

Fig. 5.2 Graphic illustration of why enteral feeding is safer and more effective than parenteral feeding: the gut is designed to digest, absorb, and distribute essential nutrients, while infusions of sterile elemental nutrients into the right side of the heart break down all safety barriers and metabolic control, and produce central vein injury

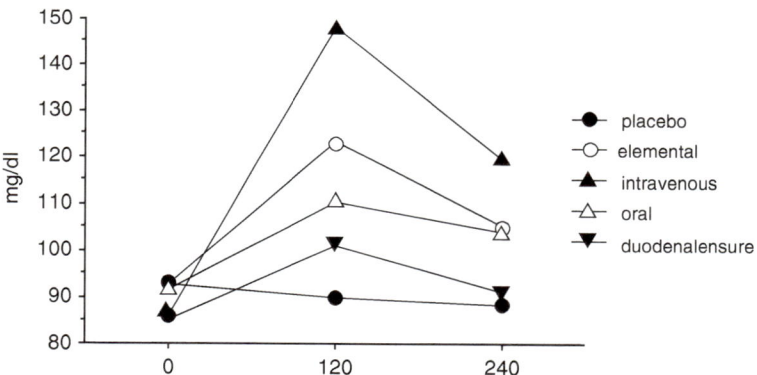

Fig. 5.3 Glycemic responses to enteral (duodenal elemental diets), oral, or duodenal infusions of a polymeric diet (Ensure) and parenteral feeding of the same quantity of nutrients. Plasma glucose responses, given as group means ± sem, illustrating the significantly higher responses to intravenously administered nutrients ($p = 0.001$) (O'Keefe et al. Am J Physiol 2003, ref. [30])

This illustrates the decreased ability of the body to assimilate glucose and amino acids when infused intravenously as compared to enterally. It also explains why hyperglycemia is virtually universal in stressed ICU patients given PN as they have the compounding problem of acute stress-induced insulin resistance. Finally, studies have shown that the utilization of infused amino acids for hepatic protein synthesis is higher if they are given by gut rather than vein [39].

TPN Liver Disease

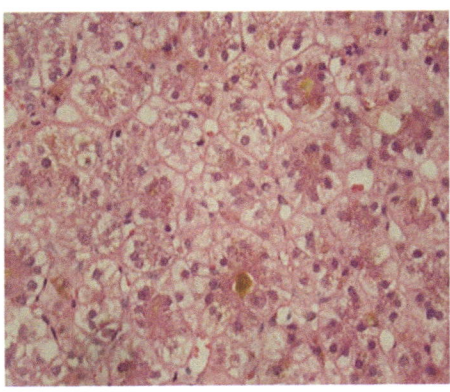 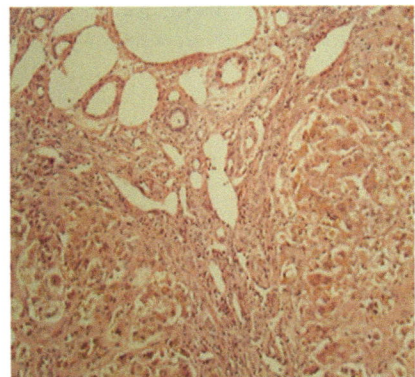

TPN Steatosis with early cholestasis

End stage liver disease demonstrating biliary cirrhosis without portal inflammation or fatty infiltration.

Fig. 5.4 Classic histological features of TPN-associated liver disease. Early changes include fatty infiltration and cholestasis (*left*), late changes include fibrosis and cirrhosis (*right*)

Perhaps the most enigmatic complication of long-term TPN is that of PN-associated liver disease (PNALD). This includes a wide variety of liver problems including steatosis, cholestasis, gall bladder dysfunction (including sludge and stones), fibrosis, cirrhosis, and liver failure. Histological features include intracellular and intracanalicular cholestasis, steatosis, periportal inflammation, fibrosis, and cirrhosis as illustrated in Fig. 5.4 [69]. While liver dysfunction, revealed by serum enzyme abnormalities, is almost universal, progression to cirrhotic chronic liver disease and liver failure is uncommon, poorly understood, and uniformly fatal unless a combined intestine and liver transplant is performed. Home PN (HPN) patients, and in particular those with short bowel intestinal failure (SB-IF), are at particularly high risk for HPN-associated liver complications because they have the major risk factors of long duration of treatment, ultrashort bowel, small-bowel bacterial overgrowth, and disruption of the bile acid pool. End-stage liver disease is more common in SB-IF infants, where survival with TPN is less than 6 months. A recent report concluded that the incidence of PNALD in infants may be as high as 50% after only 2 months of PN, and that continuation for >3 months was likely to lead to end-stage liver disease and the need for liver transplantation for survival [70]. Outcome is also poor in adults. To illustrate the evolution of PNALD, a recent review of two programs in Paris, France, noted that of the 90 home TPN patients followed from 1985 to 1996, 65% developed biochemical chronic cholestasis (>1.5× elevation of γ glutamyl transferase, alkaline phosphatase, and bilirubin) and 42% extensive portal fibrosis or cirrhosis. Twenty-two percent of all deaths were caused by end-stage liver disease. Those patients with the shortest remaining intestine and the most TPN dependent were at greatest risk. Chan et al. found the incidence of end-stage liver disease related to TPN was 15% in their home TPN patient population over 23 years of therapy [71]. Craig et al. detailed the progression of hepatic steatosis to fibrosis and eventual hepatic failure and death, based on serial liver biopsies, in a TPN-dependent patient [72].

The etiology of abnormal liver function tests is unknown, but it is likely to be multifactorial and is a consequence of the breakdown of normal digestive physiology. Numerous associations have been identified, including excessive IV dextrose; too many or too few calories from IV lipids; deficiencies of carnitine, bile acids, choline, essential fatty acids, and amino acids; a state of chronic inflammation from indwelling catheters and recurrent sepsis; and endotoxemia from small bowel bacterial overgrowth [73], but the true etiology is probably a combination of several of these factors. To illustrate the complexity, a recent study by Jain et al. [74] in a neonatal TPN-pig model showed that all animals developed cholestasis and steatosis after only 14 days [74]. In addition, plasma GLP-1, GLP-2, "ileal brake" gut peptides secreted by the ileum in response to feeding, and FGF-19, a novel hormone that represses hepatic bile acid synthesis and improves lipid metabolism and glycemic control, were suppressed compared to controls who were enterally fed. They then treated another TPN group with the bile acid, chenodeoxycholic acid, and noted a fourfold reduction in bilirubin levels and increases in GLP-1, GLP-2, and FGF-19 blood levels. Furthermore, bile acid treatment resulted in partial reversal of the mucosal atrophy associated with TPN. This all sounds very complicated: *it is*, and we can be sure that many other pathways will be identified which might equally contribute to the hepatic dysfunction associated with feeding patients by vein rather than gut. I say this because, despite the improvement of these parameters with CDCA supplementation in Jain's article, none of them returned to normal, indicating that bile acid deficiency is but one of the contributing factors to cholestasis and disturbed metabolism in TPN-fed animals.

Why Might Enteral Feeding Improve Outcome?

It has long been recognized that many of the complications associated with TPN are a consequence of bowel rest. If you don't use the gut, it fails, increasing morbidity and mortality. *The gut is designed to be fed.* If it is not fed, local and systemic complications can develop which can impair outcome from any disease.

The absence of enteral nutrients compromises the health and function of both the small and the large intestine, but by different mechanisms, summarized on Table 5.3.

Oro-enteral Feeding Prevents Gut Stagnation

Both oral and enteral feeding stimulate peristalsis, as well as salivary, gastric, pancreatic, and biliary secretion. The promotion of migrating motor complexes, as well as interdigestive contractions, sweeps luminal contents caudally, producing a

Table 5.3 Summary of the key factors explaining why the maintenance of enteral feeding improves patient outcome

The benefits of enteral feeding

Enteral nutrition

- Best supports splanchnic protein synthesis
  - O'Keefe Gastroenterology (2004)
- Prevents intestinal ischemia
  - Rahman et al. J Gastro Surg (2003)
- Maintains motility "housekeeping"
- Prevents bacterial overgrowth
- Prevents bacterial translocation and endotoxemia
  - Kotani et al. Arch Surg (1999)
- Suppresses systemic inflammatory responses
  - Wu et al. (1999); Fong et al. (1994)
- Stimulates growth factors, EGF, GLP-2, reduces permeability
  - Chen et al. (2003)

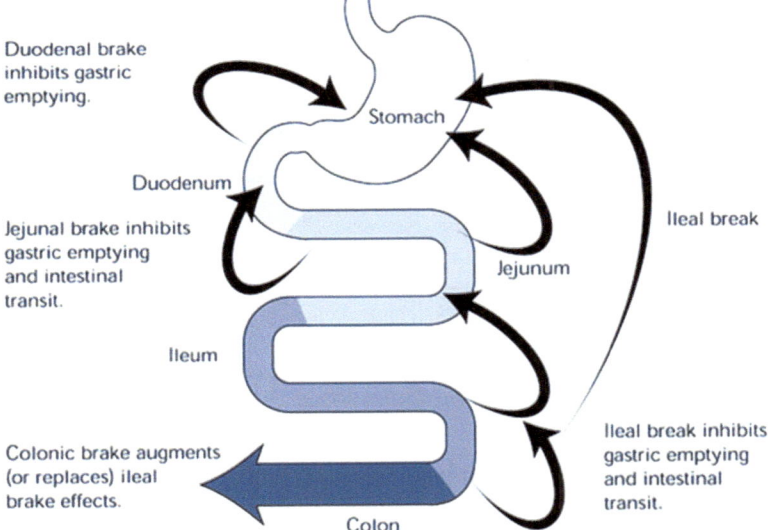

Fig. 5.5 The regulation of intestinal function. The illustration shows that at each level, the propulsion of food caudally is controlled by a balance between intestinal prokinetic motility powered by migrating motor complexes and interdigestive complexes ("housekeeping") and negative feedback loops to prevent overloading the system

motion termed "housekeeping." Furthermore, food within the small intestine stimulates colonic motility and promotes defecation through the enterocolic reflex. Figure 5.5 illustrates that the movement of food and the digesta through the gut is maintained by a series of negative feedback loops that prevent overfeeding and maintain a controlled flow caudally.

The integration of these functions is critical to maintain the sensitive balance of distribution of microbiota throughout the gut. Figure 5.6 shows the normal variation in bacterial populations down the gut. Microbes interfere with the process of digestion and absorption in the small intestine, but are critically important for absorption in the colon. The oropharynx is heavily contaminated. Populations in the stomach are dramatically suppressed by gastric acid. Post-pyloric duodenal populations are kept low by pancreobiliary secretions, and with their gradual reabsorption, populations progressively expand towards the ileum. As the ileocecal valve is passed, there is a massive explosion in population counts to allow for the fermentation and salvage of indigestible food residues.

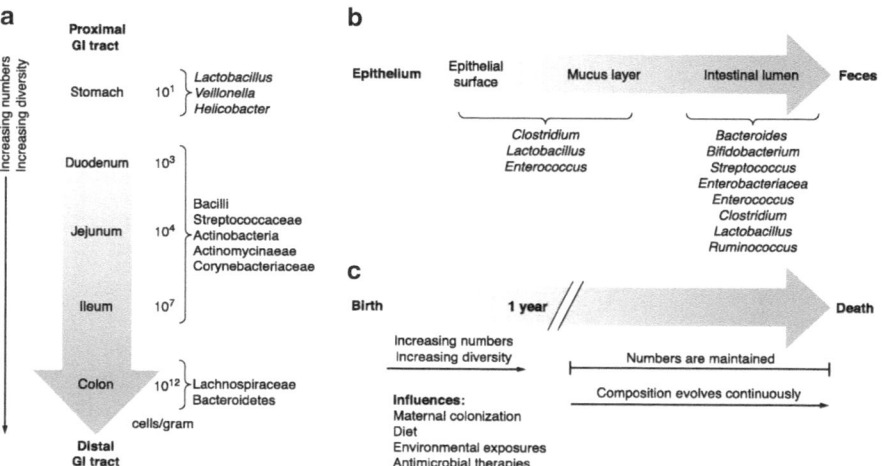

Fig. 5.6 Spatial and temporal aspects of intestinal microbiota composition. (**a**) Variations in microbial numbers and composition across the length of the gastrointestinal (GI) tract. (**b**) Longitudinal variations in microbial composition in the intestine. (**c**) Temporal aspects of microbiota establishment and maintenance and factors influencing microbial composition. Sekirov I et al. Physiol Rev 2010;90:859–904

With bowel rest, particularly if it accompanies ileus, the normal "housekeeping" by the migrating motor complexes is lost and the proximal bowel stagnates and becomes progressively contaminated by colonic organisms, leading to a condition known as *small bowel bacterial overgrowth* (SBBO). In the normal state, the bacteria within the small intestine contribute little to digestion of food, but with SBBO, fermentation shifts capitally, interfering with the normal enzymatic digestion and absorption of food in the small intestine, and resulting in maldigestion, rapid transit, increased fluid delivery to the colon, and subsequent diarrhea and malabsorption. In addition, the overgrowth produces endotoxins, which are absorbed and amplify systemic inflammatory responses [75–78]. The evidence for bacterial translocation is less compelling in man than in rats and mice [79], but it is noteworthy that most systemic infections in severe acute pancreatitis are of gut origin [80].

The absence of luminal nutrients and the almost ubiquitous use of broad-spectrum antibiotics in critically ill patients not only disturb the distribution of bacteria but also disturb the composition and function of the microbiota, leading to a condition known as *dysbiosis*. In this condition, the self-regulatory role of the healthy microbiota is lost, allowing overgrowth with potentially pathogenic bacteria, such as *C. difficile*. In a way, the gut becomes an abscess producing an acute inflammatory response, with the release of chemokines and cytokines that trigger systemic inflammatory responses. In turn, this leads to the impairment of function of distant organs such as the lungs and kidney, increasing the risk of multiple organ failure, a complex medical disorder that increases the morbidity and mortality from any form of disease [81].

Prevents Mucosal Atrophy: "Trophic" Feeding

The absence of luminal nutrients inhibits mucosal growth and results in mucosal atrophy. Studies in rats have demonstrated that mucosal atrophy increases the risk of gut permeability and translocation of bacteria into the bloodstream, illustrating the potential importance of luminal nutrients in host defense. Although translocation is less common in humans, studies have shown increased rates in critically ill patients, and it is important to note that most of the infections associated with acute pancreatitis are of gut origin [80]. The importance of "topical" nutrition is another example of compartmentation within the body, because mucosal atrophy occurs even if blood levels of nutrients are maintained by TPN. There is preferential utilization of luminal amino acids for mucosal protein synthesis as demonstrated by our enteral versus parenteral feeding studies which showed that enteral feeding with the same quantities of nutrients given enterally compared to parenterally enhanced synthesis by 80% (Chapter 3, Fig. 3.2) [31].

As discussed in Chapter 3, the preferred *energy* source for the mucosa is the amino acid glutamine, and not blood glucose [35]. Glutamine is the most abundant amino acid within the body and in the bloodstream. It is an inessential amino acid that is synthesized predominantly in muscle, but also within the mucosa, from glutamate, which in turn is synthesized from the Kreb's cycle intermediate, α-ketoglutarate. Not only is glutamine the preferred fuel for enterocytes, but it also helps maintain mucosal integrity and is a precursor for purine synthesis and therefore one of the rate-limiting factors in the turnover of rapidly dividing cells, such as the mucosa and bone marrow [40]. Considering these functions, it was originally suggested that glutamine deficiency was the cause of TPN-associated mucosal atrophy, because regular TPN does not contain glutamine for two reasons: it is an inessential amino acid that can be synthesized from glutamate, and it is unstable in storage, dissociating into glutamate and ammonia. However, the subsequent construction of TPN solutions that contained glutamine (usually in the form of a more stable dipeptide) failed to prevent mucosal atrophy—again indicating the critical importance of luminal nutrition.

Perhaps the best studies on the luminal requirements are those from Stoll's group at Baylor. Using an in vivo neonatal pig model with enteral and parenteral access, venous, arterial, and portal catheters, and an ultrasonic portal vein flow probe, they demonstrated that enteral nutrition that provided only 20% of total dietary requirements prevented protein loss from the bowel, and that 40% maintained mucosal mass [36, 37]. This might explain why in clinical practice, some have observed that "optimal" outcomes are associated with enteral infusions meeting only 50–60% of estimated needs, based on 25 kcal/kg ideal body weight/day. For example, Krishnan et al. studied the outcome of their medical ICU patients with a duration of stay >96 h, and found that the average caloric intake among 187 participants was only 50.6% of goal. However, they concluded that these goals probably overestimated needs as moderate caloric intake (i.e., 33–65% of targets; approximately 9–18 kcal/kg per day) was associated with better outcomes than higher levels of caloric intake [83].

As discussed earlier, we have shown that enteral feeding better supports splanchnic and mucosal protein synthesis than intravenous feeding [31]. Consequently, it is rational in patients with intra-abdominal injury, such as acute pancreatitis or following major abdominal surgery, to strive to use enteral rather than parenteral feeding *as this best targets the region of increased need*. This brings up two important practical management points:

1. *Intestinal anastomoses*: Surgeons are often wary of permitting enteral feeding after intestinal anastomosis. Provided the anastomosis was made securely, early enteral feeding will not only be safe, but will also *increase* the strength of the anastomosis. This concept was first suggested by Rolandelli and Rombeau in the 1980s in their study of rats with colonic transections [84]. One group was fed an elemental diet which would be totally absorbed before entering the colon, and the other a pectin-supplemented elemental diet. Results showed that anastomosis-bursting pressure was significantly enhanced by pectin (a fiber) supplementation, and that the hydroxyproline content of the anastomosis was higher indicating more intense healing.

2. *Bowel rest and enterocutaneous fistulae*: In the 1980s it was standard practice to place all patients with high output (proximal) EC fistulae on TPN and bowel rest for up to 6 weeks to achieve "spontaneous" closure. While this practice certainly reduces the flow of juice from the fistula, it compromises the health and function of the intestine as discussed above, both proximally and distally, increasing the risk of further complications. Enteral feeding, initially at a slow continuous rate, should continue to maintain mucosal health and function, and thus to support the recovery process and allow healing of the fistula. If the situation is complicated by perforation, EN should be held until the perforation either seals spontaneously or by surgery, whence EN can be restarted. The thing to remember is that if the bowel distal to a fistula is open and functional, then peristalsis will naturally propel the digesta down the bowel rather than out the fistula. If it doesn't, then surgery will be required to remove the obstruction or restore distal function. In support of this practice, a recent study on 82 patients with open abdomen management for GI fistulae and sepsis showed that early enteral feeding was associated with earlier closure of the abdomen and lower mortality [85]. It should be noted that 68% had high output fistulae treated successfully with succus entericus reinfusion distally. Finally, it must be stressed that there is *no role*

for TPN and bowel rest in the management of low output distal EC fistulae e.g. ileocolonic. First of all, TPN and bowel rest do not prevent basal intestinal secretion, and second, digestion and absorption occur in duodenum and jejunum. Stasis produced by TPN and bowel rest will simply worsen outcome by adding septic complications.

3. *Mucosal Blood Flow:* Associated with the trophic effects of enteral nutrition are increases in mucosal blood flow, and increases in trophic gut peptide release—in particular GLP-2 [86–88]. There has been a concern that enteral feeding might exacerbate intestinal ischemia, and thus precipitate gut infarction in patients with marginal blood flow. However, it is difficult to understand the rationale for this proposition, as nutrients stimulate mucosal blood flow and prevent ischemia by counteracting the effects of vasoconstricting factors, such as endothelins and selectins [89]. Furthermore, if blood flow is limiting, metabolism will be suppressed and will not be stimulated by nutrient supply. Nutrients also stimulate the release of epithelial growth factors, such as EGF and GLP-2, which independently increase tissue perfusion and preserve mucosal integrity [90].

4. *Gut Immune Function:* The intestine is our "window to the world." Every day we consume millions of live microbes and antigens that, if injected into our bloodstream, would kill us through anaphylactic shock. This risk is averted by the process of sterilization and digestion outlined above, and by the gut-associated lymphoid tissue, which encircles the lumen to engulf any remaining bacteria and to neutralize the antigenic effect of any residual antigens. Animal studies have shown that gut immune function is suppressed by TPN feeding, with enhancement of pro-inflammatory Th-1 responses and suppression of surface IgA production [91]. The key role played by enteral feeding in maintaining gut and systemic immunity has recently been reviewed by Fukatsu and Kudsk, highlighting the stimulatory effects of enteral feeding on adhesion molecules (MAdCAM-1), Th-1 responses, antimicrobial and antiviral secretory proteins (sIgA, sPLA-2, defensins), ERK phosphorylation and lymphocyte proliferation, and hepatic Kupffer cell function [32]. Furthermore, human studies have endorsed the results of numerous experimental studies [32] that have demonstrated that the inflammatory response to injected systemic endotoxin is higher in subjects fed by TPN and kept on bowel rest compared to the response when fed by gut [78].

It is these studies that provide the rationale for the use of slow enteral "trophic" feeding as soon as possible in critical illness, more for preventing septic complications than maintaining or restoring nutritional status.

Enteral Feeding and the Large Intestine (Colon)

The evolution of the digestive system is a fascinating example of our partnership with the gut microbiota and environmental microbes. Food cannot be fully digested by human digestive enzymes, but it can by our symbiotic association with the microbiota. The best example of this is starch digestion. The bulk of starch digestion is performed by pancreatic α-amylase, which is incapable of breaking down some α1–4 and most of the α1–6 glycosidic linkages. In addition, digestible starch can be partially converted into "resistant" starch by cooking and cooling. Partial digestion by pancreatic enzymes leaves behind residues consisting of linear branched oligosaccharides, known as limit α-dextrins. The digestion of remaining 1–4 (α-glucosidase) and 1–6 bonds (α-dextrinase) can be completed by enzymes embedded in the brush border of the small intestine. However, many plant glycans, commonly termed "fiber," cannot be broken down by intestinal enzymes because of their complex molecular configurations or because they are protected by plant cell walls, and pass through to the colon. This ensures that a good supply of dietary carbohydrate (30–60 g/day), which includes fiber and about 20% of potentially "digestible" starch (including "resistant" starch), is delivered to the colon to support a large and diverse range of microbes, termed the *microbiota*. The recognition that bacterial cells outnumber those of the host by 10 to 1 has alerted investigators to the importance of the crosstalk and symbiosis between the intestinal epithelium and this highly active metabolic "foreign" cell mass. Based on the sequencing of the highly conserved 16S region of rRNA, it has been estimated that there are approximately 800 different bacterial species with over 7,000 strains, with an estimated mass of 1–2 kg and number of 100 trillion [90]. It is maternally acquired at birth, and its composition is subsequently modified by environmental and host factors including breastfeeding, diet, antibiotics, radiation, and surgery. In return for a safe harbor and a constant supply of food, the microbiota penetrates the complex carbohydrate residues and releases simple sugars through their secretion of β or γ-amylase, which sustains fermentation and the production of short-chain fatty acids which play a fundamental role in the preservation of both colonic health and function [3, 33, 45]. Recent studies have shown that the microbiota participates in a wide range of metabolic functions providing a wide range of metabolites, termed the *metabolome*, that maintain not only colonic mucosal health but also general body health [93]. In addition, the microbiota is invaluable in providing "colonization resistance" against pathogenic microbiota, ensuring gut mucosal growth, motility, and angiogenesis, producing essential vitamins, for example folate and biotin [46], reinforcing the gut mucosal defense barrier, and having the crucial function of immunomodulation at the interface of the body's largest immune organ, the intestinal mucosa-associated lymphoid tissue (MALT) [44]. Most recognized is their ability to break down resistant starches and plant fibers to glycans derived from diet and endogenous sources, such as mucus, into short-chain fatty acids, thereby providing food for the bacteria and a topical nutrient source for the colon. One of them, butyrate, is the chief energy source for colonocytes [94]. Butyrate is to the colon is what glutamine is to the small intestine. Furthermore, butyrate plays a major role in the regulation of mucosal proliferation and differentiation, suppressing inflammation, colitis, and colon cancer risk [3, 33, 45]. The critical importance of luminal nutrition for the colon was revealed by the recognition that disconnection of the colon from the ileal stream led to an acute colitis, similar to ulcerative colitis, termed "diversion colitis" [95] (Fig. 5.7), that was responsive to SCFA enemas [95].

Fig. 5.7 Sigmoidoscopic
appearance of diversion
colitis in a patient

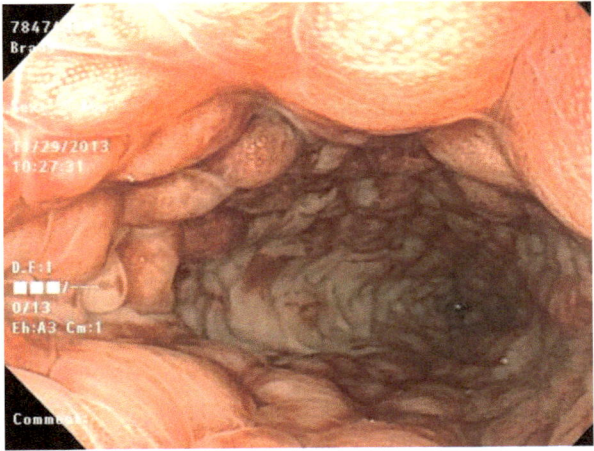

Elemental diets have the same effect on the colon as TPN has on the small intestine: the mucosa atrophies, because all is absorbed before reaching the colon resulting in the absence of topical nutrition. In an elegant series of studies in rats, Goodlad et al. demonstrated that in comparison to normal feeding with rat chow, starvation strongly suppressed colonic crypt cell production (Fig. 5.8) [96]. Feeding an elemental diet (Flexical) supplemented with the inert bulking agent, kaolin, following 3 days fast, did not restore crypt proliferation, while the addition of a mixed fiber source (hemicellulose 40%, cellulose 20%, lignin 15%, and pectin 5%) did. The restoration of the mucosal structure and function with reintroduction of dietary fiber is only possible if the normal microbiota is present [96].

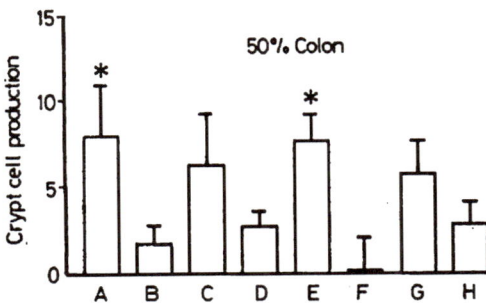

Fig. 5.8 Crypt cell production rates in the mid colon. Group A = Fed group (powdered laboratory rat diet). Group B = Starved for 3 days. Group C = Starved then refed - Flexical + kaolin. Group D = Starved then refed - Flexical + wood cellulose. Group E = Starved then refed - Flexical + Trifyba. Group F = Starved then refed - Flexical + ispaghula mucilage. Group G = Starved then refed - Powdered Standard diet. Group H = Starved then refed - Flexical (Goodlad et al. Gut, 1987, 28, 171–180)

Starvation is known to increase the risk of diarrhea presumably due to short-chain fatty acid deficiency. The problem is amplified in the critically ill who are usually fed with non-residue semi-elemental diets that effectively starve the colon, and who are usually treated with broad-spectrum antibiotics, producing a double hit on the composition and function of the microbiota. This culminates in dysbiosis, which forms a permissive environment for overgrowth with pathogens such as *C. difficile* which, in the presence of a malnourished colonic mucosa, leads to *C. difficile-associated* colitis, [97], a condition associated with high mortality rates [97, 99]. Probiotic (naturally occurring bacterial species, such as Lactobacilli and Bifidobacteria, that have been shown to have mucosal health-promoting qualities) supplementation probably helps in this situation, [99], but the best treatment is try to stop antibiotics, stop PPIs (which also promote small bowel bacterial overgrowth due to their interference with gastric acid sterilization), and provide fiber supplementation of the feeds in adequate amounts, e.g., "Benefiber" 8 g t.i.d., bearing in mind that most critical care formulae diets contain grossly inadequate quantities of fiber, i.e., <5 g fiber/l [34].

Recent studies of ours show that the *quality of tube feeding* can be improved if the semi-elemental diet is progressively supplemented with soluble fiber, even in the presence of continued antibiotic and PPI use [34]. Figure 5.9 illustrates the point that the microbiota is grossly suppressed in critically ill patients treated with semi-elemental

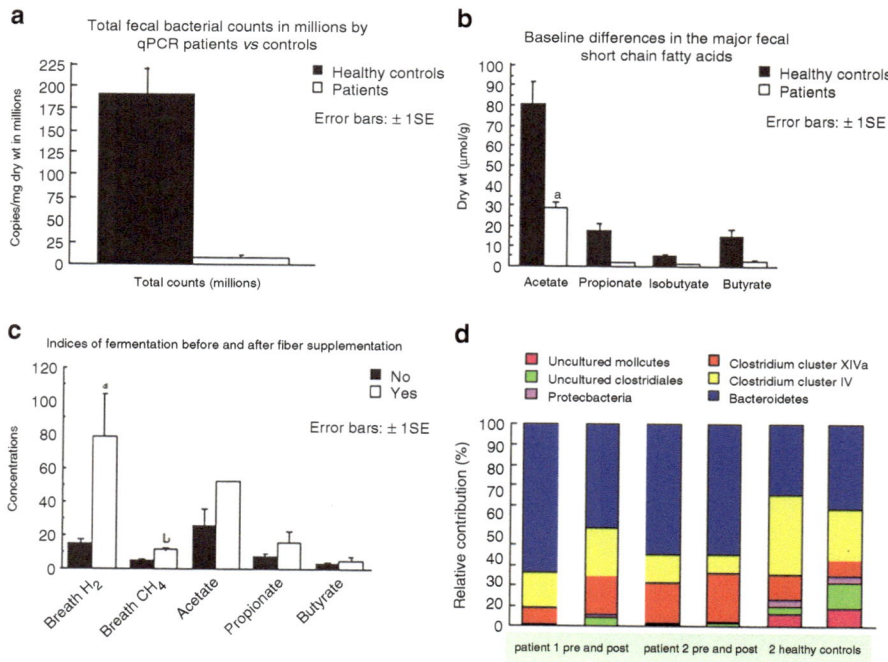

Fig. 5.9 The microbiota and their metabolites (short-chain fatty acids) in critical illness before and after fiber supplementation

diets, PPIs, and antibiotics and that this is associated with suppression in fecal short-chain fatty acid content. A more detailed analysis of the phylogenetic changes in microbial composition showed that microbial composition and diversity was also disturbed.

Fiber supplementation of the tube feeds up to 35 g/day in these patients resulted in significant increases in fecal SCFAs, but did not restore them to normal, as many continued to need antibiotics (Fig. 5.9). There was however an improvement in diarrhea in most patients given fiber supplementation. Despite the fact that the "critical illness" specific formula diet that we used was stated to contain "prebiotics" (prebiotics are food substrates, such as soluble fiber, that increase the growth of the colonic microbiota) in the form of oligosaccharides to support colonic health, the quantity was only 5 g/l, which is insufficient for the metabolic needs of the microbiota as stated above. In desperate situations where patients have been on intensive antibiotic treatment for long periods resulting in severe dysbiosis and chronic recurrent *C. difficile* colitis, the only effective treatment is to reestablish the microbiota with "fecal transplants." Here, a sample of normal stool from a pretested healthy volunteer is emulsified and delivered to the colon either by colonoscopy or nasojejunal tube [100]. Of course, this will not engraft for any length of time if the patient continues on antibiotics and non-residue diets.

The timing for fiber supplementation of tube feeds has yet to be determined. Although it would seem logical to use a fiber containing formula from word go, a recent fascinating study revealed evidence that the gut may feed the microbiota in early critical illness by a process named 'fucosylation'. Pickard et al reported in Nature that starved mice made critically ill by injection of LPS shed fucosylated proteins into the intestinal lumen [101] (Fig. 5.10). Fucose was liberated and metabolized by the gut microbiota, affecting the expression of microbial metabolic pathways with a reduction in the expression of bacterial virulence genes. This also improved host tolerance of the mild pathogen *Citrobacter rodentium*. Thus, they concluded that rapid IEC fucosylation appeared to be a protective mechanism that utilized the host's resources to maintain host–microbial interaction during pathogen-induced stress. This mechanism makes evolutionary sense as it maintains nutritional support for the microbiota during critical illness in the absence of feeding. If proven true in human studies, this would reduce the urgency of early enteral feeding in maintaining gut function.

Fig. 5.10 Fucosylation of small intestine epithelial cells (IECs) by systemic stimulation of Toll Like Receptors with systemic injection of the ligand lipopolysaccharide-4

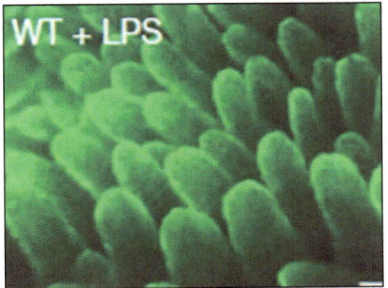

Nutritional Support Is Not a Stand-Alone Therapy

Enthusiasm for the potential for nutritional support to improve outcome and survival has led to the claim that the discipline would be better termed "nutritional therapy." This is misleading, as nearly all patients with nutritional problems in hospital have them as a consequence of an underlying disease or injury, and nutrition by itself cannot reverse the disease or injury, but supplies the body with the building blocks and energy to rebuild and recover function once specific therapy has been given to reverse the underlying problem or disease process. *Consequently, the primary aim of the medical team is to reverse the disease process with specific medications, or repair the anatomical abnormality with surgery, while the nutrition support team optimizes the healing process by providing adequate nutrients.* Nutrition is, however, therapeutic if the problem is simply starvation due to lack of food, but that is not what this book is about.

Who Needs Nutritional Support?

There are two major reasons for providing nutritional support:

1. To provide essential nutrients for the recovery from acute illness and repair from injury when body stores are depleted.
2. To maintain gut function to prevent complications.

Nutritional Support Should be Tailored to the Depth of Body Stores

In the early years of nutritional support, much emphasis was placed on the measurement of nutritional status as a way of determining the timing for nutritional intervention. The appreciation of the difficulties in defining malnutrition in critically ill patients and in knowing the degree of depletion of body stores that is limiting for organ function and host defense shifted from *improvement* or *restitution* of nutritional status to providing *nutritional support for the prevention of critical nutrient depletion* in patients that we expect to be unable to eat for a protracted period. What we still do not know is how soon should we commence nutritional support. This question is of even more concern in the obese. Can we wait longer before implementing nutrition support in the obese? The answer is probably yes with regard to calories and to a lesser extent protein, as body stores are higher, as will be discussed in more detail in Chapter 16. However, the storage of fluid, electrolytes, minerals, and vitamins is not significantly higher, and so the composition of nutritional support should be modified accordingly.

Gut Function

Even in previously well-nourished patients, the absence of enteral feeding during the first week of critical illness may give rise to more complications than the loss of nutrient stores. Again, no measurements have been made to determine how long it takes for bowel rest to cause complications, but we know well from clinical experience that the longer we wait, the more established the ileus becomes, and the more difficult it becomes to reverse. There is substantial evidence to support the use of early "trickle" or "trophic" enteral feeding (e.g., 20 cc/h of a polymeric or semi-elemental diet) to maintain gut function [102]. And if we maintain gut function, we know we can suppress systemic inflammatory responses, as reviewed above [32, 78].

The Timing of Nutritional Support

Of all the questions about the efficacy and need for nutritional support, the one that remains mostly unanswered is "when should nutritional support be started?"

There are no good studies that have examined how long you can wait before feeding a sick patient for the simple reason that it would currently be considered unethical to withhold feeding in one randomized subgroup—and the family would certainly not give consent for trial starvation! Thus, we are forced to base our judgments on what has been found in experimental animals and from extrapolations from studies on organ function in malnourished patients and starvation victims.

From the physiological studies of human starvation, we know that short-term starvation is well tolerated by the previously well nourished. Further, we are designed to survive periods of famine, and to survive critical illness without eating, for example like the example of one potential mechanism of fucolysation as described above [101] (Fig. 5.10). Experience over the past 30 years has taught us that aggressive feeding can lead to more harm than good, as both enteral and parenteral feeding have well-recognized complications. From the evidence presented in our discussion above, we will argue that nutritional support must always be designed to support the normal metabolic response, not to replace it. The question then becomes, "when does the mechanism for repair in acute illness become compromised by the lack of endogenous stores?"

To explore this question, we present an estimation of how long it would take an average 70 kg (BMI 24 kg/m²) adult male to become critically protein deficient. Of course, this begs the question, as we still do not have the tools to measure when a state of "critical protein deficiency" exists. However, from the synthesis of evidence presented above on the effects of malnutrition on gut function, we would predict that it is when the BMI dips below 15 kg/m². This represents a 40% acute weight loss, which, from the IRA hunger strikers' experience, was the degree of depletion when mortality was first documented. In an attempt to develop best estimates of how long it would take to become critically protein deficient, I sought the help of Professor John Waterlow, a renowned international expert in protein metabolism, who suggested the approach summarized in Table 5.4. Using a number of commonly

Table 5.4 Estimation of how long body protein stores will last without feeding

In health

1. Suppose initial wt = 70 kg. Ht 1.7 m. BMI 24: then muscle mass—30 kg (–43% of body wt)
2. Suppose all the loss of protein is from muscle. This is a conservative assumption, but probably not far from what really happens
3. Suppose danger point is BMI—15. Wt would then be 43.4 kg. If muscle mass is the same proportion of body wt, it would then be 18.6 kg: therefore loss of muscle = 11.4 kg
4. If muscle contains 20% protein, loss of protein = 2.28 kg
5. Calculated initial protein loss 91 g/day, estimated final loss 30 g/day, average 61 g/day
6. From 4 to 5 above, this would take 2,280/61 = 37 days

In severe necrotizing pancreatitis

1. Suppose initial wt = 70 kg. Ht 1.7 m. BMI 24: then muscle mass = 30 kg (–43% of body wt)
2. Suppose all the loss of protein is from muscle. This is a conservative assumption, but probably not fat from what really happens
3. Suppose danger point is BMI—15. Wt would then be 43 kg. If muscle mass is the same proportion of body wt, it would then be 18.6 kg: therefore loss of muscle = 11.4 kg
4. If muscle contains 20% protein, loss of protein = 2.28 kg
5. Calculated protein loss in necrotizing pancreatitis 207 g/day
6. From 4 to 5 above, this would take 2,280/207 = 11 days

after Waterlow JC (2007)

accepted assumptions (i.e., that muscle contributes 43% of total body protein in normal health, that most of the catabolic loss of nitrogen occurs from muscle, and that the rate of catabolism decreases with time) and actual measurements of rates of catabolism made by ourselves in previously well-nourished critically ill ICU patients, we first calculated it would take 37 days of starvation for an otherwise well, previously normal person, to become "critically protein deficient." However, the estimate dropped precipitously when critical illness was superimposed on the picture. Here, rates of protein catabolism were higher and did not decrease, or adapt, with time, as explained earlier in Chapter 4 (Fig. 4.1). Based on measurements of excessive urinany nitrogen losses we made in patients with severe necrotizing pancreatitis (Fig. 5.11) (similar to those reported by Shaw et al. [103]), the estimate became only 11 days until critical deficiency occurs (Fig. 5.11).

Clearly, we do not want to wait until the patient is critically malnourished, as the intervention may be ineffective and too late. In addition, less severe losses of protein may *impair the efficiency* of organ function. A more conservative estimate would therefore be to base the calculations on a drop to a BMI of 17, which we showed was associated with partial loss of intestinal and pancreatic function in hospitalized patients [28]. If we use this figure, it would then only take 8.5 days in severe acute pancreatitis. Rates of catabolism are not usually as high in other ICU patients, and catabolic losses are nearer 20 g nitrogen per day, representing 125 g protein. In this situation, we could theoretically wait 2 weeks in a previously well-nourished individual. Thus, if protein deficiency is employed as the key determinant of the need for nutritional support, it would be reasonable to wait until the second week of acute illness in a previously well nourished critically ill patient.

However, in a previously well nourished critically ill pateint, these estimates do not take into consideration the effects of starvation on gut function, where stasis and

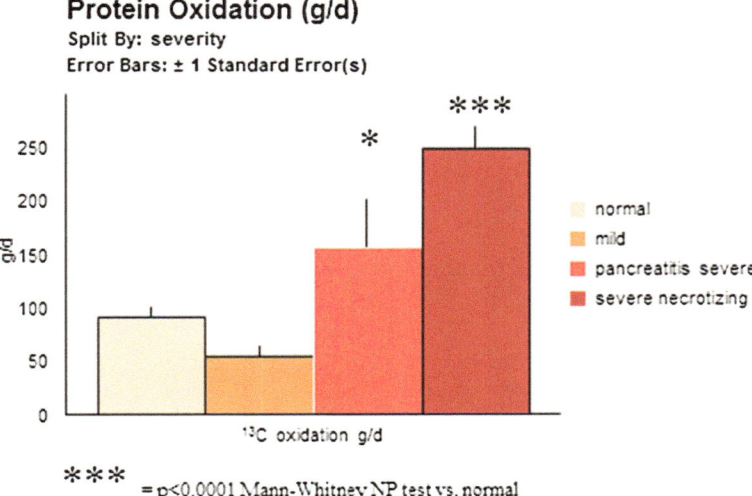

Fig. 5.11 Protein catabolic rates in patients with variable levels of severity of acute pancreatitis compared to healthy controls

bacterial overgrowth may lead to complications that worsen outcome. As discussed above, we do not know how long a critically ill patient can be starved before gut-associated complications impair outcome, but we can assume that the addition of bowel rest to starvation will reduce our estimates of how long we can wait before starting enteral feeding. What we do know is that the protein mass of the bowel can be maintained if as little as 20% of nutritional requirements are given enterally [36], and so "trophic" enteral feeding should prevent the gut-associated complications of starvation. This would suggest that enteral trophic feeding should be started as soon as the patient has been stabilized.

Recent Advances: Nutritional Outcomes Studies More Is Not Always Better

Despite the absence of trials of starvation versus interventional feeding in the management and outcome of hospitalized patients, two recent large, well-designed, randomized clinical trials have just recently been published which have finally shed some light on this subject. Up until very recently, there was a growing trend towards aggressive feeding in the ICU to prevent build up of the "negative energy gap," which was shown in *uncontrolled* clinical studies to be directly associated with both morbidity and mortality [104, 105]. This gap becomes established during the first week of ICU admission, and can be explained by combinations of the high initial rates of metabolic expenditure (catabolism) in acute illness, plus the lag in commencement of feeding due to efforts to stabilize and investigate the patient.

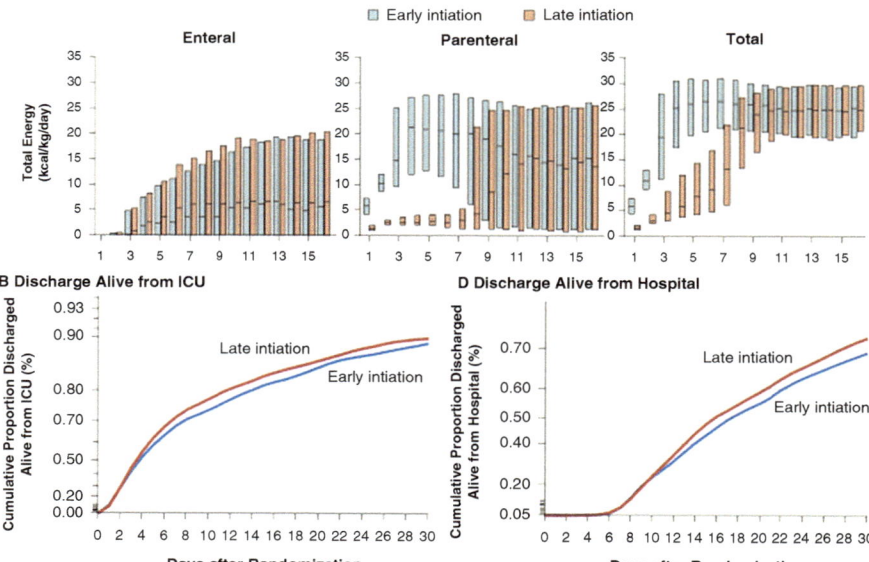

Fig. 5.12 Filing the "energy gap" with PN in the first week did not improve outcome

Furthermore, it usually takes several days to get enteral feeding to goal in the ICU. It was reasonably assumed that mortality would drop if the gap was prevented by the bimodal employment of *enteral PLUS parenteral feeding*. The initial nutrition gap could be prevented by the immediate implementation of parenteral feeding, which was continued until feeding tubes had been placed and advanced to goal with tolerance. Unfortunately, when this was put to rigorous testing by randomized clinical trial, outcome was actually worse [106], indicating that the relationship between mortality and the energy gap was not one of cause and effect! Figure 5.12 summarizes the results of this Belgian study which included 4,640 ICU patients in a randomized, multicenter trial comparing early initiation of PN (within 48 h of ICU admission—this follows the ESPEN European guidelines [107]) to late PN initiation (after day 8—this follows the ASPEN American and Canadian guidelines [108, 109]. The early group developed *significantly more ICU infections and cholestasis, which translated into significantly higher ICU and hospital mortalities*. The take-home message here is to *be wary of basing your clinical practice on the results of uncontrolled studies*. Rather, use them for hypothesis testing in adequately powered randomized controlled trials. This is the only way we will advance the quality of our clinical practice.

In the second study from the US National Heart, Lung, and Blood Institute ARDS Clinical Trials network, 500 ICU patients were randomized to early (within 48 h) "trophic" (or "trickle") enteral feeding (10–20 cc/h) for 6 days, followed by goal feeding (goal 25–30 kcal/kg/day), or "full" enteral feeding to goal as quickly

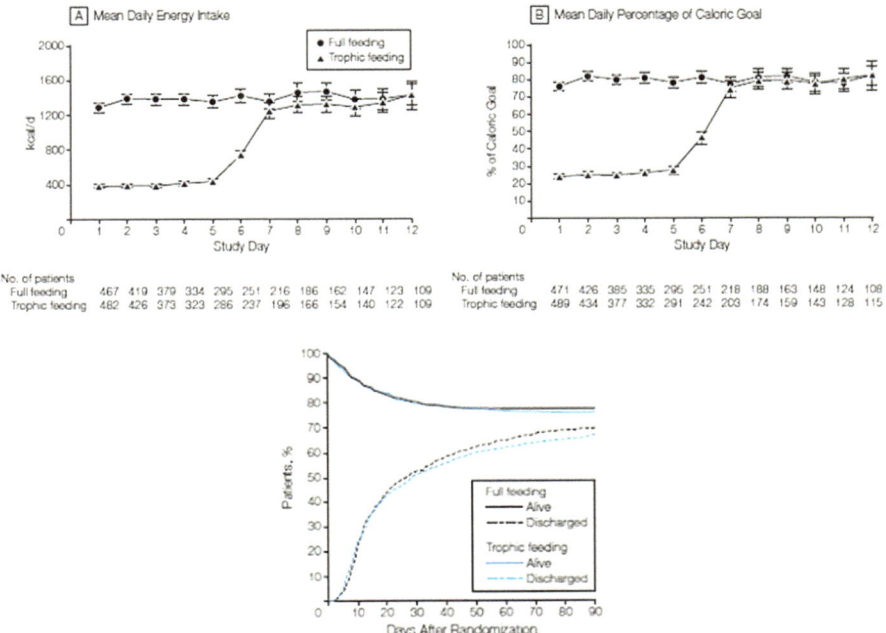

Fig. 5.13 "Full" early enteral feeding or "trophic" early feeding on outcome: no difference, more GI side effects with "full" early feeding

as possible [102]. Outcome was followed over 28 days. Figure 5.13 illustrates the chief results, which showed that there was no advantage to early aggressive "full" feeding with regard to survival or discharge. Furthermore, the full feeding group had, not surprisingly, more GI complications.

"Nutripharmaceutical" Supplements

Interestingly, the first 272 patients in the above US ARDS study were also randomized to receive a nutritional supplement containing fish oils and antioxidants (2×2 factorial design). This part of the study was subsequently abandoned [110] as the group that received the supplement actually developed a higher mortality! A similar, but much larger, well-conducted RCT in 1,223 mechanically ventilated adult patients with multi-organ failure in 40 ICUs in Canada, the United States, and Europe has just been completed to assess the efficacy of high-dose glutamine supplementation (0.5 g/kg/day alanyl-glutamine IV and 30 g glutamine enterally) or no glutamine and antioxidants (500 µg selenium IV plus EN antioxidants containing 300 µg Selenium) or no antioxidants for a maximum of 28 days (Heyland et al.). Not only were antioxidants unhelpful, but mortality was actually *higher* in the glutamine supplemented patients. Advocation for glutamine supplementation has been held by some ever since a non-randomized clinical study reported low tissue levels of glutamine in critically ill patients, leading some to postulate that glutamine was "conditionally essential" under these conditions. This has always been difficult to understand, bearing in mind that glutamine is the most common amino acid within the body and is readily synthesized from Kreb's cycle intermediates. Furthermore, the investigators failed to prove that there was a deficiency of either glutamine or antioxidants in the study patients before commencing the supplementations. The final "nail in the coffin" for glutamine supplementation was provided by another recently conducted RCT comparing a complete amino acid formulation to one supplemented with 30 g glutamine per day, where outcome was again better in the non-supplemented group (Ziegler et al.). The investigators kept the nitrogen content of the two diets the same, which meant that the study group actually got less essential amino acids and an excess of nonessential amino acid glutamine, which really does not make sense as essential amino acids are rate limiting to the synthesis of body proteins!

All of these studies support a more commonsense approach to the nutritional support of the critically ill patient. *The metabolic response to critical illness has evolved over millions of years to allow us to survive. Thus, it should be supported, not modified.* Interventions should not suppress the redistribution of body stores; they should only fortify them when stores become depleted. Further, the composition of the support should reflect as closely as possible the composition of the stores. Excessive enrichment of the support with bioactive molecules, whether they be steroids or nutrients with immune-modulating properties, such as fish oils, arginine, leucine, glutamine or antioxidants, should be avoided, as the natural inflammatory response, the metabolic response, and the maintenance of machinery and structure all demand the full spectrum of nutrients found in food and body stores for body repair, recovery, and survival, as discussed in Chapter 2.

Benefits and Risks of Nutritional Support

Benefits

1. Supports life in the depleted patient.
2. Supports the metabolic response to illness in the depleted patient.
3. Maintains organ function in the depleted patient.
4. Supports tissue repair in the depleted patient.
5. Prevents life-threatening depletion and loss of body stores.
6. Maintains gut function.

Risks

1. Enteral:

    (a) Aspiration pneumonia—life threatening.
    (b) Tube placement issues:

    - Sinusitis, nasal injury.
    - Mucosal injury.
    - Bowel perforation (rare).

(c) Overfeeding and the refeeding syndrome.

(d) Hyperglycemia.

(e) Azotemia.

(f) Hypertriglyceridemia.

(g) Diarrhea.

2. Parenteral.

(a) Central vein cannulation complications.

- Pneumothorax—life threatening.
- Air embolism—life threatening.
- Bleeding—life threatening.
- Sepsis: bacteremia, septicemia, septic shock—life threatening.

(b) Hyperglycemia—life threatening.

(c) Overfeeding and the refeeding syndrome—life threatening.

(d) Liver dysfunction, liver failure—life threatening.

(e) Azotemia.

(f) Hypertriglyceridemia.

(g) Venous thrombosis, loss of access: life threatening.

Summary

Do not prescribe TPN unless enteral access is impossible, because with enteral feeding:

1. Nutrients are more efficiently utilized for body function and repair.
2. Gut function is maintained and organ failure is reduced.
3. Systemic inflammatory responses are suppressed.
4. Central vein catheter placement complications are avoided.
5. Metabolic side effects (e.g., hyperglycemia) are less common.
6. Costs are reduced—and more lives are likely to be saved!

General Recommendations for Nutritional Support

Based on the above arguments, we can reasonably recommend the following:

1. *In all critically ill patients who are unable to eat,* correct and maintain hydration and electrolyte stability. Although this could be done by feeding tube, all such patients will have IV cannulas and IV infusions will ensure rapid correction of deficits. Remember that unless the patient is severely malnourished, *the commencement of nutrition support is never an emergency, whereas the correction of fluid and electrolyte deficiencies is.* Consideration for the early supplementation of vitamins in the form of a "happy bag" or "banana bag" (e.g., 1 l saline containing multivitamins, 2 g magnesium, 100 mg thiamin, and 2 mg folic acid) should be

made in all patients, and most especially in those with a history of alcoholism and/or chronic liver disease.

2. *In previously well-nourished individuals suffering from continuing severe illness*, nutritional support containing protein and energy should be commenced during the second week of critical illness. Although body stores would probably support the recovery process for longer than this, there is concern that death can occur rapidly once critical deficiency occurs, and we know that it is difficult, and takes time, to replenish stores in critical illness in the setting of hypercatabolism driven by pro-inflammatory cytokines and catabolic hormones. Further research needs to be done to define when stores of minerals and vitamins become functionally depleted, but in the meantime it seems reasonable to commence supplementation within the first week of inanition. *Recognizing that interventional feeding, whether it be parenteral or enteral, is not without its own complications (see below), it is perfectly reasonable to wait up to 7 days before starting complete nutritional support in a previously well-nourished patient, while resuscitating and stabilizing the patient to assess the severity of the illness and its response to therapy.* Only those patients who remain critically ill thereafter should be given interventional feeding. Ideally, the enteral route should be started as early as possible, with approximately 20% of nutritional requirements fed to maintain intestinal enterocyte functional mass and "housekeeping" motility.

3. *In malnourished patients defined by SGO or a BMI <17* with recent weight loss, feeding should be commenced as soon as possible to support the metabolic response and recovery process. Enteral feeding should always be first attempted after correction of fluid and electrolyte deficiencies, but short-term PN may be used to break the vicious cycle in the severely malnourished (e.g., BMI <15) with diarrhea due to gut dysfunction ("bridge TPN").

4. *In the obese, with BMI >30*: This is considered in detail in Chapter 16. Obesity results in increased stores predominantly of energy in adipose tissue, but also to a lesser extent in protein. Consequently, initial support should be geared towards fluid, electrolytes, minerals, and vitamins as suggested above. Complete nutrition support should be commenced as above for the previously well nourished, with the exception of restriction of glucose, e.g., 100 g glucose per day, and fat infusions, e.g., 40 g a week. Once commencing full nutritional support, *remember to never use actual body weight* to calculate goal feed rates, use ideal body weights, and consider using a formula that provides normal protein, fluid, electrolyte, and micronutrient infusion rates, and hypocaloric energy to support mobilization of body stores. A practical guide is that if hyperglycemia is induced by feeding, cut back on glucose rather than add insulin, as insulin will enhance storage and prevent the physiological mobilization of energy stores.

Part II
The Practice

Chapter 6
The Nutrition Support Team

Introduction

While nutritional support includes food modification and supplementation, it is primarily an interventional process based on enteral and parenteral feeding techniques. It must therefore be remembered that, as with any intervention, there are potential complications and it must therefore be applied, as discussed in Chapter 5, only when shown to be of overall benefit to the patient. Furthermore, the delivery is complex and important decisions need to be made to determine which feeding method and what composition of nutritional formula should be given. For all these reasons, the practice of nutritional support is beyond the capability of one person alone, and has to be managed and delivered by a nutritional team whose collective experience and skill will ensure its success in improving patient outcome. While it is feasible that a single "nutritionist" could run a nutrition support service by acting as a consultant and "subcontracting" the interventional aspects of care to surgeons and interventional radiologists for central vein catheter placements, and to gastroenterologists for post-pyloric and jejunal feeding tube placements, larger hospitals and academic institutions should collect such individuals together to form a unified team so that they can learn from each other and support each other and thus optimize the quality of care given to the patient. The creation of such teams also fosters academic excellence, providing a subdivision that has regular clinical practice and research meetings where medical and surgical fellows, residents, and students can rotate through to further their medical education and gain valuable clinical experience. The cost-effectiveness of the team approach has long been proven [111, 112], and interested parties should approach their institutional and administrative heads to obtain recognition and support in the form of time and an administrative base (office/secretary/coordinator).

© Springer Science+Business Media New York 2015
S.J.D. O'Keefe, *The Principles and Practice of Nutritional Support*,
DOI 10.1007/978-1-4939-1779-2_6

Composition of the Nutritional Team

Proper management of nutritional support requires knowledge of how food is digested and absorbed, and how it is metabolized and stored. Furthermore, knowledge of the anatomy of the gut and the venous system is required in order to facilitate enteral and parenteral access. Finally, delivery has to be closely supervised to ensure that nutritional requirements are met and to closely manage the feeding systems to make sure that they function efficiently. It is clear from this that no one person can be responsible for nutritional support. *Multiple disciplines are needed.* This fact accounted for the birth of the "Nutritional Team," a perfect example of how individuals from several lines of specialities can work together to provide optimal clinical care for the hospitalized patient (Fig. 6.1). The following represents an example of a typical team, but there are no absolute rules and the final composition should consist of the best mix of local talent available in the particular hospital center.

The Team Leader and Physician: Overall patient management has to be assumed by someone with sufficient authority within the medical center to (a) liaise with the primary-care team requesting help, and (b) to become responsible for a key part of the general management of the patient. This can create problems, as it sometimes conflicts with aspects of clinical care managed by others. For example, enteral feeding can complicate fistula and diarrhea management and affect drug absorption, and both enteral and parenteral nutrition may disturb diabetic and fluid balance control. Despite the multiple publications and resulting guidelines on the appropriate use of nutritional support, firmly held beliefs on

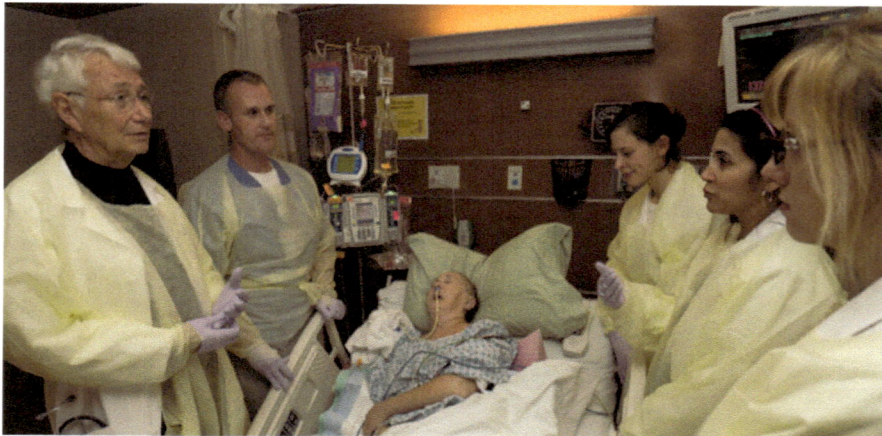

Fig. 6.1 This picture illustrates the complex management of critically ill patients who cannot eat. Nutritional management must be discussed with the primary team at the bedside to ensure integration of effort to optimize treatment and outcome

the restorative powers of nutrition in curing illness, improving quality of life, and prolonging survival remain raise serious ethical issues particularly in the aged and terminally ill. *Thus the nutrition attending has not only to be an expert in the latest nutritional techniques and feed compositions, but also a patient teacher, giving frequent "in-servicing" to nurses, interns, residents, and attendings, and sometimes a pragmatic politician, helping change regulations and codes so that state-of-the-art care can be delivered.* Unfortunately, despite considerable efforts by some to develop specific credentialing programs, nutritional support is not widely recognized as a distinct discipline and so team leaders usually belong to one of several allied specialties such as gastroenterology, surgery, critical care, endocrinology, or general internal medicine, to which the Nutrition Team then becomes administratively attached. The situation regarding clinical nutrition as a specialty is confused by the existence of three different credentialing examinations for physicians from three different organizations. These are the National Board of Nutrition Support Certification for the American Society for Parenteral and Enteral Nutrition (NBNSC; https://www.nutritioncare.org/NBNSC/index.aspx), Certification Board for Nutrition Specialists (CBNS), and Intersociety Professional Nutrition Education Consortium (ABPNS). No consensus has yet been reached on how to merge them into one body [113].

The Nurse Specialist: General patient management is usually the responsibility of an *RN or Nurse Practitioner*, as such a person is best placed to interact with the nursing staff who ultimately manage feeding delivery and identify complications. Day-to-day supervision and monitoring is extremely important to ensure appropriate feeding, and to adjust infusion rates according to tolerance and thus minimize the risk of complications. Quality nutritional care depends not only on the establishment of enteral or parenteral access, but also on the daily monitoring care to make sure what is prescribed is actually given, and to maintain the function of feeding tubes.

The Dietitian: With the commercialization of enteral feeding, there are an increasing number of regular and specialized liquid formula diets available. The provision and supply of these enteral feeding products is usually the domain of the hospital dietitian. This fact, plus the specialized knowledge dietitians have of the composition and requirements of nutrition, makes a *dietitian* another essential member of the team.

The Pharmacist: TPN is usually compounded within the hospital pharmacy and so an NSS pharmacist is, likewise, an essential component of the team to ensure that the correct balanced formulation is prescribed, admixed, and delivered to the patient under sterile conditions. Even if standardized TPN commercial admixtures are used, TPN should be treated like IV drugs, and controlled through the pharmacy. A pharmacist is also essential to manage general drug prescription as requirement dosages may differ in patients with compromised gut function and drug kinetics change when feeding is altered from intermittent to continuous.

Nutrition Consulting Service

The traditional role of the nutrition team was to provide a consulting service to deal with all nutritional problems in the hospital, from medicine, to surgery, to psychiatry. Thus, *each referral is visited and assessed at the bedside*, and then specific recommendations are made which the primary care team executes. However, nutritional problems tend to be chronic and cannot be cured like an acute infection, and so follow-up is essential. Tolerance to enteral feeding needs to be monitored, feeding rates should be started slowly and increased to goal with tolerance over time, and metabolic status has to be closely followed, particularly in patients starting on TPN. Nutritional requirements change with time and clinical condition and there is no "one fits all" solution to nutritional support. Progress needs to be followed every day, and it is essential that regular business rounds, at least twice a week, be conducted to share problems with the team and seek their resolution.

The TPN Service

Unfairly, a recent publication entitled "Death by TPN" demeaned the role of TPN in the management of ICU patients [114]. However, there is some truth in the statement if TPN is not used correctly. Unlike enteral or oral feeding, there are no protective mechanisms that prevent overfeeding, and overfeeding, like underfeeding, can kill patients. It is for this reason that many hospitals have now insisted that the use of TPN should be first approved and then managed by a group of individuals who (a) have received training, (b) have experience in its use, and (c) attend regular CME courses to keep up to date in what can be a rapidly changing field. There are several decisions that need to be made. First, it has to be determined whether TPN is indicated. *The team leader needs to visit the patient* and make a full assessment to determine whether "intestinal failure" is present and whether it can be overcome by interventional feeding tube placement. *Because TPN is easy to start, the first reaction of most primary care teams is to order TPN for patients with nutritional problems. Erroneously, many consulting physicians will claim that urgent TPN is needed because the albumin or prealbumin has dropped, when all that has happened is the hydrational status of the patient has changed, or they have developed sepsis, with "3rd space" losses. This accounts for the dramatically higher use of TPN in institutions that do not have a nutritional team.* Second, the type of venous access has to be chosen depending upon the expected duration of TPN feeding; if it is short, i.e., less than 2 weeks, PPN might suffice; if it is intermediate, i.e., 2–4 weeks, a PICC line would suffice; and if it is long, i.e., 3+ months, then a central vein catheter tunneled down the anterior chest wall would be the best choice for possible home PN. Third, it has to be determined whether the patient is at risk from *refeeding syndrome*. If so, metabolic abnormalities have first to be corrected and then TPN should be started slowly, i.e., 25%, increasing slowly over 3 days with metabolic tolerance monitored by blood testing (incl. glucose, phosphate, potassium). Fourth, the team must follow progress daily, monitoring electrolytes, glucose, and renal function until goal infusion rates are achieved and metabolic stability is proven.

The Nutrition Intervention Service

In the past, surgeons and radiologists dominated nutritional intervention, as the chief demand was for central vein access. With the increasing awareness of the benefits of enteral as opposed to parenteral feeding, the emphasis has shifted to the role of interventional gastroenterologists and radiologists in placing feeding tubes past upper GI obstructions, and into regions of preserved functional gut below the obstruction.

Recent developments in endoscopic technology have allowed us to place nasoenteric tubes even as far down as the mid-jejunum in patients in the ICU, without the need for fluoroscopy for radiological confirmation [63, 115, 116]. The use of transnasal endoscopy with endoscopes with a diameter of 5–5.8 mm allows safe placement under direct vision with minimal discomfort at the bedside, avoiding the delays and disruptions in management involved with the transport of patients off the floor to IR. Interventional endoscopy is not part of routine endoscopy provided by the average hospital GI service, but is not difficult to master with practice, and teaching videos are available (https://www.youtube.com/watch?v=YlkiY6YTnYk and https://www.youtube.com/watch?v=UjVjDkdDLW0). For example, we train our GI Fellows to be competent within a 4-week rotation on the NSS. It is therefore recommended that a gastroenterologist should be a member of the team so that he/she would have time allocated for complex tube placements within the GI lab or for "travel" to the ICU for bedside placement.

Chapter 7
Key Principles for Nutritional Intervention

Nutritional Assessment

From the dialogue in Chapter 5, nutritional assessment will play a key role in determining how and when to commence nutritional support. That having been said, accurate nutritional assessment in sick patients is extremely difficult to obtain in practice with the current tools we have, as fluid retention and losses, together with shifts between intra- and extracellular compartments, obscure the value of blood concentrations which are most commonly advocated for the nutritional assessment of nonhospitalized populations, and also limit the sensitivity of measurements based on body weights and electrical conductivity. These changes *invalidate the use of plasma protein concentrations, such as albumin, prealbumin, transferrin, and retinol binding protein* as measures of body protein status. Despite this fact, plasma albumin concentrations are probably more used as indicators for the need for nutritional support in hospitals today in the USA than any other measurement.

In support of my emphasis that *albumin should never be used as an index of protein nutritional status in hospitalized patients*, we measured anthropometrics (body weight, height, triceps skinfold thicknesses, and mid-arm circumferences) and plasma albumin concentrations in 546 general hospital patients [117]. Our results revealed that there was no association between albumin concentrations and body weights expressed as percentages of ideal nor was there an association between albumin concentrations and triceps skinfold thicknesses. Importantly, patients with the lowest albumin concentrations were shown subsequently to have the highest hospital mortality rates, emphasizing the fact that plasma albumin is an excellent biomarker of survival. In a subgroup of 50 patients receiving nutritional support (enteral or parenteral feeding containing 80–100 g/day protein, 1,500–2,400 kcal/day energy), chiefly critically ill patients in the surgical ICU, measurements were repeated after at least 2 weeks of feeding. Critically, there was no association between improvements in nitrogen balance and increases in albumin concentrations (Fig. 7.1).

© Springer Science+Business Media New York 2015
S.J.D. O'Keefe, *The Principles and Practice of Nutritional Support*,
DOI 10.1007/978-1-4939-1779-2_7

Fig. 7.1 Albumin
concentrations are not good
measures of nutritional state
in hospitalized patients, but
are biomarkers of degree of
sickness and survival

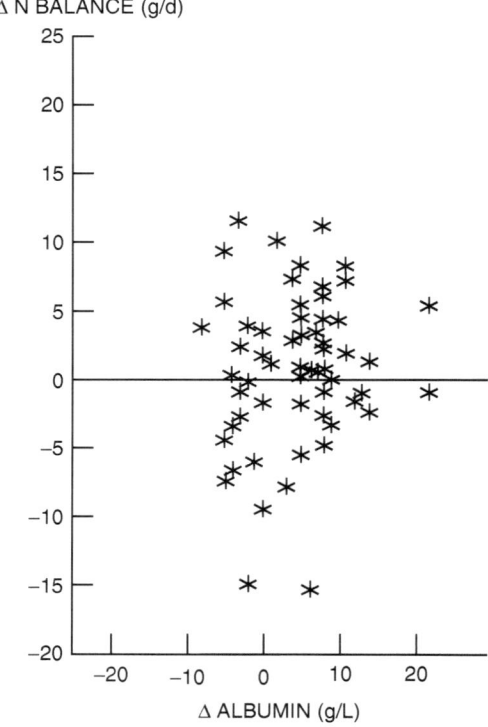

Additionally, it was noted that reductions in albumin concentrations after feeding were associated with higher mortality rates. This study confirmed our contention that the measurement of plasma albumin concentrations in hospitalized patients provides no useful nutritional information either for baseline assessments of candidates for nutritional support or for the efficacy of interventional feeding in improving nutritional status. *On the other hand, the measurement of albumin concentrations is useful in predicting the severity of illness and risk of mortality.* It has been recognized for years that albumin concentrations correlate strongly with long-term mortality (Studley, JAMA 1936), and therefore provide a good measure of the "sickness" of a patient. Some have suggested that a C-reactive protein (CRP) level should be measured simultaneously to assess the degree of stress: if the CRP is high then a low albumin is meaningless as a measure of body protein status. A good illustration of this point is a small internal study I performed many years ago when rounding with the nutrition team when I guessed the albumin concentration after physical examination and evaluation of the clinical condition of 100 consecutive new patients I was consulted on. Overall, I was within 5% of the measured value. This comes from years of clinical experience, but shows how powerful clinical judgment can be and *how important it is to examine patients at the bedside* (Fig. 7.2). This is also illustrated by Jeejeebhoy's development of the "subjective global assessment" below.

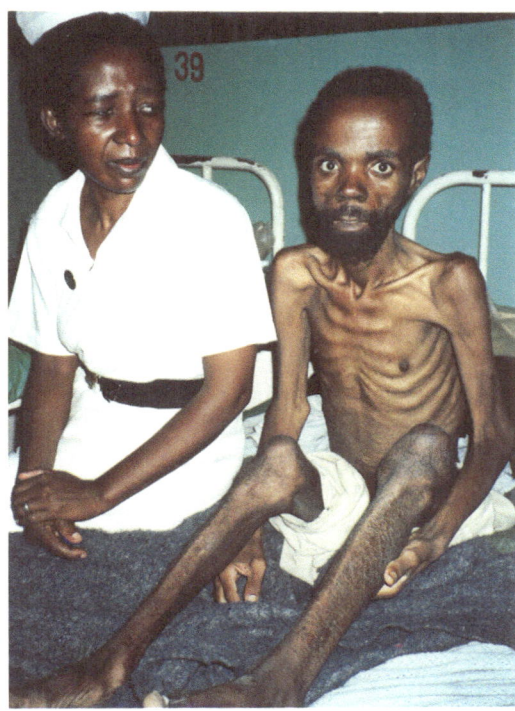

Fig. 7.2 An extreme example of marasmic malnutrition in a patient with disseminated pulmonary tuberculosis. Invasive tests and the use of complicated nutritional prognostic indices are not needed to categorize this patient at extreme nutritional risk. Protein deficiency is clearly evident from *observing* muscle wasting (plasma albumin was only mildly depressed) and fat deficiency from feeling the triceps skinfold thickness which was ~2 mm. Importantly, the protein energy deficiency was associated with multiple vitamin and mineral deficiencies, including thiamine, vitamin A, and zinc, all of which contribute to the illustrated exfoliative dermatitis. Such patients are at great risk of refeeding syndrome. Enteral feeding often exacerbates diarrhea, and the judicious use of IV infusions should initially be used to correct hydration, renal function, and electrolyte levels. Because nutritional stores are dangerously low, IV nutrition may be needed for a short period (e.g., 1–2 weeks) to provide the building blocks for digestive enzymes and absorptive cells, before conversion to enteral feeding

Alternative methods of assessment have included the measurement of anthropometric parameters, such as weight, height, triceps skinfold thicknesses (index of fat stores) and mid-arm circumferences (to calculate muscle circumference), bioelectrical impedance analysis (to calculate total body water and thus fat mass), blood vitamin levels, total lymphocyte counts, immune reactivity as shown by skin antigen testing [118], urine creatinine excretion, and the development of "prognostic nutritional indices" by combining several of these parameters [119].

In a classic study by Jeejeebhoy's group in Toronto, the group developed the concept of "*subjective global assessment*," which in essence used the physicians mind as a computer to assimilate multiple clinical parameters (no lab values) related to nutrition to categorize individual patients into (a) normal nutritional status, (b) mildly (or suspected of being) malnourished, or (c) obviously (definitely) malnourished [120, 121]. The clinical parameters included *history of dietary intake, amount of weight loss, the character of the underlying disease, functional muscular weakness or inability to work or perform daily activities, and physical signs of muscle wasting, fat depletion, edema, ascites, glossitis, and skin lesions specific to vitamin deficiencies.* In a study of 59 surgical patients, they compared the performance of their SGO to that of other commonly used measures, including plasma albumin and transferrin, delayed hypersensitivity skin testing, anthropometry, creatinine-height index, and the prognostic nutritional index [122], and showed that SGO was a more sensitive and specific predictor of a nutrition-associated complication, namely the development of an infection, after surgery, than any of the other measurements, or combinations of measurements. Of course, the criticism of this study is that there was no true "gold standard," as malnutrition is not the only cause of postoperative infection (which occurred in 42% of their patients), and there was no evidence that nutrition support prevented these infections. *Nonetheless, the concept of using your brain to guess who is most likely to need nutritional support after surgery or during critical illness is beautifully illustrated by this now classic study.* It also emphasizes *the essential need for the nutrition team to visit the patient and perform a bedside evaluation.* "Sit down rounds" are fine for reviewing progress, but are no substitute for physical evaluation.

Perhaps the most practical and useful measurement, despite its shortcomings in edematous patients, is the *body mass index* [123, 124]. The measurement of body weights has been a fundamental nursing observation since the time of Florence Nightingale. The use of mechanical-electronic beds in the ICU now permits weight measurements even in the sickest and most disabled patient. However, body weight on its own is a poor indicator of nutritional status as a patient with a weight of 65 kg could be underweight, normal weight, or overweight—depending on his/her height. Thus some correction for body size is needed: to do this we use height squared, which is related to body surface area. Heights are known by the family, and thus the calculation of BMI as kilograms per meter squared

$$BMI = Weight\,(kg) / height^2\,(in\,meters)$$

should be available in any hospitalized patient. Calculation is facilitated by the presence of numerous websites which can be looked up on your iPhone/Android (e.g., http://www.health-calc.com/body-composition/ideal-body-weight). It is generally accepted that a normal BMI falls between the values of 18.5 and 24 kg/m^2 and that values >30 indicate the presence of obesity. From our discussions and estimations of the depth of body stores in Chapter 5, we consider a BMI <17 indicative of severe depletion, and values <15 as life-threatening. Of course, weight, and therefore BMI, is also affected by hydrational status and therefore its use in nutritional assessment must be taken in conjunction with physical examination, or SGO, as measurements will be artificially high with fluid retention. For "sit down" rounds, the BMI, and not simply body weight, must be calculated to provide a rough guide to the nutritional state of the patient, but remember this is no substitute for visiting the patient and a bedside exam.

Nutritional Requirements

Normal Levels

Metabolic needs vary by age, activity level, and health status. In turn, the process of adaptation can modify these needs further. Consequently, we should not talk of specific levels, but rather of ranges, or more commonly, "safe" levels which will be on the generous side to include most of the population at large. Of course, this can be criticized in the current situation where obesity is becoming # 1 health hazard in the westernized world. For the third straight year, the incidence of obesity, defined as a BMI >30 kg/m^2, has increased in the USA such that 40% of the adult population is now obese (Centers for Disease Control and Prevention (CDC) Overweight and Obesity: 2010. www.cdc.gov/obesity/data/adult.html). The safe levels used in the USA are termed RDAs (recommended dietary allowances), but their use for the general population is at best controversial as they were designed more to prevent malnutrition within the community, than preventing obesity.

Patient Requirements

Energy

In the early days of nutritional support, it was generally assumed that requirements would be higher in acute illness because of the acute metabolic response. Patients in the ICU were commonly given 3,000 + kcal/day or 40–50 kcal/kg body weight/day by TPN [125], as classic studies had shown that glucose infusions suppressed protein catabolism ("protein sparing") as described in Chapter 4: Pathophysiology: Nutrition in Illness. Furthermore, Elwyn and colleagues showed in 1979 that nitrogen balance was progressively improved when ten depleted septic patients receiving TPN were given a constant nitrogen diet (1 g/kg/day) with increasing dextrose at approximately 15, 40, and 60 kcal/kg/day (Fig. 7.3) [126]. Unfortunately, it was soon recognized that these high glucose infusion rates often worsened outcome, as the beneficial effects of feeding were overshadowed by the complications of overfeeding, in hyperglycemia, infections, and liver dysfunction. A more scientific approach to feeding was subsequently introduced by the measurement of actual metabolic expenditure by indirect calorimetry. These studies revealed that metabolic expenditure was not as high as expected, possibly because patients were inactive, lying in bed, and often sedated. In even the sickest patients, metabolic

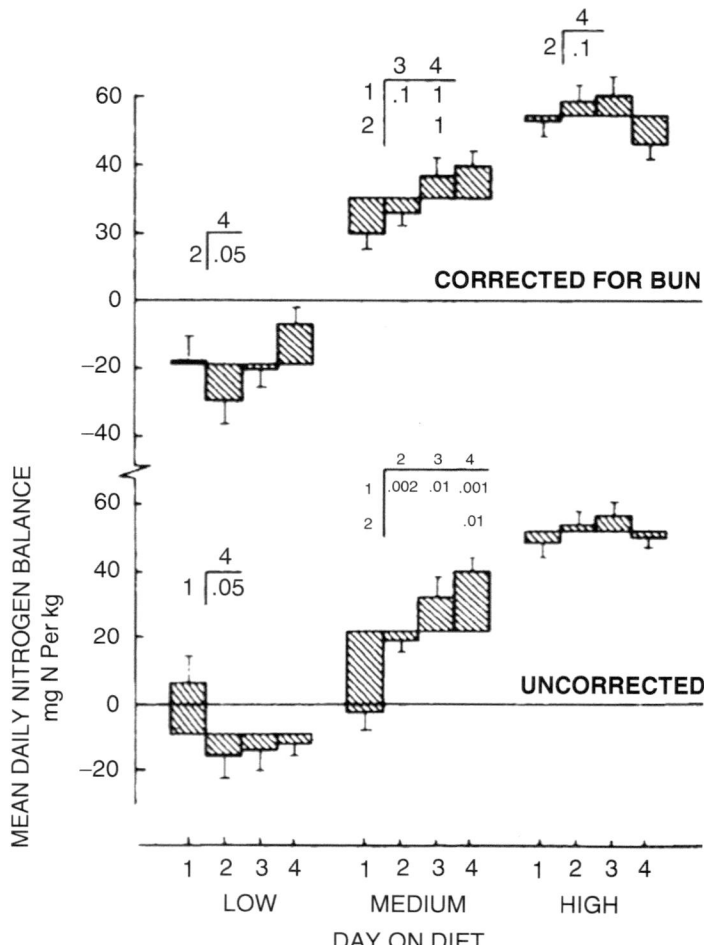

Fig. 7.3 The retention of infused amino acids increases with increasing dextrose co-infusion even in the critically ill—but so does hyperglycemia

expenditure rarely exceeded 1,800 kcal/day [127]. Consequently, current guidelines recommend a nutritional goal of only 25 Kcal/kg ideal body weight/day. It is also important to understand that this formula should be calculated on *ideal*, not actual body weight (e.g., a BMI of 24 kcal/m²). Because of the high prevalence of obesity, the use of actual weight will result in overfeeding in the majority of our patients, while in the marasmic depleted patient the use of actual body weight would impair the restitution of body stores. This point is often misunderstood, with cries of "how can you give a patient 50 kcal/kg/day?" I cite examples such as the patient in Figure 7.4 and our published article on a young male patient with immunoproliferative small intestinal disease who was admitted having lost 60% of his body weight (normally fatal depletion) and had a BMI of only 9 kg/m² (see full discussion on

Chapter 2, Fig. 2.4, p. 15). Having treated the underlying condition, he became strongly anabolic consuming over 100 kcal/kg/day resulting in normalization of his body weight in 3 months [29].

Protein

The evidence for protein catabolism in critical illness is more compelling, and of more concern as sufficient amino acid supplies are essential for host defense and organ repair. In clinical practice, estimations of loss have been calculated from the results of urine urea nitrogen (UUN) losses:

$$\text{Rate of Protein Catabolism}(g/d) = \text{UUN}(g/d) \times 1.2 \times 6.25$$

where 1.2 is the correction for urine non-urea nitrogen content (approx. 20%), and 6.25 is the conversion factor for the nitrogen content of protein. It should be noted that protein or amino acid infusions also increase hepatic amino acid oxidation rates, urea synthesis, and therefore UUN. Thus, the calculated rate of protein catabolism will be increased by feeding, and trying to match infusion rates with nitrogen losses will, in the same way we described for energy infusions and increasing energy expenditure under Nutritional Assessment above, result in "chasing your tail" and metabolic dysregulation with accumulation of nitrogenous end products (e.g., increasing BUN relative to creatinine) and acidosis in critically ill patients. Thus measurements should be made during fasting to get a better idea of what endogenous protein catabolic rates are, which, as discussed in Chapter 4: Pathophysiology: Nutrition in Illness, is what you need to know to best support the metabolic response to critical illness.

In research studies, a more accurate estimate of protein catabolic rates has been the measurement of amino acid oxidation rates with stable- or radioisotope labeling techniques. Our studies showed that mean losses after major abdominal surgery were equivalent to 100 g protein per day [50, 52], with exceptionally high losses in patients with acute tetanus of 130 g/day [53], and in necrotizing pancreatitis of 180–200 g/day [103, 128]. Interestingly, the study reported by Elwyn et al., described above, showed that nitrogen balance was achieved with only 1 g/kg/day when energy intake matched energy expenditure [126]. Based on these and other studies, a level of 1.5 g protein/kg ideal body weight/day (approximately 100 g/day for an average person) is commonly advocated for ICU patients [108, 129, 130], which is 50–80% higher than normal dietary requirements. Some advocate rates up to 2 g/kg, but the evidence for additional benefit is not there and excess is simply oxidized— further increasing "catabolic" rates, increasing BUN levels as described above, without enhancing protein synthesis.

Of course, diseases that affect nitrogen recycling will also affect requirement levels. Liver failure inhibits amino acid oxidation and urea synthesis. Consequently, plasma levels of amino acids that are chiefly oxidized in liver, such as the aromatic amino acids, increase as does ammonia, which cannot be incorporated into and excreted as urea. This disturbance of plasma amino acid pattern and ammonia accumulation has been associated with neurological disturbances and encephalopathy [131]. This led to the use of low-protein (20 g/day) and no-protein diets until it was shown that amino acid oxidation continued, at albeit slower rates, and that insufficient protein resulted in catabolism of endogenous proteins and protein deficiency. We examined this concern with isotope-labeled amino acid tracer kinetic studies and showed that even patients with fulminant hepatic failure required at least 60 g/ day to prevent progressive protein depletion [132, 133]. We showed further that aromatic amino acid (AA) metabolism was suppressed far greater than branched chain amino acid (BCAA) metabolism (because AA can only be oxidized by the liver), and that the infusion of specialized amino acid formulae depleted in AA and enriched with BCAA corrected plasma amino acid patterns and optimized the synthesis of hepatic proteins [134, 135]. These studies supported the use of "liver-specific" enteral and parenteral diets (e.g., Hepatamine, B. Braun Medical Inc. USA, IV and oral preparations available) with reduced quantities of AAs and increased content of branched chain amino acids, which will be discussed further under Liver Disease, Chapter 15. Renal failure also disturbs nitrogen metabolism and a low-protein diet will reduce the rates of increase of blood urea. But again, this leads to progressive depletion of body stores, and the recommendation nowadays is to use regular dialysis and provide normal levels of nutrition support, as will be discussed further in Chapter 15.

Fluid and Electrolytes

As a general principle, fluid balance should be measured in all patients dependent on artificial feeding, in the acute, daily; in the chronic, less frequently. The quantity of water should be adjusted to maintain normal blood creatinine levels and a urine volume of 1–2 l per day. This usually works out to 1–1.5 ml/kg ideal weight/h. Sodium intake should be adjusted to maintain not only normal plasma concentrations, but also levels in the urine >20 < 120 mmol/day. Because of renal conservation due to aldosterone, blood levels often remain normal in borderline deficiency states while urine is devoid of sodium, indicating impending critical deficiency. It must be remembered that a low plasma sodium does not necessarily mean a low body sodium; it might be explained by fluid retention and disturbed intracellular:extracellular balance, as in chronic liver disease. There is no renal hormonal-regulated conservancy for potassium and so the maintenance of blood levels alone is sufficient.

Vitamins and Trace Elements

Considerably less research has been performed on identifying ideal requirement levels for micronutrients. Much of the work has aimed at providing sufficient supplementation to preserve blood levels, which might or might not be associated with metabolic sufficiency. For example, low plasma vitamin C or folate levels may not be associated with functional impairment at the tissue level. In an early study, we found that the use of commercial mixtures of water and fat-soluble vitamins did not conform to FDA recommendations and failed to normalize blood levels of vitamins C and B_6 in 83% of patients on prolonged TPN, and levels of vitamin A and E concentrations in 40% of hospitalized patients. However, no clinical evidence of vitamin deficiency states were evident [136].

The use of TPN has perhaps characterized specific vitamin deficiencies better than any other situation because, unlike even the most impoverished food, TPN is totally synthetic and the addition of essential trace nutrients can be missed. Any mistake in prescription can result in the production of a diet that is adequate in protein and calories, but devoid of an essential micronutrient, such as a vitamin. An excellent example is one of the 6 TPN patients who developed severe refractory lactic acidosis, hyperglycemia, and Wernicke's encephalopathy associated with thiamine deficiency due to a national shortage of commercial parenteral vitamins in 1988 and again in 1996 [137–139]. He was a 19-year-old man who was discharged home on TPN because of the inability to eat because of gastrointestinal dysmotility resulting from complications of abdominal surgeries. The 2,750 ml bag of TPN contained 120 g amino acids, 600 g dextrose, 50 g fat emulsion, electrolytes, minerals, vitamins, and trace elements. Two months later he was admitted because of fever and acute neurological signs including slurred speech, diminished deep tendon reflexes, ophthalmoplegia, and evidence of cortical blindness despite a normal fundoscopic examination. Blood testing showed profound lactic acidosis (lactate 16 mmol/l, normal <1.6). Magnetic resonance imaging scan of the brain was consistent with Wernicke's encephalopathy. Catheter sepsis was excluded, and consultation with the homecare company revealed that the multivitamin preparation had been omitted from the formula for 1 month prior to admission because of the national shortage. He was commenced on IV thiamine (and the other vitamins contained within the multivitamin mix) with rapid resolution of his neurological signs. It is likely that the course of his deficiency was accelerated by the excessive quantity of glucose and amino acids in the TPN which need thiamine for the synthesis of thiamine pyrophosphate (TPP), a coenzyme essential for the catabolism of sugars and amino acids. This is a similar situation as the refeeding syndrome, which can be precipitated by high glucose infusion rates. Figure 7.4 illustrates the critical importance of thiamine in glycolysis and energy production through the Kreb's cycle. The enzyme responsible for the conversion of pyruvate to acetyl CoA is thiamine (thiamine pyrophosphate) dependent, as is the TCA cycle enzyme α-ketoglutarate dehydrogenase. With the high infusion rate of glucose in the TPN, glycolysis is amplified with high production rates of pyruvate, which cannot be oxidized and has to be converted to lactate, resulting in lactic acidosis. The other six cases presented predominantly with severe acidosis and hyperglycemia associated with low plasma thiamine concentrations. In 2000, the FDA mandated a change in the formulation of parenteral multivitamin preparations to contain more vitamin C, folic acid, thiamine, and pyridoxine.

Fig. 7.4 Metabolic
explanation for lactic acidosis
in patients fed high quantities
of IV glucose in TPN without
sufficient thiamine

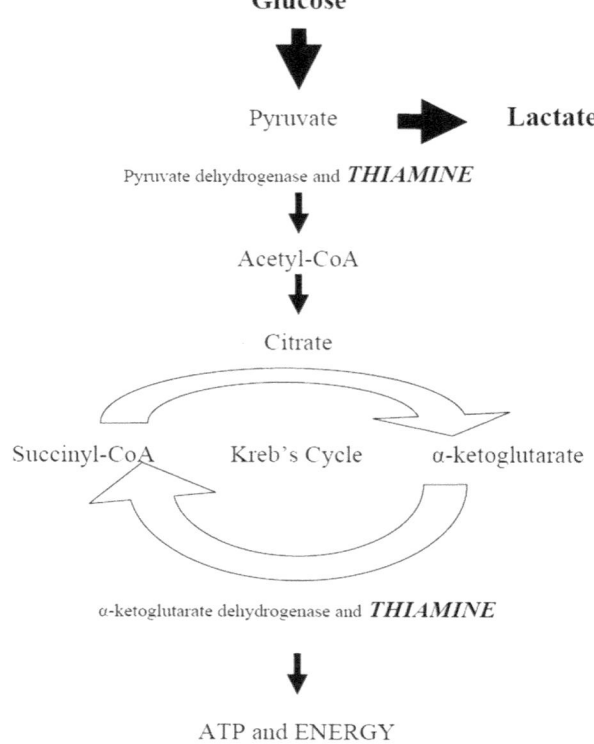

As the measurement of vitamin levels is expensive, they are rarely performed in routine hospital care, and it is assumed that the routine use of commercial additives is sufficient. We do, however, monitor micronutrient levels in our home PN patients every 6 months (B-12, folate, vitamin A and D), together with trace elements (chromium, copper, manganese, selenium, and zinc). Problems with excretion can arise in patients with liver and renal failure, and so blood levels should be monitored more frequently in such patients if the nutritional support is chronic.

The Problem of the Sick, Malnourished, Patient with "Failure to Thrive"

All too often, we are consulted to increase feeding rates because the patient remains critically ill, clinically malnourished, with muscle wasting, and low albumins and prealbumins, despite goal feeding as described above. It is imperative to resist the temptation to "vamp-up" the feeding rate (particularly in PN patients), as this will simply introduce or exacerbate metabolic complications and have no effect on body stores for the reasons outlined in Chapter 4. Metabolism during acute illness is geared to catabolism, not anabolism. To fine-tune the rate of caloric infusion, the measurement of energy expenditure by indirect calorimetry (10 min collection of expired gas to measure oxygen consumption and carbon dioxide production) is useful but bedside metabolic carts are not commonly available, and measurements are technically difficult in ventilated patients. To illustrate this point we were recently asked to reconsider our feeding rates in a severely wasted (BMI 17 kg/m^2), ventilated, 40-year-old patient who had suffered a series of complications post-liver transplant and was now chronically septic (abdomen/chest) 6 months later. He had severe gastroparesis, but some jejunal feeding had been successful via NGJ tube placement, but rates higher than 20–40 cc/h were not tolerated because of abdominal pain. His bowel dysfunction was exacerbated by his narcotic dependence. Because of his weight loss, PN had been started to achieve, together with the EN, the goal feeding rates discussed above. His estimated ideal body weight was 70 kg, indicating a goal of 1,750 kcal of energy/day and 100 g amino acids. Under pressure, the team increased his PN to 2,800 kcal/day and 120 g amino acids, which resulted in hyperglycemia, increased insulin needs, disturbed liver function, and no improvement in weight or prealbumin. Importantly, his C-reactive protein, an indicator of acute stress, increased further. Our immediate advice was to reduce his total nutrient infusions back to the original goal and measure caloric expenditure.

The measurement of metabolic expenditure by indirect calorimetry (IC), which allows calculation of caloric requirements through collections of expired air, has been available for years, but the equipment has been expensive, cumbersome, and therefore little used, apart from in research studies. The accuracy of this technique in determining needs is variable because (a) it bases its estimate of 24-h metabolic expenditure on oxygen consumption over only 10 min intervals and extrapolates these rates to 24 h, and (b) feeding increases metabolic expenditure. Thus you can be trapped "chasing your own tail", as discussed above, if you keep increasing feeding to match expenditure, a scenario which could have fatal metabolic consequences. Measurements should therefore be made during fasting to get a better idea of what endogenous expenditure rates are, which, as discussed in Chapter 4: Pathophysiology: Nutrition in Illness, is what you need to know to best support the body's metabolic response. The potential for development of more advanced global bedside digital methods of assessing continuous 24 h metabolic needs and organ function of critically ill patients is tremendous, and can be predicted to be an area of intense future research. For example, recent developments in sports medicine and body health offer exciting novel approaches, as illustrated by the development of an adhesive arm band containing multiple embedded sensors, including a 3-axis accelerometer, Galvanic skin response, and 2 temperature sensors (near body and skin). These sensors collect over 5,000 readings from the body every minute, measuring the user's motion, skin temperature, heat flux, and galvanic skin response (a sweat-related measurement). Data is stored in the device's memory until the data is extracted and analyzed (http://vancive.averydennison.com/en/home/technologies/metria/MetriaIH1.html#sthash.XNcyKi45.dpuf).

To gain insight into what was going on with our patient with failure to thrive described above, we employed this technique to assess metabolic rate and activity continuously for 7 days. An illustration of the daily printout is shown on Fig. 7.5 The average daily expenditure over this week was calculated to be 1,940 kcal/day, which was slightly higher than expected, probably because of the marked increases in expenditure associated with the occasional attempts to get the patient out of bed and into a chair—something the usual IC recorder would have missed. The record also sensed that he was not sleeping well. It was not until the fifth day that he registered small amounts of deep sleep. The accuracy and validity of these techniques in sick patients needs formal evaluation and I mention this example more for food for thought, given the weakness of most of our current techniques at measuring the efficacy of nutritional support in supporting normal diurnal rhythms which are essential for health and metabolic function, and to better examine the role of specific nutrients, such as vitamins and minerals, in improving organ function, and for answering fundamental questions raised in Chapter 5 of how much protein (or any other nutrient) can we afford to lose before organ function becomes impaired.

Finally, going back to our patient, PN infusions were reduced to providing 1,500 kcal/day in the form of 250 g dextrose, 40 g fat, and 100 g amino acids while enteral infusions added 480 kcal in the form of a semi-elemental formula, thus matching total energy expenditure rates. In the ensuing days, enteral rates were slowly increased by 10 cc each day with tolerance towards an interim goal of 60 cc/h, with reductions in regular narcotics, increased mobilization, and synchronized reductions in PN to maintain goal nutrient infusion rates. This induced severe watery diarrhea which tested positive for *C difficile* toxins. This was treated,

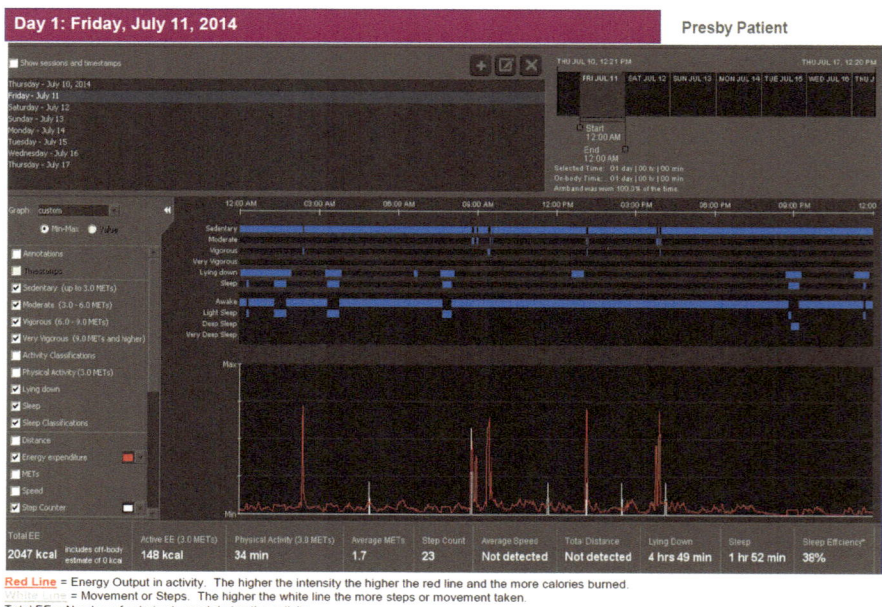

Red Line = Energy Output in activity. The higher the intensity the higher the red line and the more calories burned.
White Line = Movement or Steps. The higher the white line the more steps or movement taken.
Total EE = Number of calories burned during the activity.
Avg. METs = A grading scale to determine the intensity of an activity. 1.3 METs is = to sitting and talking; 3.5 METs is = 3.5 mph on a treadmill.
Active EE = Number of calories burned at 3.5 METs or higher.
Physical Activity = Amount of time spent at 3.5 METs or higher.

Fig. 7.5 An illustration of new developments in continuous metabolic monitoring in ICU patients. The method used to calculate the IH1 Patch data (MetaFit Solutions, Pittsburgh) comes from the heat sensor data measured per minute of the entire wearing time (7 days). Algorithms are used to calculate outcomes from the combined date of the heat sensors and the tri-axis accelerometers

not by stopping the tube feeding, but by starting oral vancomycin and progressive soluble fiber supplementation and stopping PPIs in the manner as previously described on p. 50 chapter 5, Fig. 5.10 [34]. The soluble fiber was added to the feed and given at a constant rate increasing to 18–24 g per day. After 5 days the diarrhea resolved. With intensive treatment of his underlying medical condition, he was eventually extubated and mobilized with progressive reduction in the need for narcotics, and return of appetite and normal bowel function, allowing first discontinuation of PN, then EN, and finally weaning back onto normal food. Only following discharge to a rehabilitation center did his weight begin to increase back towards normal.

The critical lesson to be learned from this case report is that it illustrates the principles outlined in Chapter 4: Pathophysiology: Nutrition in Illness and shows that it is impossible to get critically ill, stressed, patients to gain "nutritional" weight with forced feeding, and that overfeeding will adversely affect outcome by adding complications. The priority is to treat the underlying condition, medically or surgically, and to provide nutritional support to prevent critical depletion of body stores, rather than repletion of normal body stores. Once the underlying condition resolves, the catabolic response switches to an anabolic one, allowing increased feeding and spontaneous repletion of normal body stores.

A book about practice needs to be didactic; otherwise everyone will be sitting around twiddling their thumbs while the patient slowly fades away! So, from the synthesis of what has been discussed above, we suggest that patients should initially be categorized into well nourished, mildly malnourished, or severely depleted by the use of body mass calculations together with a subjective global (SGO), or clinical, assessment (for definitions, see above). Based on this, the following recommendations can be made:

Feeding Recommendations

Method of Feeding: Remember: oral feeding is best, enteral feeding is second best, and parenteral feeding should only be used if the first two options fail and the patient is shown to have gut failure (see below).

Functional Gut

1. Starting Nutritional Support

    (a) Mild-Moderate Acute Illness, expected duration <7 days:

    - *Previously well nourished* (defined by SGO or BMI >18.5): No nutrition support required, *ad libitum* diet, symptomatic medical management.
    - *Mildly malnourished*: SGO or BMI 17–18.5: dietary modification, oral supplements.
    - *Severely malnourished* SGO or BMI <17: oral supplements if tolerated, if not enteral tube feeding plus *ad lib* diet.

- *Critically malnourished*: SGO or BMI <15: combination of IV infusions to correct fluid, electrolyte, vitamin, and mineral deficiencies plus tube feeding started slowly.

(b) Severe Acute Illness: expected duration unknown.

- *Previously well nourished* (BMI >18.5): wait 5–7 days while stabilizing and investigating the patient before commencing interventional feeding. Generally, such patients cannot eat, but there is no reason to keep them NPO and oral fluids may be taken if requested. If an NG tube is placed initially as standard of care and GRVs are <400 ml/4 h, nasogastric feeding should be started at a slow rate, e.g., 25 cc/h, to maintain intestinal function. It may be kept at this rate for up to a week or progressively increased if tolerated to 50 cc/h and then to goal in successive 24 h periods if the patient is stable and making progress. *Note that "goal" is a moderate feeding rate gauged to match, not exceed energy requirements*. In the absence of fasting indirect calorimetry measurements, it is reasonable to use a goal energy infusion of 25 kcal/kg *ideal* body weight/day. To calculate ideal body weight you need to know the patient's height, and then back-calculate the weight that would give a BMI of 24 kg/m^2. Many websites can be found on the Internet that will help you achieve this (e.g., http://www.health-calc.com/body-composition/ideal-body-weight). There is no justification for using actual body weights as the goal of nutritional support in the hospital is *NOT* to maintain obesity in the obese, or malnutrition in the marasmic.
- *Mildly malnourished*: SGO or BMI 17–18.5: it is wise to commence enteral feeding as described above, or as soon as possible after the completion of the initial investigations and stabilization. In other words, nutrition support is part of the general management.
- *Severely malnourished*: SGO or BMI <17: First correct fluid and electrolyte abnormalities, with particular attention to plasma potassium and phosphate, and then assess gut function. Commence nutrition support as soon as the patient is in a stable condition. Start at the same slow continuous rate, but wait at least 24 h and recheck urea and electrolytes, plus phosphate, to avoid the **refeeding syndrome** before increasing the rate to goal with tolerance over 3–4 days.
- *Critically malnourished*: In marasmic patients (SGO/BMI <15) with multiple fluid, electrolyte, and nutritional deficiencies, tube feeding may be poorly tolerated, with exacerbation of diarrhea as described in Chapter 2 [29]. Severe protein deficiency impairs digestion and absorption and a short period of IV feeding to provide the building blocks for digestive enzymes and mucosal absorptive cells may be needed to break the vicious cycle. This has been termed "*bridge TPN.*" This should be started as soon as possible, but cautiously as above to avoid refeeding, while investigations are performed and while enteral feeding is established. Gut recovery is rapid, and so conversion to full enteral feeding should be possible by the second week.

Gut Failure

2. Starting Nutritional Support

From our calculations above, there is no need to start parenteral feeding during the first week of acute illness, unless the patient is severely malnourished with a BMI <17 kg/m². This is because the potential complications of PN outweigh the marginal benefits on maintenance or restoration of body stores. Intravenous fluid and electrolyte support alone is sufficient, to maintain normal blood values and renal function, with the addition of standard multivitamin mixtures by the end of the week.

Chapter 8
Enteral Nutrition

The Enteral Nutrition Formulae (LFDs)

There are a wide variety of standard and specialized enteral feeds available as illustrated in Table 8.1, but most hospitals select those they have the greatest demand for. *Bottom line: most patients can be managed with standard polymeric liquid formula diets (LFD) as they are "balanced" and contain all the essential nutrients.* Specialized formulae are appropriate when there is maldigestion and/or malabsorption, in severely catabolic, and in renal and hepatic failure patients. Polymeric LFDs are not only cheaper, but are also usually better tolerated. Pancreatic function is suppressed in the critically ill, but never to the degree that leads to maldigestion and malabsorption of LFDs if they are given at a constant 24 h infusion rate. *The earlier enteral feeding is commenced, the lower the risk of intolerance and the greater the chance of maintaining digestion and absorption.*

- *Polymeric:* Basically, polymeric diets are liquidized food and therefore satisfy normal nutritional requirements. They are therefore used when patients cannot eat normal food for whatever reason but have normal intestinal digestion and absorption. Several commercial products are available, varying little in composition. Usually, 1,500–2,000 ml will provide total daily nutritional requirements, but the protein:calorie and fat:calorie ratios vary making some products more useful in stressed and glucose intolerant patients. The quality of protein may also vary depending on its origin, i.e., casein (animal) or soya (vegetable). The chief advantage of polymeric diets is their low cost and palatability. Because the macronutrients are in a complex form, the formulae also usually have a low osmolarity and are therefore well tolerated. Being 'complete' they usually contain resistant starches or fiber and therefore maintain healthy colonic function, something that has now fashionably been termed "prebiotics." They are available in powder form for reconstitution (cheaper still) or as full liquids either in cans or in "ready-to-hang" plastic bags—alike TPN bags. Reconstituted formulae are particularly useful for longer term supplemental feeding, while factory-packaged

© Springer Science+Business Media New York 2015
S.J.D. O'Keefe, *The Principles and Practice of Nutritional Support*,
DOI 10.1007/978-1-4939-1779-2_8

Table 8.1 Some of the enteral feeds commonly used in hospitals in the USA

Tube feeds	Product	Vendor	cal/cc	% Pro	% CHO	% Fat	MCT:LCT ratio	Special features
Standard polymeric	Osmolite 1.2	Ross	1.2	19%	52%	29%		Ideal where intake is insufficient
	Isosource	Nestle	1.2	14%	57%	29%		
High nitrogen	Traumacal	Nestle	1.5	22%	38%	40%		
High nitrogen, low K	Replete	Nestle	1.0	25%	45%	30%		Low K with 38 mEq/1,000 ml
	Replete with fiber	Nestle	1.0	25%	45%	30%		Low K with 38 mEq/1,000 ml
High fiber	Probalance	Nestle	1.2	18%	52%	30%		
	Jevity 1.2	Ross	1.2	18.5%	53%	29%		Fructooligosaccharides
	Fibersource	Nestle	1.2	14%	57%	29%		
	Fibersource HN	Nestle	1.2	18%	53%	29%		
Electrolyte	Nutren renal	Nestle	2.0	14%	40%	46%		32 mEq K per liter
Restricted	Nepro CarbSteady	Ross	2.0	18%	34%	48%		27.1 mEq K per liter
	Novasource renal	Nestle	2.0	15%	40%	45%		28 mEq K per liter
Volume restricted	Nutren 2.0	Nestle	2.0	16%	39%	45%		
	Two Cal HN	Ross	2.0	16.7%	43%	40%		
	Novasource 2.0	Nestle	2.0	18%	43%	39%		

	Product	Vendor	cal/serv	g pro/serv	g cho/serv	g fat/serv	K+/serving	Special features
Semi-elemental	Peptamen	Nestle	1.0	16%	51%	33%	70:30	High MCT
	Peptamen pre bio	Nestle	1.0	16%	51%	33%	70:30	High MCT
	Peptamen 1.5	Nestle	1.5	18%	49%	33%	70:30	High MCT
	Peptamen AF	Nestle	1.2	25%	36%	39%	50:50	Higher MCT
	Optimental	Ross	1.0	21%	55%	25%		5.5 g arg/l, structured lipids, high MCT, FOS
	Peptinex	Nestle	1.0	20%	65%	15%	50:50	High MCT
Immune enhancing	Crucial	Nestle	1.5	25%	36%	39%	50:50	15 g arg/l
	Pivot 1.5	Ross	1.5	25%	45%	30%	20:80	13 g arg/l, very hi pro, structured lipids, FOS
	Impact	Nestle	1.0	22%	53%	25%	00.0	12.5 g arg/l, multiple studies
	Impact 1.5	Nestle	1.5	22%	38%	40%	?	18.7 g arg/l, has MCT
	Impact with fiber	Nestle	1.0	22%	53%	25%	0.00	12.5 g arg/l
Modular, protein	Beneprotein	Nestle	25.0	6 g				
	Prosource	Sysco						Liquid, individual servings
Modular, CHO	Polycose	Ross	200.0		50 g			
Modular, pro/fat	Benecalorie	Nestle	330.0	7 g			33 g	
Modular, fiber	Benefiber	Nestle	16.0					
Oral supplements	*Product*	*Vendor*	*cal/serv*	*g pro/serv*	*g cho/serv*	*g fat/serv*	*K+/serving*	*Special features*
Standard polymeric	CIB lactose free	Nestle	250	8.75	33.1	9.2		Poor taste, can only
	Ensure	Ross	250	9	40	6		Bottle
	Boost	Nestle	240	10	41	4		Can only

(continued)

Table 8.1 (continued)

Oral supplements	Product	Vendor	cal/serv	g pro/serv	g chol/serv	g fat/serv	K+/serving	Special features
High cal/high pro	CIB lactose free plus	Nestle	375	13.1	44.1	16.2		Poor taste, can only
	CIB VHC	Nestle	560	22.5	49.2	30.6		Can
	Ensure plus	Ross	350	13	50	11		Bottle
	Boost plus	Nestle	360	14	45	14		Can only
Diabetic supplement	CIB sugar free	Nestle	150	12	13	5		315 ml servings (10.5 oz)
	Glucerna shake	Ross	220	9.9	29.3	8.6		2.8 g dietary fiber and 1 g FOS
	Boost diabetic	Nestle	250	13.8	20	11.7		Good taste, FOS,
	Resource aspartame sweetened health shake	Sysco (Nestle)	300	12	34	13		6 oz serving milk based, contains phenylalanine, 3 g fiber/serving
Clear liquid	CIB juice drink	Nestle	163	6.5	34	0.3	45 mg	5.5 oz serving size
	Enlive	Ross	300	10	65	0	40 mg	Poor taste
	Resource breeze	Nestle	160.0	8	31	0	230 mg	Good taste
Milkshake	Shake-em ups	Sysco						
Dysphagia	Ensure pudding	Ross	170	4	27	5		4 oz serving, 1 g fiber, and 1 g FOS
	Boost pudding	Nestle	240	7	33	9		5 oz serving, no fiber
	Magic cups	Sysco	280.0	8	36	11		4.2 oz, frozen, melts to pudding, contains lactose
Immune enhancing	Impact advanced recovery	Nestle	340	18.1	44.7	9.2		Immune enhancing, 4.2 g arg/serv, 3.3 g fiber
Oral rehydration sol	WHO solution							

liquid formula are advantageous for feeding the immunosuppressed and criti-cally ill patients where a "closed system" reduces the risk of feed contamination. It must, however, be remembered that all tube feeds, like normal food, are non-sterile and they only differ in the degree of contamination.

- *Semi-Elemental (ED):* Here, some of the macronutrients have been predigested. The proteins are usually in small or large peptide form, the carbohydrate as maltodextrins, and the fat either low in quantity or in medium-chain triglyceride form. The advantage of these formulae is that they are easier to absorb and there-fore should have advantages in patients with compromised digestive and absorp-tive capacity. On the other hand, the osmolarity is higher and they have to be delivered at a slow continuous rate and *never* in bolus form. Semi-elemental diets are not surprisingly more expensive and are probably overused in hospital prac-tice as they are better advertised and more fashionable. It must be remembered that there is considerable digestive and absorptive reserve, such that you need to lose >90% of either function before malabsorption is encountered. Consequently, a low-cost polymeric formula is usually better tolerated even in the sickest of ICU patients *provided it is given at a slow continuous rate*. However, patients with pancreatic insufficiency are better managed with an elemental formula, but close supervision of blood glucose is mandatory, particularly in those with asso-ciated pancreatic endocrine dysfunction. Another indication is in the feeding of severe acute pancreatitis (SAP) for reasons of digestibility and minimization of pancreatic stimulation (see Chapter 13). Pancreatic enzyme secretion is reduced dramatically in SAP [128]. It must however be remembered that the use of an ED does not avoid pancreatic stimulation, but does reduce it by 50% [30].
- *Elemental:* Elemental strictly means that the diet is totally digested and can be absorbed directly. A good example of an elemental diet is a TPN solution, where protein is given as amino acids and carbohydrate as glucose (dextrose). Fat is not, however, given as free fatty acids, but as triglycerides, usually in small quanti-ties. The problem with elemental diets is that because they are broken down to their constituents, they are hyperosmolar, and if given at a fast rate will precipi-tate diarrhea. Vivonex (Nestle Nutritionals) is the most commonly used elemen-tal diet consisting of 15% of energy as protein—in the form of free amino acids, 82% as carbohydrate as maltodextrin, and 3% fat as safflower oil. The results of early studies showing that free amino acids are absorbed less well than peptides [140] together with concerns about the hyperosmolarity have led to the preferred use of the semi-elemental formulae described above.
- *Immune-Enhancing Diets* (*IEDs*)*:* The modern nutritionist is not satisfied with using nutrition intervention simply as a "support" system, while medical practice takes care of the underlying cause of the nutritional problem: he/she seeks to use specific nutrients to *treat the disease process*. The recognition that glutamine is essential for immune and small intestinal function, and that arginine generates nitric oxide that is essential for macrocyte function and blood flow has led to the development of LFDs enriched with these substances, termed IEDs. Enthusiasm

for their use was initially stimulated by the results of several small sized studies and their meta-analyses [141, 142], while more recent reviews have been negative [109, 143]. While glutamine enrichment is generally safe, unless the patient has liver failure in which case it could exacerbate encephalopathy, it must be remembered that it is an inessential amino acid that can be synthesized by the body from glutamate, which, in turn, is synthesized (by transamination) from a Krebs cycle intermediate a-ketoglutarate. Thus giving an excess of an inessential amino acid will result in a reciprocal reduction in essential amino acid intakes, or excessive nitrogen intake, and nitrogenous breakdown products are potentially toxic. Secondly, arginine enrichment may exacerbate the inflammatory response in septic patients [143]. A thorough review of the literature led the Canadian group to conclude that diets supplemented with arginine and other select nutrients not be used for critically ill patients [109]. Consequently, few ICUs routinely use IEDS. My personal view is that the most common nutritional problem in ICUs is inadequate feeding of *food*, which consists of a wide spectrum of essential nutrients, *including* glutamine and arginine. Consequently, outcome can be best improved by the provision of a balanced nutritional composition—which is, after all, what we evolved to survive on.

Enteral Access Techniques

Enteral feeding is used when patients cannot eat sufficient to meet requirements, when they are at risk of complications through not eating, and when they have functional GI tracts. The reader is referred back to the last section (Chapter 5) where much time was spent defining what "gut function" is and how it can be enhanced. The key point to remember is that ileus, or absent bowel sounds, or high gastric residuals do not necessarily translate into gut failure, and commencement of slow continuous enteral feeding may restore gut function. The chief problem with any form of naso-enteric feeding is that it is unsightly and uncomfortable, and given the option, many patients would opt for IV feeding. *However, it must be emphasized that EN vs. PN is not a patient choice, and PN must never be employed because the patient refuses EN.* It must be acknowledged that the long-term use of nasoenteric feeding can produce nasal damage, sinusitis, and sialorrhea. It is therefore our practice to convert, if practically possible, per-nasal feeding to per-cutaneous if patients require enteral feeding for periods longer than 4 weeks. The most common approach is to use endoscopic placement (or alternatively, radiologic or surgical placement), either directly into the stomach (PEG), or via the stomach into the intestine (PEG-J), or on the rare occasion to place the tube directly into the intestine (PEJ) (see Chapter 8).

Enteral Access

Although the placement of specialized enteral and parenteral feeding tubes or catheters can be performed by persons without specialized knowledge of nutritional support, just like the placement of PICC lines is generally performed by technicians as a service, it is helpful to either have someone who is attached to the team, or who develops a special relationship with the team, to place difficult tubes for enteral or IV access. For enteral access, it is advisable to have a *gastroenterologist* (remember, I am biased, but remember the role of the gut is to absorb food and one of the chief consequences of gut disease is disturbance in nutrition) as a team member or an associate so that he/she can develop skill through experience in placing tubes by endoscopy and/or fluoroscopy to improve nutrition. As diseases of the gut most commonly result in feeding disorders and the need for nutritional intervention, most GI divisions should have someone with an interest in nutrition support. Similarly, it is important to develop an association with a GI surgeon for surgical percutaneous or laparoscopic jejunostomy placements in patients with obstructed upper GI tracts. Previously, we developed relationships with vascular surgeons to place tunneled subclavian catheters, but nowadays it is conventional to associate with an enthusiastic interventional radiologist (IR) who has the skills and techniques to place enteral or parenteral tubes anywhere in the body you choose!

Nasogastric (NG)

The most common form of enteral access is the placement of NG tubes by nursing or house staff. Although this is usually easy, it can be difficult in sick patients, and can be associated with life-threatening complications arising from "blind" misplacement or aspiration of feeds. Consequently, a strict protocol needs to be adhered to before any tube is used for feeding, as outlined below. If the problem is simply anorexia, a nasogastric feeding tube is all that is needed. Provided gastric emptying is satisfactory, feeds can be given in bolus form in volumes up to 500 ml given 6 hourly (safer 350 ml/4h), as the stomach is designed to retain volume and slowly deliver it to the intestine via the pyloric "valve." It must always be remembered that the usual gastric emptying rate is 1 kcal/min and the maximum 2–3 kcal/min. Thus, a standard liquid formula diet, which contains 1 kcal/ml, will empty at a maximum rate of 180 ml/h— hence it is always wise to limit NG infusion rates to <150 ml/h or boluses to <500 ml/4 h. In critically ill patients, gastric emptying is usually delayed and so slower rates should be used, not exceeding 100 ml/h, and resting volumes (gastric residual volumes or "GRVs") should be checked regularly (4–6 h). To increase tolerance, feeds should be given as slow continuous infusions rather than bolus. Simple measures to promote gastric emptying and to prevent reflux and aspiration, such as elevate head of bed and the use of prokinetics, should be employed (see below).

Fig. 8.1 Transnasal
endoscopic view of an NG
tube placed in the trachea,
note bifurcation

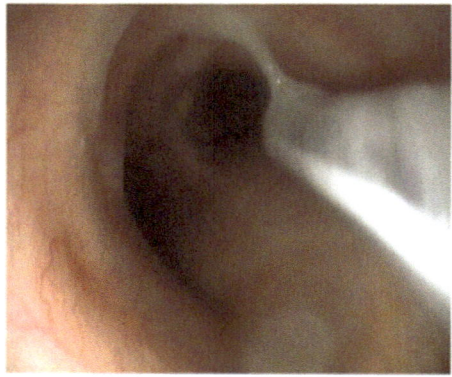

Benefits: Nasogastric feeding is the most common and oldest form of interventional feeding. Its attraction is that requires little skill, and can be placed by the nursing staff on admission allowing *early enteral feeding*. In patients with chronic disorders with chronic malnutrition, feeding can be given in intermittent bolus form during the day, as this is easier on nursing staff and appropriate for rehabilitation units.

Complications are associated with "blind" bedside placement and include misplacement in the tracheobronchial tree, mucosal injury with bleeding, and/or perforation. It is also not uncommon for the tube to be left in the lower esophagus, again increasing the risk of aspiration. In the extreme situation, the tube can be malpositioned in the tracheobronchial tree, as illustrated in Fig. 8.1. The patient was admitted with vomiting and a history of chronic pancreatitis complicated by pseudocyst. An NG "Salem" sump tube was placed at bedside and the patient treated with opiates for abdominal and chest pain, and sent for endoscopy in the morning. Remarkably, he complained of neither breathlessness nor cough! Transnasal endoscopy was used, anticipating the need for placement of a double-lumen nasogastric decompression jejunal feeding tube. As is our protocol, the NG tube was followed beyond the retropharynx and shown to be in the right main bronchus as shown in the figure! Once removed, the stomach was examined. The outlet was compressed by the pseudocyst and the stomach contained >2 l of bile stained fluid. Clearly, the risk of aspiration was extremely high. Luckily feeding had not been initiated. This case report serves as a warning that bedside placement of NG tubes *must* be accompanied by *(a) making sure 50–60 cm of tube goes in easily and without resistance, (b) that insufflation of 60 cc of air is well heard (with bubbling) in the epigastrium on auscultation, and (c) that an X-ray is taken to confirm correct placement before any feeding is commenced.*

Although NG feeding is understandably associated with a higher risk of reflux and micro-aspiration [144–146], it is surprisingly effective in providing enteral feeding even in some of the sickest patients in the ICU [147–149] *if the following anti-reflux measures are imposed*:

Measures to Minimize Aspiration Risk in NG-Fed Patients

1. *The head of the bed should be kept elevated 30–40° to the horizontal (semi-recumbent position).* This rule may have to be broken in ICU patients where frequent positional changes are required, but there is good evidence that ventilated patients are at high risk of vomiting and aspiration if they are rotated to prone position for hypoxia [150]. However another study found that if GRVs were low, patients tolerated feeding well even in the prone position [151]. Recent studies have shown that the use of nasogastric feeding together with continuous lateral rotational therapy in patients kept at 30° reduced the risk of ventilator-associated pneumonia in ICU patients compared to non-rotational management [152].

2. *Feedings should be started slowly and given continuously (20–25 ml/h). Note*: there is little point in starting with feeding rates slower than this as physiological secretion is way above this rate, e.g., 80–160 ml/h.

3. Bolus feeding should be avoided until good gastric emptying has been confirmed.

4. *Gastric residuals should be checked every 4 h.* If residuals are repeatedly over 400 ml it is best to place the feeding tube past the pylorus. However, if this is difficult, emptying can be improved by the use of prokinetics (e.g., metoclopramide 10 mg IV q6h) and acid secretion inhibitors (e.g., IV PPIs, pantoprazole). In patients on narcotics, Narcan 10 mg added to the feed is said to be effective, but is not commonly used for concern about other side effects—it is always better to try and wean the patient off narcotics.

The meaning and definition of high gastric residual volumes (GRV): Until recently, a GRV level of 250 ml was generally accepted as the cutoff level for "safe" NG feeding. However, a recent Spanish study has shown that there is no increased risk of aspiration in ICU patients if 500 ml is used as cutoff [153]. This has persuaded the ASPEN and American Society of Critical Care Medicine to recently revise their guidelines to 500 ml [130]. One recent study showed that aspiration was no more common in ventilated ICU patients whether a cutoff of 200 or 400 ml gastric residual volume (GRV) was used, and that gastric residuals were remarkably low (mean of 31 ml) in patients with proven aspiration [154]. This implied that aspiration pneumonia is more commonly a result of inhaled pharyngeal secretions. However, another more worrying concern is the lack of reliability of GRV volumes. For accurate measurement, the tip of the tube has to be in the "sump" of the stomach, which may vary with position, and the tip has to be free of the mucosal folds for suction to be successful. Although gastric emptying is reduced in any form of critical illness, it usually continues with a higher emptying volume, and provided the feed is given at a rate equal to or below that rate, NG feeding can be remarkably well tolerated by most ICU patients. Despite the discussion above of the results of controlled feeding trials, it would seem logical that the risk of feed aspiration would be higher in NG-fed patients. Indeed, the most recent published meta-analysis of 15 randomized controlled trials concluded that post-pyloric feeding reduced the risk of aspiration pneumonia [155]. However, earlier meta-analyses have failed to show significant differences [156], and so the benefit of post-pyloric placement must be small and suppressible by the implementation of good management practices. As previously discussed, a recent study has shown that resting and food-stimulated CCK responses are increased in ICU patients, providing a humoral explanation for delayed gastric emptying [157]. Consequently, duodenal feeding can be expected to worsen gastric emptying, indicating the potential need for simultaneous gastric decompression. Prokinetic agents, such as metoclopramide, or erythromycin, should be used in adequate IV doses (e.g., metoclopramide 10 mg IV 8 hourly) to increase gastric emptying and thus enhance feed tolerance [158]. If residuals continue to be high, the feeding tube should be placed passed the pylorus, short term PPIs should be used to suppress gastric secretions, and continuous gastric decompression should be considered.

Nasoenteric

Post-pyloric Placement

Post-pyloric placement can be performed by specialized nursing staff or the "enteral tube team" but the sicker the patient, the lower the success rate, as gastric emptying decreases progressively with the increasing severity of illness. Failure at manual placement means referral either to IR or to gastroenterology for endoscopic/ fluoroscopic-guided placement.

Benefits: Increases feeding capacity in patients with poor gastric emptying, such as those patients with critical illness or diabetes [145]. If tubes are placed >40 cm down the jejunum past the ligament of Treitz, enteral feeding can be given without stimulating the pancreas—an optimal approach for the management of patients with severe acute pancreatitis [159–161]. However, it must be remembered that the avoidance of pancreatic secretion will impair digestion and so an elemental formula feed should be used when feeding at this level.

Complications: More invasive procedure, therefore more risk of mucosal injury particularly if attempted manually. The regulatory role of the stomach will be bypassed, potentially resulting in overfeeding, with diarrhea, distension, bloating, and discomfort. It is imperative to remember that bolus feeding must NEVER be used. This is appropriate for the stomach, but not the small intestine, which is designed to receive slow constant infusions of emulsified food from the stomach. Boluses of feed injected into the jejunum may produce "dumping" symptoms. Likewise, tube flushes should not be the same in the stomach and intestine: while gastric tube flushes (or "hydration fluids") with 100–200 cc of water are commonly well tolerated, jejunal flushes should be restricted to 25 cc/4 h. Contaminated feeds are more likely to cause GI disturbances with post-pyloric infusion, as bacterial suppression by gastric acid is lost. Consequently, a sterile feed delivered through a prepackaged "closed" system should be employed.

Placement

- *Manual*: Many large hospitals have formed an enteral feeding team consisting of nurses with specialized training and experience in feeding tube placement. This undoubtedly increases success and reduces the risk of complications. Such personnel become good at not only placing NG feeding tubes, but also post-pyloric placement. A number of bedside techniques have been published. Transpyloric migration is facilitated if 500 cc of air is injected into the stomach when the tip of the feeding tube is in the antrum. This stimulates gastric emptying and the tube can then be gently advanced through the pylorus, after having turned the patient on his/her right side. This is usually effective in patients with normal motility and anatomy, but will fail if there is gastroparesis, distortion, or compression of upper GI tract.
- *Interventional Radiology*: In patients with distortion or dysmotility of the upper GI tract, the next step would be to send the patient to interventional radiology (IR) for post-pyloric guidance. The downside of this approach is that it interferes with patient management, which could be a critical issue in patients needing ICU management. Secondly, there are usual delays of 24–48 h before the procedure can be accommodated. The alternative is to use endoscopy, which can be performed immediately, if necessary, at the bedside in ICU patients, or in the endoscopy suite in more stable patients.
- *Endoscopy*: (*a*) *Per Oral*: Traditionally, a regular 27 French upper GI endoscope is used. The duodenum is cannulated as far as possible and then a guide wire is placed through the endoscope and advanced under vision down the duodenum and then, blindly, around and past the ligament of Treitz. The endoscope is then withdrawn leaving the guide wire in position. This leaves the proximal end of the guide wire emerging from the patient's mouth, and another awkward procedure is required to transfer the wire through the nose before the feeding tube can be deployed. To do this, a slim (e.g., 6 French) 12 in. length of tubing is passed down the nostril into the retropharynx where it is grasped with a pair of forceps and pulled out of the mouth. The proximal end of the guide wire is then threaded through the distal (oral) end of the small tube and pushed through so that it emerges from the proximal end of the small tube out the nose. The small tube is then pulled out of the nose and the guide wire is straightened, allowing passage of the feeding tube through the nose, through the stomach, and down the duodenum. Other endoscopic techniques are to first place the feeding tube down the nose and into the stomach, and then to pass a regular EGD scope into the stomach. When the tip of the tube is identified, it is grasped with an endoscopic biopsy forceps or snare and dragged with the endoscope through the pylorus and as far down the duodenum as possible. In our experience, this rarely works as the best placement will only be within the duodenum and the tube commonly come back into the stomach with the endoscope. One solution is to use an endoscopic clip to tether the tip of the tube to the duodenal mucosa, but this produces mucosal injury.

Transnasal Endoscopic Placement of Feeding Tubes

- This is what we prefer, because

    (1) It obviates the need to perform another uncomfortable procedure at the end
        of a *per* oral endoscopic feeding tube placement to hook the feeding tube
        through the nose,
    (2) Because it is easier to cannulate compressed or stenosed segments of bowel
        under direct vision, and
    (3) Because it is safer to see where you are going.

We use a standard ultra-slim 5.8-mm EGD endoscope (made by all the major
endoscope manufacturers) that will permit transnasal intubation of the GI tract [116,
162]. The smaller 5.0-mm endoscope may also be used, but it is less versatile as it
only has one hand control, with up–down and no side to side tip movement.
Placement of the guide wire through the endoscope is the same as described above,
but this time the wire will emerge out of the nose with the endoscope, thus negating
the need for an additional uncomfortable procedure. The most effective way of
ensuring placement of feeding tubes far down the jejunum is to use the combination
of *transnasal endoscopy with fluoroscopy*, as the guide wire position can be manip-
ulated under fluoroscopy into a confirmed position far down the jejunum. However,
this is only suitable for patients who can be transported to the endoscopy suite. In
other patients in the ICU, the deployment of the guide wire beyond the ligament of
Treitz and down the jejunum has to be done blind, which is usually not that difficult
with practice. This technique is relatively easy for the average endoscopist to learn.
Our GI fellows in training are usually competent after 4 weeks working with us.

The Nasogastric Decompression–Jejunal Feeding Tube (*NGJ*): A teaching video
recording has been placed on U-Tube for further details on endoscopy and placement of NGJs (https://www.youtube.com/watch?v=YlkiY6YTnYk and https://
www.youtube.com/watch?v=UjVjDkdDLW0). We find this procedure particularly
useful in feeding patients with acute severe pancreatitis in the ICU without the need
to transport them out of the unit, as it bypasses the compressed upper GI tract and
permits placement of the tip of the feeding tube >40 cm past the ligament of Treitz
where feeding does not stimulate pancreatic secretion, thereby proving *enteral feeding without pancreatic stimulation* [159]. However, as discussed earlier, the method
is also useful in any ICU patient with persistently high GRVs, and in any patient
with gastroparesis and gastric outlet obstruction, where placement of the J-tube not
so far down, at or around the ligament of Treitz, is sufficient [116]. Examples of
these problems and their solution with NG-J placement are discussed at the end of
this chapter. We use a double-lumen tube (NG-J), which contains a shorter, thicker,
outer tube, which is left proximal to the obstructed segment in order to provide
proximal gastric decompression (Fig. 8.2). Two examples in the USA are the
"StayPut" (Nestle Nutritionals, MN), which is a fixed system with an 18 Fr gastric
decompression tube and a 9 Fr J-tube that will reach the ligament of Treitz which is
most useful in general ICU patients, and the "Kangaroo-Dobhoff" system (Covidien-
Kendall-Tyco Products, MA), which has a 16 Fr 97 cm outer gastric decompression
tube and an inner 9 Fr 170 cm adjustable jejunal extension that permits non-stimulatory

Tube-Within-a-Tube System

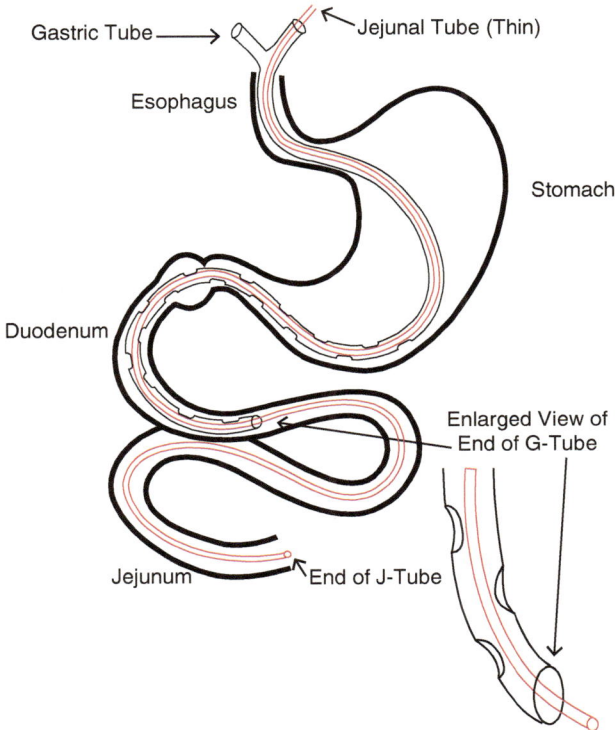

Gastric Tube ⟶   ← Jejunal Tube (Thin)

Esophagus

Stomach

Duodenum

Enlarged View of
End of G-Tube

Jejunum   ↖ End of J-Tube

Fig. 8.2 The NG-J feeding tube system illustrating the double tube within-a-tube conformation allowing proximal GI decompression and distal feeding into the unobstructed jejunum

mid-jejunal (>40 cm) feeding in patients with acute pancreatitis with gastric decompression (Fig. 8.2). *It is critically important to decompress the upper GI tract if there is compression and obstruction of the antrum or duodenum.* If there is accumulation of fluid in the stomach proximal to the obstruction, the patient will vomit and the whole system is likely to be dislodged. In a similar way, it is an ideal method of providing enteral feeding for patients with chronic pancreatic disorders and pseudocysts who also have compressed and distorted upper GI tracts and where pancreatic stimulation is best avoided. They are commonly diabetic, which adds gastric dysmotility and exacerbates the defective gastric emptying. These patients are usually mobile, allowing placement in the GI lab with fluoroscopic assistance. Other common indications are post-partial gastrectomy and post-Whipple's procedure, when there is functional impairment of gastric emptying resulting in vomiting after meals. Although many feeding tube systems come with a guide wire included in the kit, in our experience it is preferable to use specialized ERCP-type guide wires (e.g., JAG-wire, Wilson-Cook, NC) as they are much easier to manipulate through the loops of small intestine distal to the ligament of Treitz and do not kink. As with all procedures, the more frequently these tubes are placed, the easier it becomes. There are specific tips. For example, when withdrawing the endoscope it is very important to make sure that no loops of redundant guide wire are left within the stomach otherwise the whole system simply rolls back into the stomach when the feeding tube is advanced. Secondly, it is useful to reintroduce the endoscope through the opposing nostril while feeding the feeding tube over the guide wire and to watch the progress of the tip of the tube straight down the greater curve and through the pylorus. This ensures the feeding tube and guide wire take the shortest route to the pylorus and that there are no gastric loops.

We published our initial experience with these placements (chiefly StayPuts) in 57 ICU patients in 2003 [162]. All patients had been referred to us for TPN as they had high GRVs associated with respiratory failure, acute head injury, and acute pancreatitis. Placement was successful in >90% and TPN was avoided in 77%. As an additional bonus, previously unrecognized esophageal and gastric pathology was identified in 60% of patients. Recently, we updated our experience with double-lumen (NG-J) tubes anchored in place with nasal bridles, but this time we only used the Covidien adjustable tubes (Kangaroo-Dobhoffs), as the majority of patients needed pancreatic rest and so the J-tube was placed approximately 40 cm down the jejunum [116]. The study included 50 consecutive patients with obstructions chiefly due to complicated severe acute ($n=31$) or chronic cystic pancreatitis ($n=11$). The chief outcome parameters are shown in Table 8.2. Duration of subsequent feeding ranged from 1 to 145 days, median 25 days, and 19 patients were discharged home (HPN, see Chapter 10) with their tube feeds. Only 1 patient could not tolerate feeding and needed to be converted to parenteral feeding. Average tube life was 14 days, replacement being needed most commonly for kinking or clogging of the jejunal tube (56%) or accidental dislodgement (24%). The obstruction resolved spontaneously in 60% allowing resumption of normal eating. Of the patients with severe acute pancreatitis or pancreatic pseudocysts, pancreatic rest resulted in resolution of the disease without surgery in 87%, and need for surgery in the remainder was put off for 31–76 days. Seven patients died, most from complications of acute pancreatitis between days 1 and 31. We concluded that NGJ feeding provided a safe conservative management for critically ill patients with upper GI obstructions, reducing the need for surgery and parenteral feeding.

Table 8.2 Analysis of final outcome parameters

Outcome	
Duration of jejunal feeding, median (range)	25 (1–145)
Individual feeding tube life span, median (range)	14 (1–124)
Weaned back to normal food, no. (%)	30 (60)
Converted to percutaneous endoscopic gastrostomy/jejunostomy or surgical gastrostomy-jejunostomy tube, no. (%)	4 (8)
Home parenteral nutrition, no. (%)	1 (2)
Surgery, no. (%)	8 (16)
Died, no. (%)	7 (14)

Fig. 8.3 Illustration of a double-lumen nasogastric decompression (note bile-stained fluid being aspirated) and jejunal feeding tube (the smaller one going through) anchored in place with a nasal bridle clipped onto the tube at the nose with tape straddling the nasal septum

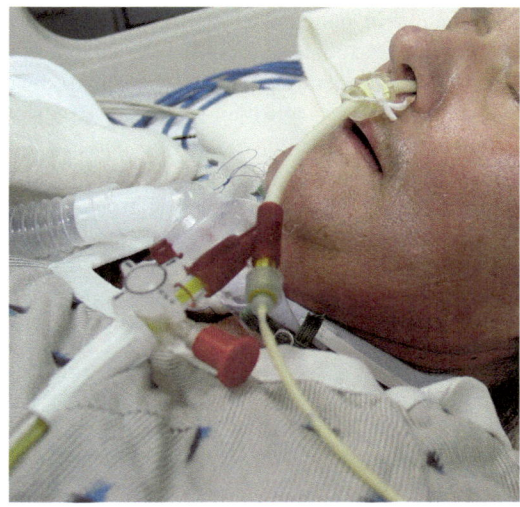

The Nasal Bridle

One of the most frustrating things in interventional feeding tube placement is to struggle to successfully place the tube and to be told the next day that "the tube fell out"! Many of the patients we place tubes in are confused and disorientated and it doesn't take much effort to dislodge a tube fastened to the nose with a piece of tape. The development of nasal bridles was, therefore, for us a divine event, as it increased the life span of the average feeding tube in ICU patients from days to weeks. We currently use the AMT bridle (Applied Medical Technology, Inc., Brecksville, OH 44141 USA) that consists of two 10-cm four French flexible plastic probes with magnets at the tips of both and a thin cotton tape attached to the other end of one. After lubrication with xylocaine-containing gel, the probes are passed up each nostril until they pass the end of the septum, whence a "click" can be felt, indicating interconnection of the two magnets. The tube without the tape is then pulled out, dragging the other with the tape out. The tape then forms a bridle around the septum, and the two ends are clamped onto the feeding tube to secure it in place (Fig. 8.3). Initial fears about septal injury have not been realized, and we have some patients who go home with the bridles and feeding tubes for months on end [116].

Percutaneous

Endoscopic Gastrostomy (PEG)

Indications: The indications for PEG placement are the same as those for enteral feeding detailed above, but, because the procedure is invasive, necessitating perforation of the bowel, and has significant potential complications, its use should only be *considered* in patients who will require enteral feeding for longer than 4 weeks. Continuing nasoenteric feeding beyond that time is uncomfortable and unsightly for the mobile recuperating patient, and can produce nasal injury and sinusitis. However, gastroenterologists must not simply act as technicians when asked to place PEGs, as their complications can be severe and life-threatening. Every attempt should be made to wean patients off enteral feeding and back onto food before contemplating PEGs. Although serious complications are rare in stable patients, they become increasingly more common in critically ill and debilitated patients. It must be stressed that the placement necessitates perforation of the bowel which can lead to intra-abdominal infections and bleeding. Sometimes, the family or nursing home demand PEG placement to ease the care of chronically debilitated patients, but remember that many patients will strongly resist placement—for good reasons— even if their food intake is low. Eating may be one of the few pleasures remaining for them. Any experienced gastroenterologist can place PEGs, but they must be aware of the potential risks and benefits, and only proceed if there is good evidence that the procedure *will improve nutrition and quality of life.* For example, they should never be placed in the terminally ill for maintaining feeding, as there is no evidence that maintaining feeding in this situation improves quality of remaining life or survival: in fact it might do the reverse by introducing complications. PEG feeding should also be avoided in the elderly with advanced dementia, who have lost the will to eat and outcome is poor. It is a bitter pill for the family to often accept that starvation is part of the dying process, but patients must be allowed to die with dignity, and not assaulted with invasive or disfiguring procedures. This will be covered in more detail in Chapter 17. The reader is referred to the vast literature on this subject [163, 164].

Placement: As mentioned above, the gastroenterologist must remember that he/she is not simply a technician, and prior to PEG placement the past medical and surgical history needs to be taken, the abdomen must be examined carefully to illicit signs of previous surgeries that might have altered their anatomies, and to feel for masses that might impair percutaneous access. It is also important to avoid placement in patients with active infections; better to get the infection under control beforehand. PEGs should also be delayed in patients with recent histories of myocardial infarction, and in patients where anticoagulation cannot be temporarily held. The procedure requires sedation and, in patients with poor respiratory reserve or cardiac failure, may result in respiratory or cardiac arrest. Consequently, it is our practice in such patients to use monitored anesthesia care so that maximum sedation can be used in safe, expert hands. Controlled studies have shown that a single IV dose of broad spectrum antibiotics (e.g., 1 g cefazolin), given immediately before the procedure, reduces the risk of more serious invasive infections [165]. A full diagnostic esophagogastroduodenoscopy (EGD) must first be performed to exclude the possibility of mucosal disease, such as gastric ulceration, and to ensure there is no gastric outlet obstruction or impairment due to the presence of distal disease. The urgency of placement must be reconsidered if ulceration is detected: it is better to postpone placement when significant ulceration (i.e., ulcers with depth) is found and to treat appropriately before trying once more. On the other hand, PEG placement might be important in the presence of superficial ulceration to commence feeding and stimulate mucosal repair, or to improve drug delivery. Infection at the abdominal incision site is universal, but usually mild, resolving with time. Placement complications such as perforation or fixation of the colon, liver, or spleen can be minimized if PEG placement is only attempted when there is good transillumination of the light on the end of the endoscope through the abdominal wall, and if a CT scan is performed beforehand (this is almost done as routine in sick patients nowadays!) to make sure there is a "window" of access to the stomach. After PEG placement, a repeat endoscopy must be performed immediately to check the position of the internal bumper and the tension between the internal and external bumpers, and to inspect for complications such as bleeding. If it is too loose, the internal bumper might migrate and create an obstruction; if too tight, a "buried bumper" may occur when the bumper is pulled beneath the mucosal surface.

Systems: A wide variety of commercial PEG systems are available. The sizes commonly used range between 18 and 28 French. In general, small diameter tubes should be avoided in patients with poor gastric emptying and the need for intragastric medication administration. If a jejunal extension is required (PEG-J), for example in patients with gastroparesis, then a wider tube will be required (e.g., 24 French), enabling cannulation with a smaller diameter (e.g., 16 French) jejunal (J) tube. In patients with severely distorted upper GI tracts, it might be necessary to use a 28 French tube as this allows cannulation with a 5-mm endoscope and placement of a guide wire well down the distorted small intestine for jejunal tube placement in a similar fashion to that described for NGJs. The placement of J extensions is described below.

The risks of PEG placement can be reduced if the following safeguards are maintained:

1. Use monitored anesthesia care in unstable patients.
2. Provide prophylactic antibiotics.
3. Always perform a complete EGD to rule out the presence of disease. Active deep ulceration should ideally be treated before PEG placement.
4. When placing the PEG make sure that good transillumination of the endoscope light through the anterior abdominal wall is seen with the overhead lights darkened. Simple palpation of the abdomen looking for indentation of the gastric wall is not good enough for PEG siting, as the colon can be transfixed between the stomach and the anterior abdominal wall and finger palpation will still be seen.
5. Avoid placement in patients with ascites or on peritoneal dialysis. If a PEG has to be placed in a patient with ascites, make sure the fluid is drained beforehand and the abdomen is lax.
6. Avoid placement in head injury patients who have had a VP shunt placed within the past week.
7. Ensure that a coagulopathy is not present and that the patient is not on anticoagulants. Subcutaneous heparin should be held at least 6 h prior to the procedure.

If platelets are reduced below 50,000 cells/cm, provide platelet cover at the time of placement.

8. Do not perform the procedure single-handed. Use an endoscopic assistant (GI fellow or GI colleague) to help with placement so that sterility is maintained. Four hands on deck!
9. After insertion of the PEG, re-endoscope to check final placement and to detect complications.
10. Do not overtighten or undertighten the internal–external bumper system. The internal bumper should be flush with the mucosa and should swivel easily.

Management: Many of the late complications of PEGs can be avoided with good nursing practices. Initially, the incision site should be covered with gauze for protection and the external tube fastened to the abdominal wall with a Stat-Lock as shown in Fig. 8.4 to prevent pulling. We usually advise initial q4-h water flushes, but bolus feeding can be started by 8 h in stable patients, with good intestinal function. Leakage of the feed is unusual in this circumstance, as normal motility will propel the feed down to the duodenum, rather than out the PEG orifice. The site should be examined daily to make sure the external bumper is not too tight and that there is no infection or discharge, and cleaned with an antiseptic. With time, 4–8 weeks, the gastrocutaneous passage becomes epithelialized and becomes established by fibrosis such that if the tube is pulled or falls out, another can be safely replaced at the bedside without re-endoscopy. However, the hole closes over rapidly

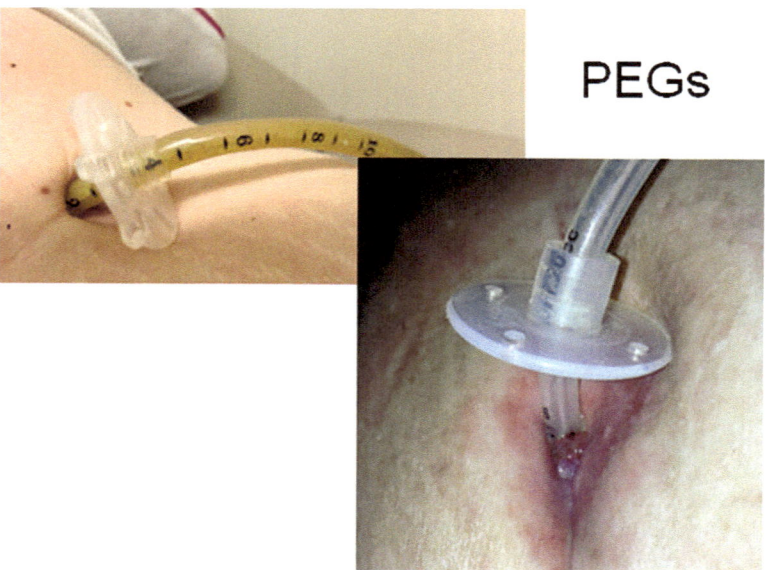

Fig. 8.4 *Left*: Well-healed insertion site, managed with soap and water toilet, daily dry dressings if necessary. *Right*: Healed with "granulation" tissue associated with mucoid discharge. Treated with initial and then monthly applications of silver nitrate until fibrosed, barrier crèmes, daily re-dressings until dry

and so a replacement should be placed asap, within 6–8 h. In an emergency, any simple tube, such as a Foley's catheter, can be used. If there is ever any difficulty inserting a replacement tube, it is mandatory to check the position by X-ray after contrast injection, before restarting tube feeding. Within the first month of placement, loss of the tube will necessitate replacement by endoscopy, as there is a real chance of misplacement of the manually inserted tube into the peritoneum. Healed exit sites are best cleaned with soap and water and kept dry and protected by loose gauze dressings. Some patients continue to have a serous discharge associated with "granulation" tissue as shown in Fig. 8.4. This is best treated by monthly applications of silver nitrate, contained in swabs at the end of sticks, until the red tissue retracts and the skin around the hole becomes totally healed as in Fig. 8.4.

Percutaneous Radiological Gastrostomy

Gastrostomy placement can be performed relatively simply by interventional radiologists. However, due to manpower reasons, IR usually are only asked to place tubes when endoscopy is impossible because of stomal, pharyngeal, or esophageal obstruction, or when PEG fails, for example due to failure to observe endoscopic transillumination. Generally the technique is based on (a) the insertion of a needle into the lumen of the stomach for inflation under fluoroscopic or ultrasound guidance, (b) the placement of "fasteners," i.e., small needles with tethers that can be deployed once inside the stomach, which hold the stomach wall against the anterior abdominal wall while (c) a trochar with graduated dilators is used to pierce the two layers, ultimately allowing (d) the placement of a gastrostomy tube with an inflatable internal bumper.

Surgical Gastrostomy

This is the classic method of gaining gastric access for feeding or decompression. Numerous comparative studies have been performed which have compared endoscopic to surgical gastrostomy placement, and all indicate that the endoscopic method is a quicker and less complicated approach to take. However, the procedure is simple and we usually refer all patients in whom safe endoscopic placement cannot be performed.

PEG-J

As mentioned above, this consists of the passage of a secondary feeding tube through the PEG and through the pylorus into the duodenum or proximal jejunum. With practice, this procedure is fairly easy to perform, but again a skilled assistant is essential, as you need four hands. The first step is to place a PEG as described above. Next, the provided guide wire is placed through the PEG tube and grasped with endoscopic forceps. The forceps are then shortened to the end of the endoscope and the tip of the endoscope is advanced with the wire through the pylorus as far down the duodenum as possible (4th part). It is always important to cannulate the duodenum before this procedure is performed to know where you are going, because the first part of the duodenum is often deformed in patients with gastric outlet obstruction needing J-tube placement! Blind advancement can injure the duodenal cap mucosa with the tip of the forceps and guide wire. Once the final position in the duodenum is achieved, the secondary jejunal feeding tube is passed over the guide wire from outside the body through the PEG, holding the wire taught to prevent looping in the stomach. It helps to advance the biopsy forceps slightly forward of the endoscope so that the tip of the J tube can be observed under direct vision to have reached the end of the guide wire where it is held by the forceps. Once the J-tube tip is seen, the biopsy forceps are slowly fed through the end of the endoscope while the endoscopy is synchronously pulled back from the duodenum into the stomach, leaving the biopsy forceps, guide wire, and J tube well down the duodenum. When the endoscope is looking at the pylorus, the guide wire is released from the forceps, and the forceps are pulled out of the endoscope. The endoscope is then brought back to the PEG internal bumper to check that the J tube goes *direct* from the internal PEG bumper to the pylorus, without looping in the stomach. This is good placement, and the endoscopy may now be safely withdrawn. The alternative is to perform the "exchange" and guide wire release when the endoscope is still well down the duodenum, but the J-tube often sticks to the endoscope and flips back into the stomach when the endoscope is withdrawn. In some patients with gastroparesis and large stomachs, the position of the internal PEG bumper is often facing the esophagus rather than the pylorus, and no matter what you do, the J tube will loop within the stomach before entering the pylorus. This is bad placement, as the whole tube will shortly fall back into the stomach. In this situation it can be helpful to loosen the external bumper of the PEG tube and to push the tube 5–10 cm into the stomach so that the bumper now faces the pylorus. Another alternative is to use a 28 French PEG tube and then use an ultra-slim 5.0-mm endoscope (NB: not the one we use for transnasal endoscopy which has a diameter of 5.8 mm, which is too big) which may be passed directly through the PEG and advanced through the duodenum for deployment of the guide wire and feeding tube, akin to the method described above for NG-J placement. The endoscope is then withdrawn, leaving the guide wire in the jejunum, and the J-tube is then passed over the guide wire, through the PEG and past the pylorus into the jejunum. With the rapid advancement of endoscopic technology, it can be predicted that this form of endoscopic-assisted placement will become standard with time.

Direct PEJ

In some patients with gastroparesis or surgically altered anatomy, the J-tube of a PEG-J frequently recoils back into the stomach, necessitating repeat endoscopies for repositioning. In others, a gastrostomy is impossible due to surgical resection. In these situations, a feeding jejunostomy will be needed. Most commonly this is performed surgically by open or laparoscopic technique, but it is always worth first performing an upper GI endoscopy to pass the tip of the endoscope as far as possible down the small intestine to try and detect abdominal wall transillumination, so that a direct PEJ can be placed [166]. Percutaneous endoscopic jejunostomy (PEJ) placement consists of an endoscopic procedure very similar to PEG, but involves the direct placement of the percutaneous tube into a loop of small intestine that lies immediately below the abdominal wall allowing clear transillumination of the endoscope tip through the abdominal wall after the loop is distended with air. The use of direct PEJ is more risky as the small bowel is more mobile and of smaller size, and satisfactory transillumination is not often seen. The same precautions used for standard PEG placement need to be imposed. A smaller diameter (e.g., 16–18 French) PEG tube is preferable, but systems up to 22 French often work well and do not obstruct the lumen if tethered correctly.

Surgical Jejunostomy

This is the most common form of percutaneous jejunostomy used as it is often placed at the end of a complicated abdominal surgery when there is concern that upper GI function may be impaired by the surgery and take a while to return, for example after a partial gastrectomy, a Whipple's procedure, or any other form of complex esophageal, gastric, duodenal or pancreatic surgery. Under direct vision, a loop of small intestine is approximated to the abdominal wall and the tube is tunneled caudally to maintain position and facilitate motility.

Laparoscopic Jejunostomy

With the increasing use of and expertise in minimally invasive laparoscopic surgery, laparoscopic placement of feeding tubes is becoming more popular. The indications are those for PEJ, namely the need for long-term access and home enteral feeding, and the advantages over PEJ are that it doesn't rely on abdominal transillumination of the bowel lumen and therefore is possible in a wider population of patients.

Recent Developments: Situations Where Enteral Feeding Should Now Be Used Instead of TPN

Dysmotility and Ileus

Classically, ileus, or "paralytic ileus" as it is commonly termed, occurs in patients following major abdominal surgery and also from critical illness. It is evidenced by the absence of bowel sounds, the typical X-ray appearance of distended intestinal loops of bowel with or without air fluid levels, nausea and vomiting, and the absence of stooling and flatus. For years, the dogma was not to give any oral or enteral feeding to patients with ileus until bowel sounds were heard, and flatus is passed. This actually perpetuated the problem, as the most effective treatment for ileus is the resumption of feeding. This practice was finally debunked by the classic study of Waldhausen et al. in 1990 [167]. During major abdominal surgery, they inserted electrodes into the stomach, jejunum and colon allowing them to pace the electrical conductivity of the intestine in the recovery period.

Remarkably, basic electrical activity showed no changes in frequency after surgery and the electrical activity was poorly associated with the presence of absence of bowel sounds. A number of studies have subsequently shown that postoperative ileus is not equated with intestinal failure, and that bowel function and nutrient absorbing capacity may be suppressed, but not absent [168]. For example, intraoperative percutaneous jejunostomy feeding tube placement allowed enteral feeding to resume within 24 h of major surgery with good tolerance and absorption, and controlled trials have shown that most patients tolerate oral intakes immediately following more moderate forms of surgery [169, 170]. Figure 8.5 illustrates a patient admitted to hospital with vomiting, abdominal pain, ARDS, and ileus due to severe acute pancreatitis. Many would consider this intestinal failure, and prescribe NG decompression, NPO, and TPN. A double-lumen NGJ tube was successfully placed by transnasal endoscopy as shown in the X-ray enabling simultaneous gastric decompression and the commencement of slow continuous (25 ml/h) jejunal feeding. Ileus resolved within 24 h, stooling returned, and TPN was never needed. The critical importance of this observation is that there are an accumulating number of

Fig. 8.5 Patient with severe acute pancreatitis, admitted with radiographic ileus: NG-J feeding tube has been positioned

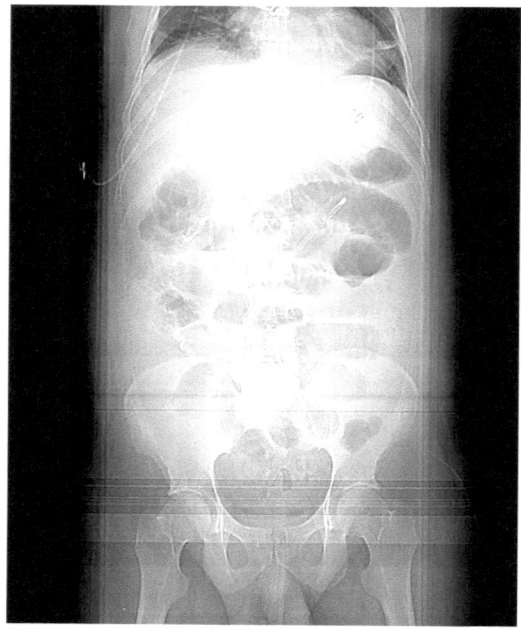

Table 8.3 Investigations of early enteral feeding in medical and surgical patient populations

Author/journal	Study parameters	Study design	Outcome
Marik PE [78], 2001/CCM	Feeding < or >36 h	15 studies	↓ Infections
		753 patients	↓ Length of stay
Lewis SJ BMJ [79], 2001 (surgery patients)	NPO versus <24 h	11 studies	↓ Infections
		837 patients	↓ Length of stay
			↑ Vomiting risk
Heyland D JPEN [80], 2003 (medical ICU)	<24–48 h	8 studies	Trend to ↓ infections and mortality
Lewis SJ [81], 2009 (J GI Surgery)	<24 h	13 studies	Decreased mortality
		1,173 patients	
Doig GS [82], 2009/Int Care Med (critically ill patients)	<24 h	5 studies	Decreased infection and mortality
Osland EJ [83], 2010/WJ GI Oncology (GI surgery with resection)	<24 h	15 studies	45% decrease in morbidity
		1,240 patients	
Doig GS [84], 2010/Injury (trauma patients)	<24 h	3 studies	Decreased mortality

studies that suggest that early enteral feeding improves outcome in ICU-ventilated patients (Table 8.3), and so attempts at enteral feeding, initially at a slow rate with NG suction, should not be delayed by X-ray or clinical evidence of ileus.

The etiology of ileus following abdominal surgery and in non-surgical critical illness is similar and equally complex, as recently reviewed by Caddell et al. [171]. As they suggest, a problem with multiple potential causes will have multiple potential treatments, as illustrated by Fig. 8.6. Prokinetic agents such as metoclopramide and erythromycin are effective in the short term in improving gastric emptying, but long-term use is impaired by decreased efficacy and side effects. Our experience is that virtually all these patients can be fed enterally, if a feeding tube is placed past the ligament of Treitz (i.e., in the jejunum) and provided gastric decompression is maintained. This remains one of the most distressing battlegrounds with some traditional surgeons who continue to demand PN for their postoperative patients with ileus! Education works, and the above references should be distributed. The use of an NGJ tube ensures safe gastric decompression while jejunal feeding can be started slowly (20 cc/h) and advanced with tolerance, with the resultant resolution of ileus.

Inflammation, electrolyte abnormalities, edema, neurotransmitter changes and opiates all play a role. For this reason, the treatment of ileus is also complex, but improvement can be expected from any form of treatment that removes the underlying disease and promotes recovery. In practice, early enteral feeding and the minimization

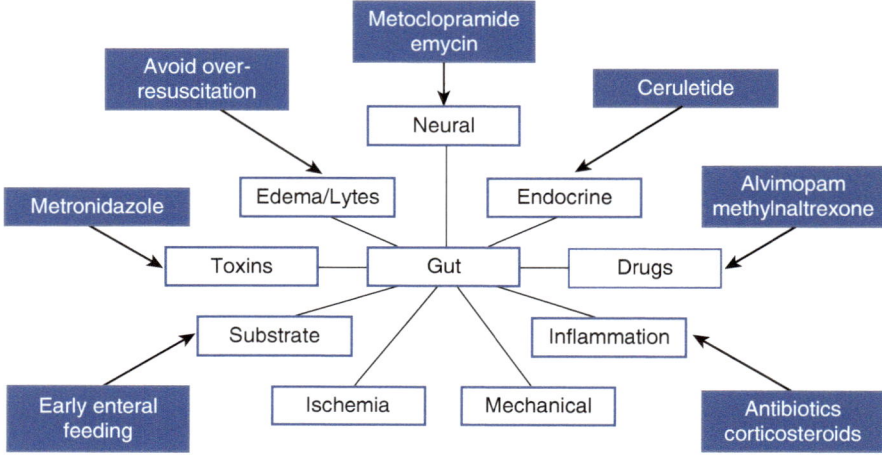

Fig. 8.6 Upper GI dysfunction in critically ill patients has multiple causes, and therefore multiple treatments (Caddell et al. [171])

of narcotic use are probably the most effective forms of treatment, as luminal nutrients stimulate secretions and peristalsis, prevent intestinal inflammatory cytokine production and bacterial overgrowth, and maintain gut function. This accounts for the change in current practice to *start enteral feeding early but slowly*, in the course of the hospitalization. As gastric emptying is most commonly disturbed, it is best to place a feeding tube post-pyloric and commence feeding with a regular polymeric diet at a slow rate (20–25 cc/h) the day following major surgery or on admission to the ICU with any form of critical illness. As reviewed earlier, this rate may be continued for the first week providing what has been termed "trophic feeding," to maintain gut function and mucosal integrity. Colonic function is the last to return and so early consideration, i.e., by the end of the first week, of the addition of a soluble fiber source (e.g., wheat dextrin 10–20 g/day) to the feeding schedule is wise.

Gastric Outlet Obstruction

Perhaps the most common indication for TPN up until recently was poor gastric emptying and high NG aspirates associated with critical illness. Gastric emptying is slow, as is general gut motility, in most ICU patients. Fraser and colleagues have shown that CCK levels are commonly increased in ICU patients, and jejunal feeding will increase levels further [157], leading to further reductions in gastric emptying. These physiological observations, coupled to experience in practice, have lead us to advocate the use of double-lumen feeding tubes "NG-J" tubes as described above (e.g., "StayPut," Novartis; "Kangaroo-Dobhoff," Kendal), with a distal jejunal feeding tube and a proximal gastric decompression tube. Our first experience with

Table 8.4 Illustration of the wide variety of patients with upper GI dysfunction (gastroparesis) treated successfully with NGJ feeding tube placement (O'Keefe et al. [115])

Group median values of the 51 patients, plus range in brackets[a]								
Subgroup	n	%	Age (year)	Procedure time (min)	Initial success	Duration of feeding (day)	Hospital stay (day)	Deaths
Respiratory failure	15	29	50 (41–82)	15 (14–31)	14/15	10 (3–54)	33 (10–78)	5/15
Head injury	14	28	41.5 (18–50)	18 (13–25)	13/14	9 (2–21)	25 (5–71)	4/14
Acute pancreatitis	17	33	45.0 (18–77)	30 (20–45)	14/17	7 (1–90)	21 (4–181)	2/17
Sepsis	2	4	31.5 (18–45)	17 (10–24)	2/2	8	19.5 (19–20)	2/2
Cardiac failure	1	2	40	18	1/1	13	66	0
Liver failure	1	2	52	20	1/1	5	23	0
Abdominal surgery	1	2	59	20	1/1	7	14	0

[a]Demographic data of the 51 patients included in the study, summarizing procedure results (group median [range]) and outcome

placement of double-lumen tubes by transnasal endoscopy (Fig. 7.3) was reported in 2003 on 51 consecutive ICU patients referred to us for TPN, because of failure to be able to use the gut because of "high gastric residuals and ileus" [162]. The demographics are summarized in Table 8.4 showing the variety of underlying conditions associated with disturbed upper GI function.

Initial placement was successful in all apart from five patients with massive gastric dilatation and acute pancreatitis complicated by duodenal compression who required fluoroscopic guidance. In confirming correct tube placement, there was a near-perfect concordance between re-endoscopy and X-ray (45/46) indicating that there was no need to confirm placement with abdominal X-rays. Figure 8.7 illustrates correct placement, with the arrows marking the stomach, the pylorus, and the ligament of Treitz. Previously unrecognized upper gastrointestinal tract pathology was detected in most patients, with acute gastritis in 47, superficial gastric ulceration in 24, and erosive esophagitis in 5. These results led us to conclude that endoscopic placement of these feeding tubes in the ICU is quick, effective, and minimally disruptive of intensive therapy. In addition, it can reveal unrecognized pathology, which potentially could lead to improvements in overall medical care [162]. Our most recent published experience on 50 further ICU patients, predominantly with gastric outlet obstruction due to severe necrotizing pancreatitis, endorses this view, with only one patient failing enteral feeding and needing PN [116].

Fig. 8.7 The endoscope has been withdrawn from the patient and the double-lumen feeding tube ("StayPut," Novartis) has been passed over the wire, through the nose, and into the correct position with the outer gastric aspiration ports within the gastric sump (*arrow top right*), the internal jejunal tube passing through the pylorus (*left arrow*) and going through the ligament of Treitz (*right lower arrow*) into the jejunum

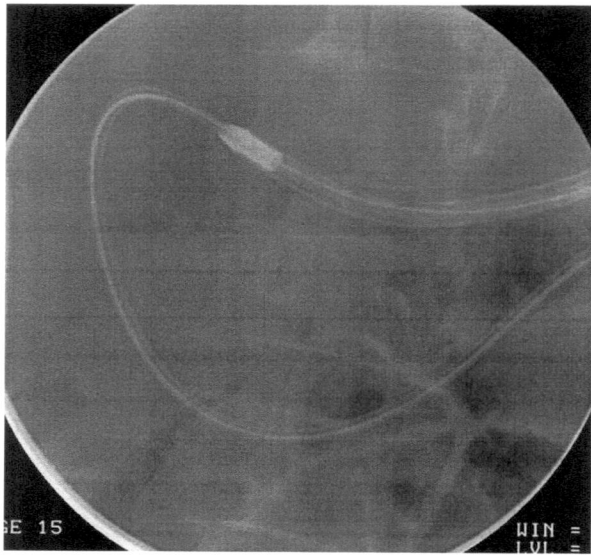

Secondly, masses in the esophagus, stomach, and duodenum, or masses outside the lumen causing extrinsic compression, can compress the upper GI tract, causing obstruction. However, the bowel distal to the obstruction remains functional—if it can be accessed. The classic example is patients with acute pancreatitis or chronic pancreatitis with large pseudocysts producing extrinsic compression of the upper GI tract (Fig. 8.8). Barium studies performed on these patients commonly demonstrate "high-grade" obstruction of the outlet of the stomach or the duodenum. Great care has to be taken when attempting intubation in these patients, as the stomach is usually full of fluid and gagging may precipitate aspiration. Attempts at manual/bedside or even radiological placement of feeding tubes through the obstructed segment usually fail in this situation. The use of endoscopy allows the compressed segment of bowel to be traversed by the endoscope using direct vision. Once past the obstruction, the distal bowel is seen to be open and functional with active peristalsis, allowing placement of a guide wire through the endoscope into the functional bowel. As previously described under NGJ feeding above, the endoscope is then retracted leaving the guide wire straddling the obstructed segment. A feeding tube may then be fed over the guide wire from the nose into the functional bowel allowing resumption of full enteral feeding, with no need for TPN. At the same time, it is critically important to decompress the bowel proximal to the obstruction, as secretions will collect inducing nausea and vomiting, which might dislodge the jejunal feeding tube and lead to aspiration. In more chronic conditions, a percutaneous endoscopic jejunostomy (PEJ) can be placed directly into the patent bowel distally. Alternatively, if the patient requires surgery, a surgical jejunostomy may also be placed to gain access to functional bowel.

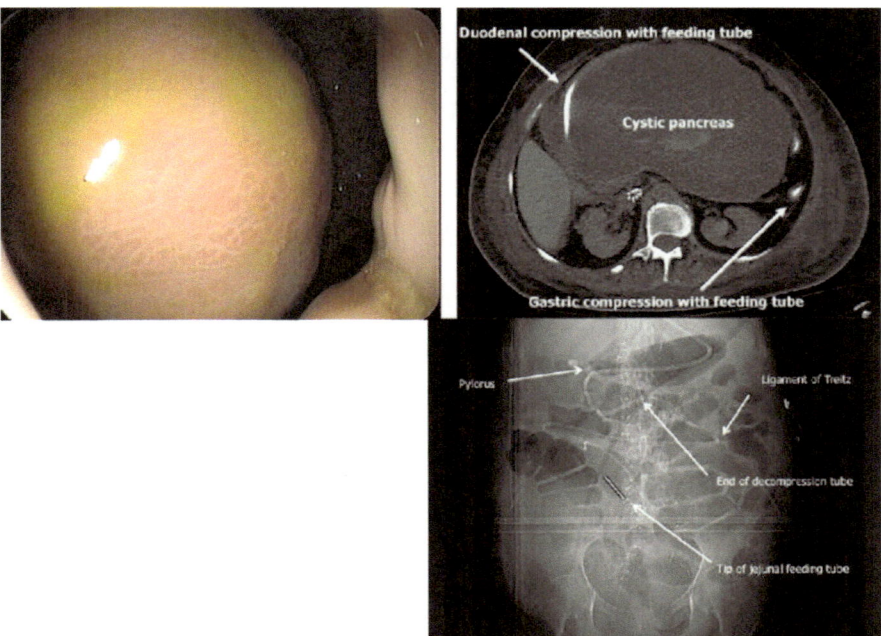

Fig. 8.8 Examples of gastric compression due to extrinsic compression by pancreatic masses and the restoration of gut function by transnasal endoscopic placement of a double-lumen nasogastric decompression jejunal feeding tube (NG-J). (**a**) endoscopic view of a large pancreatic pseudocyst compressing the stomach, (**b**) CT scan of the same, (**c**) successful placement of an NG-J feeding tube with tip 40 cm past ligament of Trietz

Severe Diarrhea

Critically ill patients given tube feeding frequently develop diarrhea, but the composition of the feed is rarely to blame. As has already been discussed under *Why Might Enteral Feeding Improve Outcome?* (Chapter 5, p. 42) diarrhea is usually a consequence of disturbed microbiota due to the combined effects of antibiotic therapy, PPIs, and bowel rest [34, 97]. As discussed in Chapter 5 (p. 48), recent studies have shown that the microbiota are essential for the maintenance of colonic function and health. In critical illness, they suffer a double hit from (a) the almost universal use of antibiotic therapy and (b) the use of non-residue tube feed formulae that derive them of their nutrition [34]. PPIs also disturb the composition of the microbiota and can precipitate diarrhea [172]. Diarrhea or loose stools are particularly common in patients at commencement of feeding. *It is extremely important not to hold the feeding until the diarrhea resolves as this starves the microbiota further exacerbating dysbiosis and adds to the rate of nutritional deterioration.* With continued feeding at a slow rate of 20–40 cc/h, the microbiota slowly recovers and the diarrhea usually improves after 3 days, allowing advancement in feeding rate to goal. If the diarrhea continues, efforts should be made to restrict antibiotic and PPI use, and to investigate other common causes of diarrhea, for example the use of sorbitol-containing liquid medications. In patients who need continued antibiotic therapy, it is important to add a probiotic to support the microbiota.

Gastroesophageal Reflux and Aspiration Risk

Although the presence of a feeding tube in the lower esophagus and stomach reduces the competency of the lower esophageal sphincter, reflux is chiefly caused by factors such as sepsis, trauma, drugs, body position, gastroparesis, esophageal dysmotility, and obesity. Aspiration in this situation is, however, preventable, even in nasogastrically fed patients, by the adoption of strict management protocols, as detailed under NG feeding above. Consequently, there is *never* a need for TPN in this group of patients.

Chapter 9
Parenteral Feeding

Indications

The indication for parenteral feeding is simple: when nutritional support is needed and enteral feeding is not possible. *The absolute indication is in patients with permanent intestinal failure where patients will become progressively more malnourished and die unless PN is started.* These patients will need permanent home parenteral nutrition (HPN). However, intestinal failure is rarely a black and white issue, and the majority of patients referred for nutritional support have partial loss of intestinal function as a consequence of critical illness. The intestinal failure usually remits as the underlying disease is successfully treated and PN can be delayed if nutritional stores are sufficient.

Definitions of Intestinal Failure

- *Permanent Intestinal Failure* "results from obstruction, dysmotility, surgical resection, congenital defect, or disease-associated loss of absorption and is characterized by the inability to maintain protein-energy, fluid, electrolyte, or micronutrient balance." [173].
- *Temporary intestinal failure*: This is defined as "reversible intestinal failure due to obstruction, dysmotility, surgical resection or disease-associated loss of absorption and is characterized by the inability to maintain protein-energy, fluid, electrolyte, or micronutrient balance." The urgency of starting PN in this situation in critically ill patients depends upon the nutritional status of the patient and the degree of intestinal failure. Such patients commonly can tolerate *some* enteral feeding, and the question then becomes "how much negative nutrient balance can be tolerated without impairing organ function?" As discussed in Chapter 5, we will assume that the loss of body stores associated with a drop in BMI <17

© Springer Science+Business Media New York 2015
S.J.D. O'Keefe, *The Principles and Practice of Nutritional Support*,
DOI 10.1007/978-1-4939-1779-2_9

results in significant impairment of organ function, and that in severe illness it would take approximately 7 days for a previously well-nourished patient to become functionally protein deficient. *Consequently, it would be reasonable to start all patients with a nonfunctioning gut and a BMI <17 on PN. In others, with a BMI >17, it would be reasonable to wait 7 days focusing on treatment of the underlying medical or surgical condition, restoring fluid and electrolyte balance, correcting micronutrient deficiencies, and achieving enteral access, before starting PN. Note* that the commencement of TPN—and nutrition support in general—*is never an emergency* and it can generally wait until after the weekend or after a holiday while the general condition of the patient is optimized, e.g., correction of fluid and electrolyte balances.

Nutritional Support of the Critically Ill Patient

Acutely ill patients cannot eat normally for a variety of reasons, e.g., altered mental status, ventilation, nausea and vomiting, and anorexia. The excessive and premature use of TPN in this subset of patients in the past led to metabolic and infective complications that counteracted the potential benefits of IV nutrients [174, 175]. As discussed in Chapter 5, patients with mild acute pancreatitis did worse if they were given TPN [61], and the classic VA "preoperative TPN" study showed that TPN only helped those who were malnourished to begin with [64]. This, together with the recognition of the importance of maintaining gut function, is responsible for the dramatic drop in the use of PN and rise in interventional tube feeding over the past 15 years. For example, between 2000 and 2005, PN use in one surgical trauma ICU fell from 26 to 3% [176]. The problem with EN is, however, that in clinical practice it is difficult to achieve goal infusion rates because it is started slowly to assess tolerance and tolerance is reduced in critically ill patients. This inevitably leads to an "energy gap," particularly in the first few weeks of illness. This has raised concern, as outcome studies have shown that energy gap is a predictor of poor outcome and ICU mortality, and led to the increasing use of PN to "top up" nutrient provision [177]. However, as discussed in Chapter 5, there is no good evidence from randomized controlled trials that "PN top-up" improves outcome; in fact the most recent RCT suggests that it may be detrimental, as complications were added without improvements in outcome [106]. From a physiological point of view, it would be logical to avoid forced feeding in patients with sufficient stores (i.e., BMI >17) and to accept hypocaloric enteral feeding, or IV fluid and electrolyte support alone. Indeed, some studies have shown that optimal outcome is achieved when enteral infusion rates of only 15–20 kcal/kg/day are given [83]. Extrapolating from pig model studies, we know that at least 20% of nutritional requirements need to be given enterally to maintain intestinal mass and function [36] and human studies have shown that PN complications may be suppressed by partial enteral feeding [178]. Thus, there is good theoretical evidence to support the concept and use of "trickle" *or* "trophic" enteral feeding, i.e., infusion rates of 20–25 ml/h, to reduce complications, while the deficit is made up with PN *only* in depleted patients (i.e.,

BMI <17 kg/m^2). Based on these observations, the following pragmatic guidelines are recommended:

- *Previously well-nourished patients defined by SGO or with a BMI >20*: Resuscitate with IV fluids and electrolytes and then continue daily infusions to maintain fluid balance, renal function, and to correct electrolyte and micronutrient deficiencies. Monitor gastric function by NG tube decompression. If 24 h volumes are <1,000 ml, start polymeric tube feeding at 25 cc/h and measure 4 h gastric residual volumes. If volumes are consistently <250 cc/h, increase feeding rates by 25 cc/h each day until goal is achieved over 3–5 days as described below under NG feeding. Only consider PN supplementation if the patient is unable to tolerate >50% of requirements enterally by the second week of illness.
- *Malnourished patients defined by SGO or a BMI <17*: Manage as above, but supplemental PN during the first week once cardiopulmonary and metabolic stability has been achieved.
- *In the mildly malnourished patient* (i.e., BMI 17–20): Use either approach, depending upon the general clinical picture using SGO.

- *Preoperative feeding in the patient with reversible intestinal failure*: Should you "feed up the patient" with TPN before surgery, or simply stabilize them and perform the surgery to relieve the cause of intestinal failure so that normal eating can resume? Based on the literature, we have come to the following practice guidelines:

  - *In previously well-nourished* (SGO/BMI >20) patients, simply correct fluid, electrolyte, and micronutrient deficiencies and proceed to early surgery to relieve the obstruction so that they can resume eating. At the time of surgery, place a jejunostomy feeding tube if there is any concern that GI function will remain impaired after surgery.
  - *In the malnourished patient* (SGO/BMI <17), do not attempt to "normalize" a patient's nutrition before corrective surgery. Correct fluid, electrolyte, and micronutrient deficiencies, and then start PN before surgery and operate after 7 days. Following surgery, stimulate gut function with trickle feeding to prevent ileus and progress to full enteral via nasoenteric or surgical percutaneous jejunal feeding tube while tapering off PN. This will correct underlying metabolic deficiencies, provide the essential building blocks for tissue repair, and minimize the risks of prolonged PN.
  - In the mildly malnourished patient (i.e., BMI 17–20) use either approach, depending upon the general clinical picture as shown by SGO, e.g., in a previously well patient, operate; in a patient with chronic illness (e.g., alcoholic disease), provide nutritional support for a week before elective surgery if possible.

- *Note that accurate nutritional assessment is difficult in the critically ill, as discussed in Chapter 7, and that BMI must be used in conjunction with a thorough clinical examination and assessment, as in the subjective global assessment (SGO) that includes history of dietary intake, amount of weight loss, the character of the underlying disease, functional muscular weakness or inability to work or perform daily activities, and physical signs of muscle wasting, fat depletion, edema, ascites, glossitis, and skin lesions specific to vitamin deficiencies. For example, some healthy people normally have BMIs of 18, and fluid retention will weaken the value of BMI in the detection of nutrient depletion in the critically ill.*

IV Access

Parenteral nutrition solutions are generally hypertonic as they are elemental in character. Consequently, they have to be infused at a slow, and therefore continuous, rate into a large vessel with a high blood flow rate to rapidly dilute the nutrient solution and thus avoid coagulation and thrombosis complications. Access can be made by direct puncture of a central vein (e.g., subclavian) or by inserting a long catheter up a peripheral vein into a central vein, termed a peripherally inserted central catheter (PICC). However, short-term (approximately 1 week) peripheral vein infusions can be used if a high lipid-low dextrose emulsion is used which significantly reduces the osmolarity, termed peripheral parenteral nutrition (PPN). *A cardinal rule in patients requiring long-term TPN is to reserve the use of the catheter for TPN alone* to reduce the risk of contamination and sepsis. However, in the ICU this is often impractical, as patients need multichannel catheters for life-support measures, and catheters are frequently changed or exchanged.

Central Vein Placement

This is the preferred method for TPN delivery if it will be needed longer than 7 days.

In unstable ICU patients, an internal jugular approach is most commonly used with the placement of a multiple-channel catheter so that the other ports can be used for resuscitation, pressure measurements, and medications.

For longer-term use, it is preferable to use a Seldinger over-the-guide wire technique under sterile conditions in the OR, or in the radiology suite with the aid of fluoroscopy, to ensure that final catheter tip placement is at the juncture of the superior vena cava and the right atrium.

In home TPN patients, a "tunneled" *single-lumen silicone central vein catheter is best.* This consists of the initial placement of a percutaneous-central vein catheter by Seldinger technique, followed by the creation of a subcutaneous tunnel to tether the catheter down under the skin. The preferred placement is the subclavian approach, with a ~10 cm subcutaneous tunnel down the anterior chest wall to a position that can be easily seen by the patient to enable him/her to see the catheter better without the use of a mirror during IV hookups. Single-lumen silicone catheters (e.g., "Hickman," "Groshong," Bard. Boston, USA) last longer, and come with a mesh "hub" that is buried within the subcutaneous tunnel. Initially the catheter is kept secured by suture, tape, or adhesive dressing (e.g., "OpSite," Smith and Nephew, St. Petersburg, FL, or "Tegaderm" 3M, St Paul, Mn), but after 6 weeks the hub becomes fibrosed to subcutaneous tissues and held in place, obviating the need to skin sutures, thus improving comfort and reducing the risk of skin infections. The chief advantage of subclavian-chest wall tunneled catheters is that they are easier to handle for patients at home as they are easier to see and manipulate with two hands during connecting and disconnecting their own TPN infusion. This also reduces the risk of accidental contamination of the lines and connections. Another alternative for long-term home use in physically active patients is to implant an injectable port (e.g., "Port-A-Cath," Smiths Medical, Dublin, Ohio) subcutaneously on the chest wall. While preferred by many active patients, the drawback of these catheters is that they require percutaneous needle access every week, and if they become infected, they need surgery to remove, drain, and treat.

In certain situations, such as in patients with superior vena cava syndrome, the subclavian vein cannot be accessed. In these cases, the inferior vena cava can be accessed via the femoral vein and the catheter exit tunneled under the skin up onto the lower abdominal wall, again facilitating access. There is no hard evidence that infection rates are higher with femoral catheters, provided they are looked after well. Use of the hepatic vein or transthoracic cannulation of the right atrium has also been described in desperate cases of "vanishing venous access" [179].

Peripheral (PICC lines)

Today, this is the most popular approach to in-hospital TPN for noncritically ill patients because long peripheral lines can be placed by specially trained technicians on the floor, obviating the need for transport to special suites in surgery or radiology. Because of the risk of long venous thrombosis, such lines should be only used for 3–6 months, and changed prospectively to Hickman-type catheters in patients likely to need long-term parenteral support.

Feed Formulation: The TPN Prescription

Standard vs. Customized Bags

Giving parenteral nutrition is more of a science than giving enteral feeding. This is not only because parenteral nutrition is traditionally formulated in the hospital pharmacy according to the patient's specific needs, but also because metabolic tolerance to PN is less than EN because it is unphysiological and breaks down the natural protective mechanisms discussed in Chapter 5. For example, an excess of PN will result in serious metabolic complications, whereas an excess of EN will result in clinical warning signs, such as vomiting or diarrhea, before metabolic complications can occur. Consequently, PN orders should be written or approved by persons with specialized knowledge, such as the Nutrition Team. That having been said, there is increasing use of **"standardized" formulae**, particularly in Europe, as it has

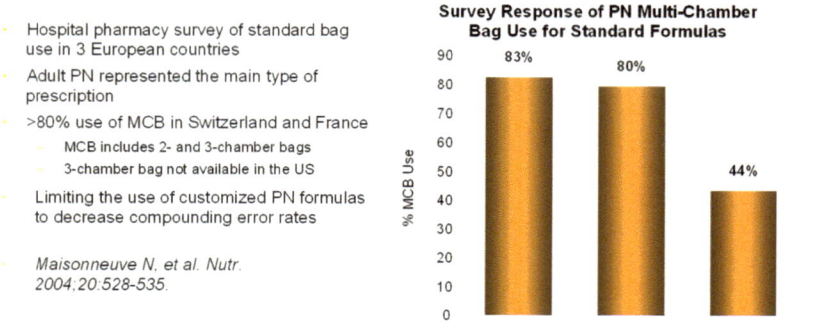

Standard Bag PN Formulations
Are Widely Used in Europe

- Hospital pharmacy survey of standard bag use in 3 European countries
- Adult PN represented the main type of prescription
- >80% use of MCB in Switzerland and France
  - MCB includes 2- and 3-chamber bags
  - 3-chamber bag not available in the US
- Limiting the use of customized PN formulas to decrease compounding error rates

  Maisonneuve N, et al. Nutr. 2004;20:528-535.

Survey Response of PN Multi-Chamber Bag Use for Standard Formulas

COMPOSITION OF THE MAIN PARENTERAL NUTRITION FORMULA USED IN SWISS, FRENCH, AND BELGIAN HOSPITALS

	Switzerland (n = 36)		France (n = 32)		Belgium (n = 27)	
	Mean ± SD	Min–max	Mean ± SD	Min–max	Mean ± SD	Min–max
Volume (mL)	1479 ± 312	1000–2190	1650 ± 605	200–3000	1864 ± 638†	1000–2580
Non-protein calories (kcal)	1376 ± 410	296–2184	1315 ± 610	47–2480	1444 ± 459	778–2184
Amino acids (g)	76 ± 23‡	40–134	45 ± 25	2–80	50 ± 31†	7–90
Lipids (g)	53 ± 27	0–100	57 ± 31*	0–100	73 ± 24†	40–100

Fig. 9.1 Standard PN bag formulae

been shown that three basic formulae, one example being 1,200 kcal, 80 g amino acids, and 40 g fat plus basic electrolyte and micronutrients, can cover most of the needs of most *stable* patients in hospital (Fig. 9.1) [180], which is not surprising as we use enteral feeds with a standard composition all the time. In the USA there are a number of standard bags commercially mixed and marketed by Baxter Nutritionals Chicago, USA, named "Clinimixes." We find two compositions useful for starting and maintaining patients on when our pharmacy is unable to mix for us, particularly at weekends:

Vol (ml)	Amino acid g	Dextrose g	Kcal	Na mEq	K mEq	Mg mEq	Ca mEq	Phos mM	Acetate mEq	Cl mEq
2000	85	100	680	70	60	10	9	30	140	78
2000	100	300	1,470	70	60	10	9	30	160	78

The advantage of this approach is that commercially admixed solutions or emulsions are less likely to contain composition errors, and they save pharmacy costs for preparation. They also allow "batch" prescription to cover weekends and holidays for stable patients. As we will discuss in Chapter 10, home PN patients, who, by definition, are stable, become established on a relatively fixed PN composition, allowing bag mixing and delivery to the home once a week, where the bags can be stored safely refrigerated.

Customized Bags

In unstable patients, prescriptions need to be reviewed and rewritten every day. It should be a team function, involving the primary care team, the NSS physician and coordinator (e.g., nurse or dietitian specialist), and the PN pharmacist. *The patient must first be seen and examined, and the results of specific investigations and past history reviewed.* Next, routine labs need to be studied. These should include electrolytes, BUN, creatinine, LFTs, magnesium, and glucose, in order to obtain essential information about fluid balance, renal function, liver function, and metabolic status. Albumin, and prealbumin, concentrations are often asked for, but their values do not influence the final PN prescription as they bear no relation to body protein stores in hospitalized patients as discussed in Chapter 7 (p. 71). It must be remembered that plasma protein concentrations are not synonymous with plasma protein synthesis rates, as they are strongly influenced by hydrational status and flux rates between body compartments. A persistent depression in plasma albumin correlates best with the severity of illness, no matter what the cause, and is one of the best predictors of survival as discussed in Chapter 7. A sudden drop commonly signifies developing sepsis. LFTs, in particular alkaline phosphatase, AST and bilirubin need to be reviewed at least weekly as PN can induce or exacerbate abnormalities, which are easily correctible in the early stages by alterations in management discussed below, noting that a progressive increase in AP and AST may signify overfeeding or underlying sepsis.

In general terms, these are the guidelines for PN composition and needs:

- *Volume*: in patients with normal renal function, start with 1.5–2.0 l per day and then adjust in concert with other IV or oroenteral fluids to maintain a urine output of approximately 1.5–2.0 l/day.
- *Energy*: Requirement for most hospitalized patients, including those in the ICU, is no more than 25 kcal/kg *ideal body weight* per day. However, because of fears of metabolic tolerance in sick and particularly in malnourished patients, it is important to always err on the side of safety and commence at about 50% of estimated requirements and to monitor metabolic tolerance closely, checking blood glucose, potassium, phosphate, acid-base, urea, and creatinine before increasing to goal. Severely malnourished patients, BMI<17, are at risk of refeeding syndrome because they are deficient not only in macronutrients but also in vitamins, such as thiamine, and minerals, such as phosphate, which are needed to completely oxidize glucose to ATP to fuel organ function. It is wise to not only start slowly, i.e., 25% of energy requirements, but also preload with thiamine and phosphate even if initial blood levels are normal, which they usually are. However, as mentioned in Chapter 5, thiamin deficiency rarely occurs on its own, even in alcoholics, and supplementation with the complete spectrum of multivitamins is judicious. The bulk of energy is given in the form of glucose, particularly initially, but a proportion should be provided in the form of fat, or lipid, not only to prevent essential fatty acid deficiency but also to control hyperglycemia without insulin infusions. Although there is concern that high lipid infusions may suppress immune function, it must be remembered that our metabolism was designed to run on a mixed energy source of glucose and fatty acids,

and an excess of either one could impair metabolic function. Usually, up to 25% of calories are given as lipid emulsion, which comes to 20–40 g/day.

- *Amino Acids*: The goal is 1.0–1.5 g/kg *ideal body weight*/day, but again start slowly at 50% and increase to goal, provided blood urea remains within the normal range. The urge to counter protein catabolism with higher infusion rates should be avoided, as this simply generates more urea and metabolic stress as described in Chapter 7. Bringing the underlying disease under control by medical or surgical therapeutics and treating sepsis best curbs protein catabolism.

- *Electrolytes*: Usual needs are 60–150 mEq of sodium and 40–100 mEq potassium per day, but requirements vary with disease. For example, potassium needs will be higher in patients with vomiting and diarrhea and lower in patients with renal dysfunction. Remember that there is far more flexibility with sodium than potassium, as there are hormonal mechanisms, namely aldosterone, that conserve sodium but not potassium. *Consequently, a better indication of sodium sufficiency is gained from measuring urine sodium rather than blood sodium*: plasma sodium can remain normal with virtually no sodium in the urine. The anion most used is chloride, but acetate can be partially substituted if blood chlorides are high or if bicarbonate levels drop. For most of the other electrolytes, a standard replacement is used and blood levels followed to assure sufficiency (Fig. 9.2).

- *Minerals*: Hypomagnesemia is common in hospitalized patients, particularly in those with GI disease, as the body pool is small compared to that for calcium, and additional supplements are important not only to avoid muscle dysfunction and tetany, but also to improve potassium retention. Iron concentrations and binding capacity is commonly low in critically ill patients, but ferritin may be high in patients with liver disease. Because of the concern that iron may increase bacterial infections, supplementation is usually reserved for those who display iron-deficiency (hypochromic) anemia. Serum zinc levels are also difficult to interpret as levels vary with stress, but low concentrations should be treated with additional supplementation.

- *Vitamins*: There is not much science behind how we handle vitamin requirements in clinical practice: we generally assume a standard requirement, and give the same dose to everybody as discussed in Chapter 7. These quantities were determined from "safe" infusion levels gauged to cover requirements for most hospitalized patients; consequently, most are given in excess. Blood levels can be measured, but analysis is expensive, and there is a poor correlation between blood concentrations and functional sufficiency. The exception is in alcoholic patients with confusion where the detection of low levels of thiamine and nicotinamide may provide a diagnosis. Such patients require multivitamin supplementation in addition to high levels of infusion of thiamin as discussed above.

- *Trace elements*: Trace element deficiency rarely occurs in patients who can eat, or are fed enterally, as complex foods contain adequate supplies of these elements. However, the initial development and use of TPN in patients with severe intestinal failure revealed for the first time classic trace element deficiency syndromes, as the diet was "synthetic," and each essential nutrient had to be added to the final sterile mixture. Good examples were in patients who needed TPN for periods exceeding a year: zinc deficiency producing scaly skin rashes (acroder-

PN Indication:	Dosing Wt (kg)		Ht (cm):
Service: must choose one (PUH only)	☐ SBTx	☐ TST	☐ Other

VOLUME/RATE INFUSION	☐ Total Volume of _____ ml / day
	☐ Continuous over 24 hours at _____ ml/hour
	☐ Cycle over _____ hours
	_____ ml/hr for the First hour, _____ ml/hr over the next _____ hrs, _____ ml/hr during the last hr

BASE SOLUTION	☐ CENTRAL	☐ PERIPHERAL (can be infused through peripheral vein)
	☐ Dextrose _____ gm per BAG	☐ Dextrose _____ gm per BAG
	☐ Amino Acids _____ gm per BAG	☐ Amino Acids _____ gm per BAG

LIPIDS 20%	☐ None						
☐ 2 in 1 Volume:	☐ 100 ml (20 grams)	☐ 200 ml (50 grams)	☐ 250 ml (50 grams)	Frequency:		☐ M W F
Infusion period: 12 hours						☐ Other _____
☐ 3 in 1 Volume:	☐ 100 ml (20 grams)	☐ 200 ml (50 grams)	☐ 250 ml (50 grams)	Frequency:		☐ Everday
						☐ Other _____

☒ Parenteral nutrition **MUST** be administered through a dedicated infusion port and filtered with a 0.22 micron filter for 2 in 1 solutions (dextrose and amino acids only) and 1.2 micron in-line filter for 3 in 1 (dextrose, amino acid and lipid containing solutions)

ALL ADDITIVES ARE PER BAG

ELECTROLYTES		Average Adult Electrolyte Requirements per 24 Hours
Calcium Gluconate	_____ mEq (4.65 mEq = 1gm)	
Magnesium Sulfate	_____ mEq (8 mEq = 1 gm)	Sodium 60-150 mEq
		Potassium 60-150 mEq
Potassium Chloride	_____ mEq	Phosphorus 20-45 mMoles
Potassium Acetate	_____ mEq	Magnesium 10-15 mEq
Potassium Phosphate	_____ mMol (3mM of KPO4 contains 4.4 mEq K)	Calcium 10-20 mEq
		Caution: To prevent precipitate
Sodium Chloride	_____ mEq	{ [2 X Calcium (mEq)] + Phos (mMol)} /
Sodium Acetate	_____ mEq	[volume(ml) /1000] } must be =or < 45
Sodium Phosphate	_____ mMol (3mM of NaPO4 contains 4 mEq Na)	

OTHER ADDITIVES					
☒ Standard Multivitamins (MVI-12 10ml)	☐ Zinc	_____ mg	☐ Regular Insulin	_____ Units
☐ Standard Trace Elements (MTE-5 Conc 1ml)	☐ Selenium	_____ mcg	☐ Famotidine	_____ mg
☐ Thiamine 100 mg	☐ Chromium	_____ mcg	☐ Other	_____
☐ Folic Acid 1 mg	☐ Copper	_____ mg	☐ Other	_____
☐ Ascorbic Acid _____ mg	☐ Manganese	_____ mg		
☐ L-Carnitine _____ mg				

(BLOCK Print TPN Specialist Name)	TPN Specialist Signature	Pager #
(BLOCK Print) Nutrition Support Attending Name:	Physician Signature:	Pager #
DATE/TIME:		
Order Set Faxed to Pharmacy by: (name / time)		Unit:

Fig. 9.2 An example of a daily TPN order form

matitis), selenium cardiomyopathy and myositis, copper neutropenia, anemia, and muscle weakness, and chromium glucose tolerance [181]. However, since the addition of trace element mixtures to the PN formulation became standard practice, these syndromes are rarely seen, and if they are seen, it is usually in the picture of severe malnutrition and multiple nutrient deficiencies. In long-term HPN patients, it is usual practice to check blood levels for zinc, selenium, chromium, manganese, B12, vitamin A and D (25 OH-D3), folic acid, vitamin C, and carnitine at the commencement of HPN, and then once stable 1–2 times per year and to adjust levels of supplementation accordingly.

To ease prescription, a standard "TPN form" is generally used, as illustrated in Fig. 9.2.

The Management of PN Complications

The chief complications associated with PN, discussed earlier in Chapter 2, are hyperglycemia, catheter-related sepsis, venous thrombosis, and liver disease.

1. *Hyperglycemia*: Sick patients are in a state of acute stress. This alters the hormonal balance, increasing blood glucose concentrations. The combination of this disturbance plus the fact that glucose tolerance is lower if the same amount of glucose is given IV or enterally [30] accounts for the almost universal observation of hyperglycemia in PN-fed critically ill patients. Studies from the Netherlands suggested that "tight glucose control" with the aggressive use of insulin infusions reduced mortality rates in critically ill patients [59], but more recent studies from other units have raised concerns that the risk of hypoglycemia might outweigh any overall benefits [182]. It is therefore pragmatic to accept mild hyperglycemia up to 150 mg/dl, and only intervene if values exceed this level. In general, do not exceed a total energy infusion rate of 25 kcal/kg ideal body weight/day. Reduce glucose to 70% of total calories and use lipid for the balance. Only then, use insulin, either in the form of a subcutaneous sliding scale or as a continuous IV infusion. Once levels are controlled, it is safe to add 2/3 of the daily insulin given directly to the PN bag so that it is infused with the nutrition as this is more physiological. Note that sudden discontinuation of the PN after you do this, or in any patient receiving injectable insulin, may result in hypoglycemia, as the action of insulin continues after the glucose infusion has been metabolized. *Cyclical PN infusions must be tapered before discontinuing for this reason.*
2. *Catheter-Related Sepsis*: This is the most serious short term complication. The infecting organism is most commonly a skin bacterium, such as *Staphylococcus epidermidis*, resulting from contamination during tube connections and bag changes. Classical presentation is fever, sweats, rigors, and/or chills with increased WBC plus bands, but in the immunocompromised patient, symptoms may be lacking and blood culture alone may be positive. In ICU patients, blood, urine, and sputum should be sent for culture and the catheter changed immediately, sending the tip also for culture. Broad-spectrum antibiotics are generally started while awaiting the return of culture with sensitivities; however the sepsis will generally settle with withdrawal of the catheter alone. It's like removing a splinter.
3. *Venous thrombosis*: In short-term PN patients, this is rarely a significant problem, but in hypercoagulable patients, it is wise to add 1,000 units of heparin/l of PN as prophylaxis.
4. *Liver Disease*: Mild liver dysfunction, as indicated by disturbed LFTs, is common in PN-fed patients, and of minor consequence, as it usually reverses when the patient gets better or when normal feeding is resumed. However, a small proportion of patients on prolonged TPN progress to permanent liver damage with fibrosis and ultimately cirrhosis, as discussed below for HPN patients. Although CT scans can suggest this progression, diagnosis has to be confirmed

by biopsy. Biopsy is not without its own complications, so it is useful to have guidelines as to when this should be attempted:

(a) *Elevated liver enzymes (e.g., SGOT, LDH, AST, AP) <2x above upper range of normal*: avoid excess PN calories, reduce to <25 kcal/kg ideal body weight/day, keep lipids <40 g/day. Try to maintain some bowel function/nutrition with sips or "trickle" feeding, both to prevent bacterial overgrowth and maintain some portal nutrient flow.

(b) *Exproportionate increase in AP*: Do as above, but in addition check ultrasound scan of gall bladder and biliary tree to exclude obstruction.

(c) *Increase in enzymes >x3 above the upper limit of normal range, or associated increase in bilirubin*: As for 1, above. In addition if available, check resting metabolic rate by indirect calorimetry to fine-tune energy balance. If no response, or with progressive jaundice and cholestasis without biliary obstruction, refer to hepatology for work-up, e.g., serology and liver biopsy.

Chapter 10
Nutritional Support at Home

Home Parenteral Nutrition (HPN)

Dudrick's now classic studies in the 1960s, which showed that Beagle pups achieved normal growth and development on TPN alone [60], first demonstrated that life was possible in patients with permanent intestinal failure. Since that time, thousands of patients with permanent intestinal failure have survived to lead remarkably full lives, and many of us have HPN patients who have survived over 30 years despite intermittent problems with *septic, metabolic, thrombotic, and hepatic complications*. Figure 10.1 illustrates one of our patients receiving PN at home, assisted by his wife dating back to the early 1980s. He had developed intestinal failure due to the loss of most of his small and all of his large intestine through repeated resections for complicated Crohn's disease. With home support, he survived over 30 years living in South Africa, running his own business. With careful management protocols, the risks of complications can be minimized, and the chief cause of mortality is the underlying disease. However, a small proportion of patients unfortunately develop "TPN failure" (see below) and will die unless they receive a successful small bowel transplant, usually including a liver.

Indications

The chief indication for HPN is permanent intestinal failure, due to loss of bowel, i.e., short bowel, or inability to use the bowel, as in chronic intestinal obstruction [73]. A typical breakdown of the patient populations is illustrated in Table 10.1,

© Springer Science+Business Media New York 2015
S.J.D. O'Keefe, *The Principles and Practice of Nutritional Support*,
DOI 10.1007/978-1-4939-1779-2_10

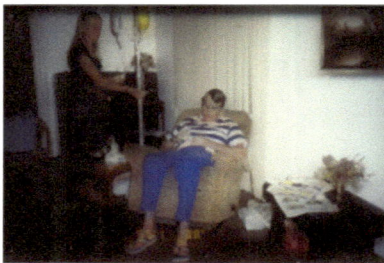

Fig. 10.1 Illustration of home parenteral nutrition management. For this to be successful, both the patient and their home spouse/companion have to be fully trained in the "no touch technique" and aseptic techniques during PN bag "hook-ups" at night and disconnections in the morning

Table 10.1 Composition of HPN population

Short bowel 63%
• IBD (chiefly Crohn's disease): 35%
• Infarction: 30%
Chronic obstruction 36%
• Radiation: 14%
• Neoplasm: 8%
• Pseudo-obstruction: 6%
• Surgical complications: 8%

based on the Mayo Clinic program in the 1990s, which included 63 patients at that time [183]. Short bowel syndrome continues to be the most common indication. Loss of bowel was previously most commonly due to Crohn's disease, but now mesenteric infarction is now becoming a more frequent with our aging population. The main variable is cancer: hospitals that specialize in oncology will have a much higher proportion, as illustrated by the Oley Foundation data, where 40% of their national HPN patient database had cancer [184, 185]. The issue of HPN and cancer is controversial. No study has shown that either the quality of life or survival is improved with HPN in the terminal cancer patient. In fact, morbidity may be higher as TPN complications are added without survival benefit. It is different, however, in the case of a malnourished patient with treatable cancer, where short-term use may be useful to replenish stores prior to chemotherapy, radiation or surgery. HPN is also indicated in patients with slow-growing tumors, such as ovarian cancer, which often results in chronic intermittent obstructions of the intestine. An increasing proportion of patients are now sent home on TPN from the hospital for short term HPN, e.g., 3 months, to improve their nutrition and allow restitution prior to further complicated abdominal surgery for unhealing fistulae or wound dehiscence. For example, patients recovering from complex abdominal surgeries with enterocutaneous fistulae, open abdominal wounds, or disconnected bowel are often initially at too high a risk for further surgery to restore intestinal continuity. *Note* that it is generally unjustified to continue HPN in this set of patients longer than 3 months, as complications begin to outweigh benefits, and the primary object must always be to restore gut continuity so that patients can be weaned back onto normal food.

Catheters

Peripheral (PICC) Versus Tunneled Central Catheter (CV) Placement

The catheters used for central venous access are similar to those described for short term PN in the hospitalized patient above, but with important differences due to the fact that these lines are more critical for the patient's survival and are considered "life-lines."

PICC: Patients on HPN require long-term intravenous access that is safe and easily accessible. Peripherally inserted central catheters (PICC) can be used for 3–6 months, but ideally should be changed to a central catheter after 2 months in any patient who is expected to need long-term HPN. Mobility is a problem, and every time the arm moves, so does the tension on the catheter. As discussed earlier (Chapter 9, p. 119), they are also more difficult for the patient to "hook up" to TPN at home because one arm, the one with the catheter in, is dysfunctional. The advantages of PICCs are that they are easier to replace and specialized non-physician teams can be trained to place them on the floor. Consequently, it is common practice to use PICC lines for high-risk patients with recurrent frequent catheter infections until they become stabilized.

Central: This is the preferred method for HPN patients. Specialists in interventional radiology or vascular surgeons most commonly perform placement using strict aseptic techniques. As mentioned above, tolerance to central catheters is higher because thrombus formation and venous occlusion is lower in large veins with high flow rates. First choice is the subclavian approach as it is more comfortable for the patient and the clavicle protects the line. Further, tunneling from this position down the anterior chest wall is easy. Tunneling is important as it allows the patient to better see and handle the catheter during TPN connections and disconnections. Long-term catheters (e.g., Hickmans) have a fibrinous cuff, which is positioned within the subcutaneous tunnel. With time, the cuff becomes fibrosed under the skin, fastening the tube into position. At this time, usually after 6 weeks, the suture holding the catheter to the skin can be safely removed, increasing comfort. Less movement of the catheter translates into less local and systemic infections, and longer catheter lives.

Replacement catheters can be changed over a guide wire to maintain the same position, but it is always preferable to use the other side, or a different site, particularly if the catheter is being changed because it is infected as risk of introducing infections is high, and the tunnel is usually colonized. Furthermore, progression of internal thrombosis will occur. In patients with loss of catheter function because of thrombosis, the patency of the superior vena caval should be investigated before catheterization. Partial areas of thrombosis can be penetrated and dilated by IR with ultrasound or venographic guidance if an alternative site can not be not identified. If this fails, then the catheter can be placed in the IVC via the femoral veins. These lines should also be tunneled away from the groin region and onto the lower abdominal wall. In the extreme situation of vanishing venous access, transhepatic cannulation of the hepatic vein or direct cannulation of the right atrium have also been described in desperate cases [186], but if this stage is reached, it is time for a small bowel transplant.

Catheter Type

In critically ill patients, central catheters with multiple ports are used to facilitate the multiple IV infusions they need. However, in stable patients requiring long-term HPN, catheters with as few ports, usually single, as possible are preferred to reduce the risk of infection. *Remember, two ports double the risk of infection!* The most important consideration is that the catheter is easy to see and access. Our preferred catheter is a single-lumen silicone catheter with implantable subcutaneous cuff (e.g., "Hickman," Bard Access Systems, Salt Lake City, UT) that can be tunneled under the skin for about 4 in. from its penetration site. Single lumen is important as it simplifies management and reduces luminal stasis and the need for multiple flushes. Less instrumentation translates into reduced infection risk. Polyurethane catheters may be used, but they preclude the use of alcohol locks. For stable, active, patients, subcutaneous access devices, such as the Port-a-Cath® (Smiths Medical MD Inc, St Paul, Minnesota) may be preferable for stability and cosmetic reasons. However, local skin problems are more common as they require needle access changes once a week, and the port has to be removed surgically if it gets infected.

Formulation

Table 10.2 illustrates the average PN composition of our HPN patients in the 90s. Today, we rarely use more than 300 g dextrose, 100 g amino acids, or 40 g fat per day as excess calories from either source increase the risk of liver dysfunction, and excess amino acids simply enhance urea synthesis and urine nitrogen losses. Daily nutrient and fluid requirements vary depending upon the cause of intestinal failure. Patients with short bowel and high stomal losses have high fluid and electrolyte requirements (often >3 l/day), while chronically obstructed patients have lower volume requirements (<2 l/day). On the other hand, IV nutrient needs are commonly lower in SBS patients as digestion is well maintained and absorption by the residual intestine, even if most of the jejunum and ileum are lost, is often significant, and liver complications are less. It is not commonly appreciated that much of the

Table 10.2 Home parenteral nutrition average composition as used in the Mayo Clinic program in the 90s (Burnes and O'Keefe [183])

TPN daily requirements
- Volume: mean 2.4 l (range 0.5–6.0)
- Glucose: 274 g (46–531)
- Amino acids: 67 g (0–85)
- Fat: 21 g (0–100)
- Sodium: 176 mEq (37–695)
- Potassium: 86 (30–220)
- Chloride: 210 (60–760)
- Acetate: 103 (0–200)

protein, carbohydrate, and fat digestion and absorption is complete by the time it reaches the proximal jejunum. Up to 1,000 kcal of energy can be salvaged in SBS patients who have preserved colonic function [187]. For these reasons, and because portal nutrients may be important in maintaining hepatic health and function, we no longer impose dietary restrictions in SB-IF patients. In fact, part of the adaptation to short bowel is increased appetite and hyperphagia (Chapter 11, p. 156).

The principles of HPN management are to adjust fluid and electrolytes to maintain a 24-h urine output >1,000 ml/day and a urine sodium content of 40–80 Meq/day while maintaining normal blood concentrations of creatinine, potassium, magnesium, phosphate, bicarbonate, and chloride. Remember that plasma sodium can remain normal, when the urine contains *no* sodium due to hormonal (aldosterone) conservation. Macronutrients are adjusted to maintain a normal body weight (i.e., BMI 18–24 kg/m^2) and renal function (BUN 18–24). Although essential fatty acid requirements can be met by adding lipid to the dextrose and amino acid solutions only once a week, fat is a normal part of food and it is logical to add 20–40 g daily.

The remainder of the admixture consists of standard quantities of micronutrients, vitamins and trace elements. Fat-soluble vitamins such as A, E, and K are stable in TPN lipid solutions, although vitamins A and K are affected by sunlight. Because blood concentrations poorly reflect biological sufficiency and costs of analysis are high, they are normally only measured 6 monthly in HPN patients. Plasma carnitine is easy to measure and carnitine supplements can be added in patients with LFT disturbances while adjusting the caloric content and dextrose:fat ratio. Calcium management is difficult because blood levels are maintained during dietary insufficiency at the expense of bone mineral stores. Consequently standard quantities of calcium and vitamin D are added, but it is advisable to monitor bone mineral density with DEXA scanning annually in patients at risk—and advise patients to sit in the sun whenever possible! Other common additives include insulin, H-2 blockers, and heparin, according to disease state. Octreotide can also be added, especially for patients with high-output enterocutaneous fistulae, but there are potential pitfalls. The manufacturer discourages its use in TPN solutions because of the formation of glycosylated octreotide conjugates that decreases its efficacy. Generally, however, octreotide is stable in TPN bags for 24–48 h. Additionally, octreotide can affect the activity of insulin and vice versa. There are no clinical trials that have verified these claims, but *in vivo* insulin and octreotide can affect one another's bioavailability. For these reasons, it is better to avoid mixing the two in TPN solutions.

Management of HPN

General Principles: HPN can not only be life saving, but also remarkably successful in restoring lifestyle and productivity in patients with permanent intestinal failure. On the other hand, if it is mismanaged, it can be disastrous. To be successful, patients should be managed in an academic environment by a team that has a large collective experience in the principles and practice of HPN. The team involves the hospital based "core" group which includes a specialist physician and coordinator (usually a specialty nurse, dietitian, or pharmacist), the home care team includes a home-care company who prepare and deliver the PN solutions according to the directions of the core physician, and provide visiting nurses to help with catheter care and management of the cyclical infusions. Last but not least, the team includes a home physician who looks after the patient on a day-to-day basis and takes regular blood tests, sending the results to the core physician for evaluation. Recognizing the complexity of this service, we have recently published a more detailed review of this process and how it should be run successfully (Fig. 10.2) [188].

In general, patients must be shown to be metabolically stable and established on cyclical feeding before they leave the hospital. Secondly, they must have received instruction from the person supervising HPN in IV administration, line care, and monitoring for signs and symptoms of complications *before* they leave hospital. Home planning is facilitated by the use of forms, such as the one on Table 10.3. Once home, the core team manages HPN, in conjunction with a home care company and the patient's local physician, or PCP. Generally, the home-care company, admixes the PN bags in batches (e.g., 7 days worth) and delivers them to the home where they are stored in a refrigerator prior to use. As vitamins are less stable, the patient adds them to the bag prior to use. The home-care team supervises catheter-care and dressings, as well as drawing weekly blood tests, principally BUN, creatinine, glucose, sodium, potassium, magnesium, CBC, and LFTs. The results are shared with the hospital team and PCP. As many patients live long distances from the hospital, it is essential to have a PCP (or local gastroenterologist) in the team for the patient to report to in case of complications. However, alteration of the PN should *only* be made by the hospital team to avoid conflicting advice and management. Complications should also be managed by the hospital team with the PCP's help. Patients should be educated that at the *earliest suggestion of fever*—even if they think it is just a cold or flu—they should report to their physicians, or better still, go to the nearest emergency room to have blood cultures drawn. With time, patients become experts in their own care and can advise others, such as ER personnel, on what should be done and who should be contacted for advice. For example, they

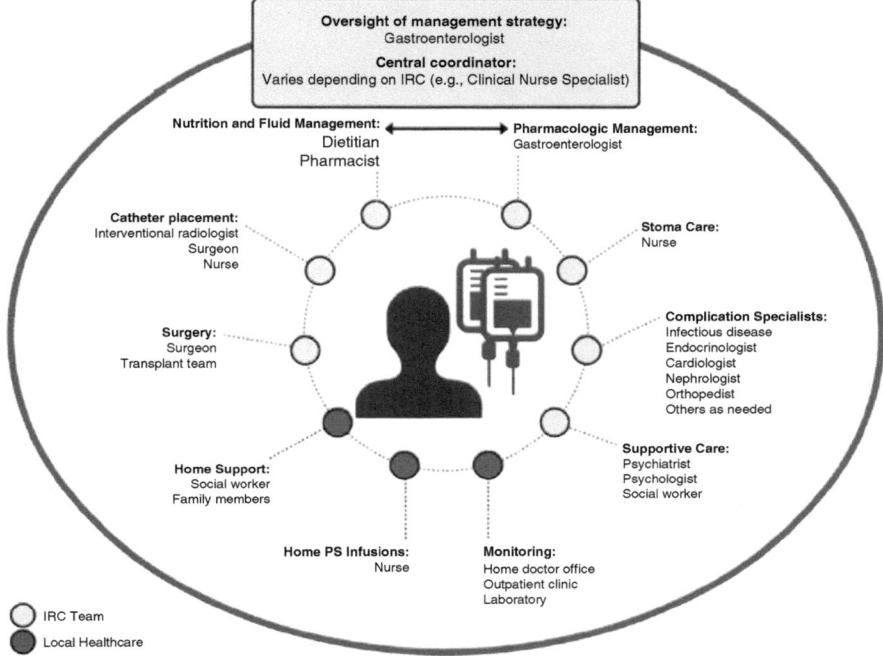

Fig. 10.2 Illustration of the complexity of HPN management. Success can only be achieved by a multidisciplinarian approach involving hospital and homecare specialists. IRC=intestinal rehabilitation center

know that oral antibiotics are totally ineffective in treating suspected line sepsis as they are not abosorbed, and that they should be referred back to the core hospital group in the event of complications.

Generally, HPN is run over 8–12 h at night so that the patient can disconnect during the day and participate in normal activities. The two major long-term concerns are catheter infection and venous thrombosis. Infections usually arise from contamination of the catheter and infusion lines during bag changes, and the *risk of infections is directly related to the standard of catheter care* [189]. Risk is also related to the number of "breaks" in the system, and the catheter should only be used for HPN. As stressed above, only use single lumen catheters.

Catheter Locks: When not being used, the catheter is capped (note modern catheters self seal) after flushing the catheter with sterile saline solution, with or without heparin. Recent studies have shown that the frequency of recurrent catheter infections can be reduced if the "lock" solution consists of 30–70% ethanol [190]. Unfortunately heparin is not compatible with alcohol, so choices need to be made in each individual depending upon which risk is highest.

Table 10.3 An example of a standardized HPN discharge form

Parenteral nutrition discharge orders	
(*Not* for implementation while in the hospital)	Imprint patient identification plate here
1. Laboratory studies to be taken by the home care agency, frequency as directed by HPN team; usually once a week until stable	
Panel #1 (date)	Panel #2 (date)
Glucose, sodium, potassium, chloride, CO2, BUN, creatinine, calcium, phosphorus, magnesium	Protime, triglycerides, total bilirubin, alkaline phosphatase, GGTP, SBPT, albumin, CBC
Fax results to nurse coordinator and/or HPN physician:	
2. Nutritional support service nursing assessment form	
Complete and fax weekly to : HPN nurse coordinator	
3. Glucose monitoring	
Urine dipstick: all patients must check urine for glucose at home using dipstick 1 h *before* TPN is completed and 1–2 h *after* completion of TPN	
	Blood glucose monitor: indicated for TPN patients with history of glucose intolerance, IDDM, NIDDM, or those who receive insulin in TPN
Yes	No
	Check 1 h *before* TPN completed and 1–2 h *after* completion of TPN
Parameters that require immediate notification of the HPN team: any abnormal blood, result plus	
Urine dipstick:	Blood glucose:
1/2% or >500 mg/dl after completion of TPN	<60 mg/dl after completion of TPN
1% or >1,000 mg/dl while TPN infusing	>250 mg/dl while TPN infusing
4. Central line care:	
Change central line dressing twice weekly. Report temperature elevation of ≥101.5 °F and any redness, swelling, tenderness, leakage, or drainage at site to home-care agency and HPN management team	
5. Records	
Record oral intake of meals and fluids, stomal and stool losses and urine outputs as instructed on the following dates and return to the home care agency and HPN team	
6. Follow-up appointment	
Yes	No
A follow-up appointment has been scheduled on… at…with the HPN physician, Dr…	
7. TPN prescription written on parenteral nutrition order form	

(continued)

Table 10.3 (continued)

Parenteral nutrition discharge orders	
An inline filter (1.2 µm) will be used for all total nutrient admixture prescriptions	
8. Other	
Physician signature	Date:

Anticoagulation: Thrombosis risk can be diminished by the use of heparin locks and by the addition of heparin to the PN bag (1,000 units/l). Low-dose oral warfarin (e.g., 1–5 mg/day remembering that most will be malabsorbed), not designed to get the INR into the therapeutic range, may also be effective in reducing risk [191]. It should be noted that central vein thrombosis is not usually treated like DVTs, with full anticoagulant therapy as the risk of fatal embolism is small. However, patients with coagulopathies, in particular those with antithrombin III, protein S, protein C, and factor V Leiden deficiency who developed short bowel due to intestinal ischemia, should most certainly be fully anticoagulated. Similarly, those with "vanishing venous access" should also be fully anticoagulated.

Catheter Protection: Patients should be taught to cover the insertion site with a non-occlusive dressing and cleanse it with hydrogen peroxide and/or an iodine solution every 3 days. The use of plastic waterproof dressings, such as Tegaderm (Nexcare, 3 M, St Paul, Mn), allows showering. Some active young patients also use special waterproof sleeves and protective devices to submerge during bathing and swimming. Although submersion adds risk, the risk is counterbalanced by quality of life considerations. The Oley Foundation is a consumer society founded specially for HPN patients and is an invaluable resource of helpful, practical, information and networking. All HPN patients should be encouraged to link up the Foundation: The Oley Foundation, 214 Hun Memorial, MC-28, Albany Medical Center, Albany, NY 12208-3478, phone 1-800-776-OLEY, (www.oley.org).

Quality of Life: Perhaps the greatest challenge is quality of life. The dependency on IV infusions, plus problems associated with the underlying disease—e.g., ileostomy/jejunostomy bags, and excessive frequent diarrhea—severely limits lifestyle and reintegration back into normal society. A major advance was to cycle the TPN infusions, so that they were given over 8–14 h at night when the patient was asleep, allowing clamping of the catheter during the day so that normal activities could be performed.

Although HPN is a last medical resort for patients with intestinal failure, it is a life-sustaining treatment [73]. There have been advancements in catheter technology and formulation to allow for greater mobility and participation in the normal activities of daily life, but studies have shown that HPN is often associated with a poor quality of life (QoL) [192]. Studies have revealed that although many patients have somatic complaints related to the underlying disease, HPN dependence often leads to anxiety and depression due to lack of freedom and limitations in social life [193]. In addition, many patients are dependent on analgesics for their underlying condition. QoL does improve, however, the longer a patient is stable on HPN.

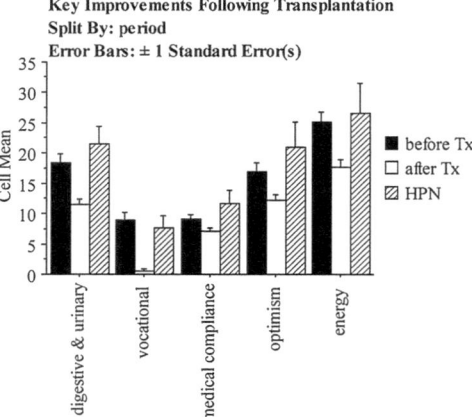

Fig. 10.3 QoL assessments were no different between HPN patients and pre-transplant patients, but following transplantation all these domains improved to significantly ($p < 0.05$) higher levels than those measured in HPN patients

In general, younger patients can adapt to their changed circumstances better and thus achieve a better QoL. In our experience, only 10–20% of HPN patients returned to work full-time [183]; however, this figure might be misleading because in the USA many HPN patients can work, but have to establish "disability" to qualify for Medicare to sustain their coverage. Accurately assessing QoL in HPN patients is difficult because it is unclear whether changes in QoL are due to the underlying disease or the problems associated with the performance and maintenance of HPN. Comparative studies have suggested that QoL is comparable to that of end-stage renal disease patients on dialysis [194].

Examination of the change in QoL in patients following small bowel transplantation should give information on the impairments of QoL due to IV infusions and chronic diarrhea and malabsorption. For this reason we followed a cohort of 46 small bowel transplant patients following successful transplantation for 1–3 years [192]. The results showed, in a validated self-administered QoL tool containing 26 domains and 130 questions, significant improvements in 13 of the domains (Fig. 10.3).

Complications: Prevention and Treatment

Complications can be contained if a strict protocol of management is imposed, and mortality is more closely related to the underlying disease than these complications. However, about 10% of patients develop serious advanced complications, which result in *TPN failure*. Although this is defined by Medicare as:

1. Impending or overt liver failure with increasing bilirubin, liver enzymes, spleen size, INR, reduced platelet counts, varices, stomal bleeding, hepatic fibrosis, and cirrhosis.

2. Thrombosis of central veins, namely two of the subclavian, jugular, or femoral veins.
3. Frequent catheter-related sepsis, with more than two episodes per year of *life-threatening* bacterial infections, or one episode of fungemia associated with shock and ARDS, and
4. Severe recurrent dehydration.

It is really only one and two that comprise TPN failure, a condition where death will occur unless an intestinal, and possibly hepatic, transplant is conducted successfully.

Methods to Reduce Complications and Improve Quality of Life

Catheter Sepsis: This is by far the most common and disabling complication, which often accelerates the development of other complications. It results in sickness, disability, and recurrent hospitalizations, culminating in escalating health care costs and deterioration in quality of life. Infections are thankfully usually mild, due to contamination with skin commensals, such as gram-positive, coagulase-negative, *Staphylococcus epidermidis*, and are easy to treat, but contamination with other organisms, e.g., gram-negative organisms or fungi, can result in septic shock, ICU admission, and death. With "good techniques," patients can remain infection free for years, as illustrated by our HPN experience at the Mayo Clinic (Table 10.4) where 10 of our 41 patients had *never* had a single catheter infection over a mean follow-up time of 5 years (range 1–15.5 years), while 7 had suffered from more than 3 septicemias/year in a mean of 6.5 years (range 2–15 years) [189]. An analysis of risk factors for recurrent catheter infections identified associations with younger age (more physically active), underlying Crohn's disease, ultrashort bowel with end-jejunostomies, central venous thrombosis, poor hygiene, and smoking. The results suggested that early preventative measures, such as maintenance of hydration, long-term anticoagulation,

Table 10.4 Catheter-related sepsis: comparison of characteristics of frequently infected and never infected HPN patients. Fischer's exact test: *$p < 0.05$, **$p < 0.005$ O'Keefe et al. JPEN [188]

	No infections	Frequent >3/year
n	10/41	7/41
Duration HPN (months)	61 (14–174)	77 (24–180)
Age (years)	67 (14)	45 (12)*
Jejunostomy	1	7**
Thrombosis	0	5*
Crohn's	0	5*
Catheter care	Good	Poor 3/7

decontamination of catheter hub, and the use of alcohol locking solutions, should be considered in patients with the combination of Crohn's disease and jejunostomies to decrease the risk of frequent septicemias. There is no doubt that recurrent infections, and their treatment with long courses of IV antibiotics, increases the risk of more serious infections with resistant organisms and fungi, which, in turn, increases the risk of other HPN complications such progressive venous thrombosis and liver disease, with the end result of "TPN failure." The following principles will help reduce risk:

Prevention: The principles behind prevention have given under Management above. It cannot be underemphasized that recurrent infections are strongly related to the quality of catheter-care, and so the most effective method of suppression is *training* the patient and family member in aseptic techniques. As recommended above, patients with recurrent catheter-sepsis should be not only retrained in catheter management best practices, but also instructed in the use of an alcohol-lock. A 30–70% solution of ethanol is injected into the catheter after use and then capped. The volume needed to fill the catheter needs to be known (make sure the person who places the catheter gives you this information) to reduce excessive spillage into the systemic circulation. Note that alcohol locks are incompatible with the plastics contained within some catheters, e.g., PVC. This is an additional reason why we favor the use of silicone single lumen catheters, such as the Hickman. Again, it is crucial that patients should be educated that at the earliest suggestion of fever, or even vague flu-like symptoms, they should report to their physicians, or better still, to come to the emergency room to have blood cultures drawn. It is better to be safe than sorry, as late treatment is more difficult and more dangerous.

- Avoid line-breaks: Minimize the number of infusions and the use of additives or injectables. The TPN line must be reserved for TPN alone, unless there is a life-threatening situation.
- Use subclavian venous access and tunnel the line under the skin to a position on the anterior chest wall that can be easily seen and handled by the patient, thus reducing the risk of contamination during line connections and disconnections.
- Use a single-lumen catheter: *Double lumens double the risk of contamination.*
- In patients with frequent recurrent infections, flush the catheter with saline, then lock catheter with 30% alcohol solution when not in use.
- Control hyperglycemia: Insulin may be added to the PN solution in diabetics, but then infusions must be tapered at the end to prevent rebound hypoglycemia. In type 2 diabetics, and the obese insulin-resistant patients, avoid insulin addition and reduce glucose and total calories, relative to amino acids. Do NOT use PN to maintain obesity!!
- Look after the catheter carefully. Redress the catheter site twice weekly, check for redness and discharge and report changes. Do not let the end of the catheter dangle down to the abdomen, especially when the patient has a stoma as this provides a generous source of infecting organisms (see Fig. 10.4). When disconnecting and reconnecting catheters to bags, rub each end with an alcohol swab for at least 30 seconds x2 before reconnecting taking extreme care not to touch the connection ends with fingers or other surfaces.

Fig. 10.4 Illustration of the greater risk of IV catheter contamination in patients with high-output fistulae: keep the tip of the catheter covered and taped to the chest!

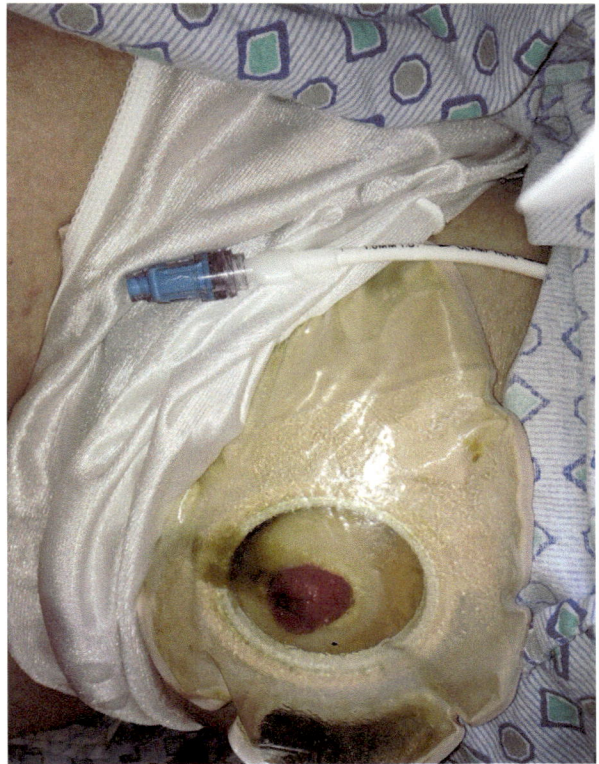

Detection and Treatment of Catheter-Related Sepsis

The classic presentation of catheter sepsis is the development of fever and chills, often associated with PN infusions. However, it can be much less dramatic, presenting as "flu-like" symptoms, with headache, body aches, and a general feeling of being unwell. Unfortunately this often results in delayed treatment as symptoms disappear with the use of simple analgesics. Less commonly still, it may be asymptomatic and detected by an unexplained rise in WBC. For these reasons, and because the earlier catheter related sepsis (CRS) is treated the better the outcome, patients are advised to report all changes in condition to their PCP, who should report them to the hospital team or take blood tests for CBC, metabolic profile, renal function, and blood cultures—which should include fungal cultures in recurrent or unusual presentations. To detect CRS:

- Take blood cultures from catheter and a peripheral vein.
- Check for other sources of infection, e.g. urine, chest.

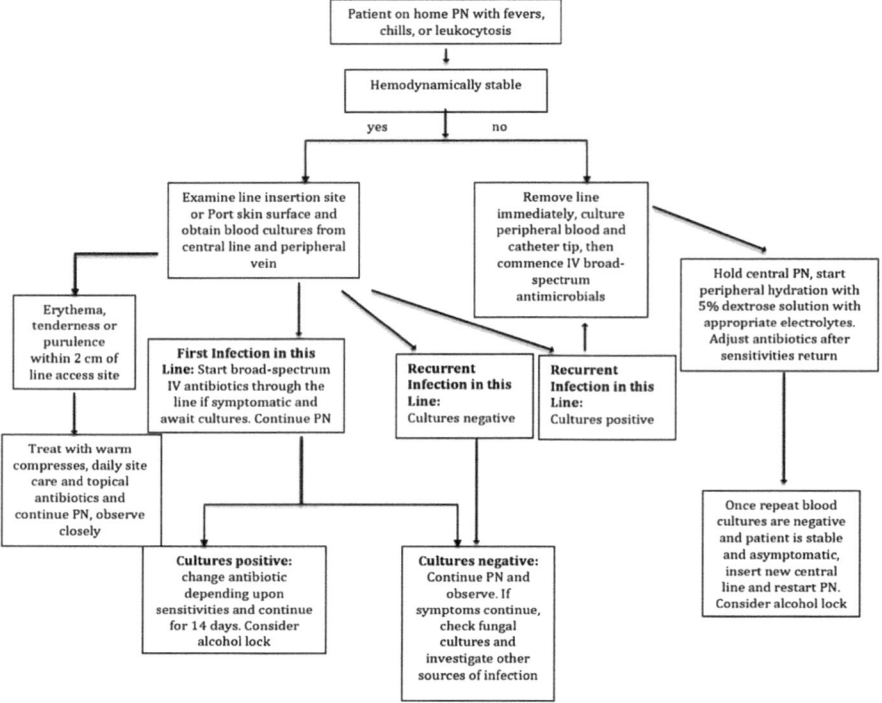

Fig. 10.5 Algorithm for the investigation and treatment of catheter-related sepsis

- If first infection with this catheter and patient stable:

    - Start IV broad spectrum antibiotic (usually vancomycin as it covers the usual organisms and can be given bid, check creatinine/renal function).
    - Continue usual cyclical TPN.
    - Change antibiotic according to culture results and sensitivities, if necessary.
    - Continue IV antibiotics for 2 weeks.

- If recurrent infection in same catheter or if patient in septic shock:

    - Pull catheter, start peripheral IV fluids.
    - Start IV broad-spectrum antibiotic.
    - When culture results and sensitivities are available, change antibiotics if necessary.
    - Reinsert central vein catheter at a different site after 3–4 days or when stable.
    - Recommence TPN. Usually PN is held until the patient's condition stabilizes rather than waiting for negative blood cultures which can be misleading.

However, in severe infections including fungal infections, patients can be safely managed without PN until all blood cultures are negative

Metabolic Complications: As discussed earlier, the utilization of IV nutrients is less efficient than enterally delivered nutrients, and so high blood levels can be expected with excessive infusion rates. Glucose can be used as an indicator of metabolic tolerance as it is simple to measure and monitor. Its levels should be controlled as discussed in Chapter 9 under "The Management of PN Complications." Insulin will also suppress amino acid and triglyceride levels, but it is probably better to monitor triglyceride levels at least 4 h following cessation of the TPN infusion as dispersal is slower than glucose. Electrolyte abnormalities (e.g., K^+, Mg^{+++}) are common and easy to correct by titrating blood concentrations with IV infusions, with the exception of sodium, which has a large distribution volume and is influenced by hydration status. In addition, normal plasma sodium concentrations are maintained in deficiency states by aldosterone. Consequently, urine concentration provides a more sensitive indicator of body status and should be monitored, especially in new patients. Aim to keep urine sodium excretion between the ranges of 40–100 mEq/day. Calcium sufficiency is also difficult to monitor as normal blood levels are maintained by release from bone stores. Patients at risk, such as those who are chronically malnourished, have chronic illness, or have been treated with steroids, should have periodic DEXA scans to assess calcium reserve.

Thrombotic Complications: "Vanishing venous access" is a frightening situation as it threatens the lifeline. As previously discussed, the presence of any foreign body within the lumen causes chronic inflammation and trauma to the vein, which leads to thrombus formation, which will progress with time to venous occlusion. In addition, a fibrin sleeve, also increasing venous thrombosis risk, will cover any catheter that has been in for several months. In some—but not all—patients, the superior vena caval system becomes progressively obliterated (Figs. 10.6 and 10.7), necessitating access via the inferior vena cava. Once the IVC thromboses, extreme measures such as direct atrial catheterization and transhepatic cannulation become necessary as discussed earlier. Of all the causes of "TPN failure," vanishing venous access is arguably the most dangerous as it makes the only long-term solution—small bowel-liver transplantation—technically difficult.

Prevention

- Avoid the long-term (>2 months) use of PICC lines: the smaller the vein, the slower the flow, the higher the risk of thrombosis.
- Use heparin locks.
- In patients with coagulation disorders (for detection, see above under "Anticoagulation"), use full warfarin anticoagulation. Remember that short bowel patients malabsorb warfarin necessitating higher dose levels to achieve anticoagulation.
- In patients with established central vein thrombosis (for detection, see above under "Anticoagulation"), use full-dose warfarin anticoagulation, i.e., INR 2–4.
- In all others use low-dose warfarin: e.g., 5 mg/day, without keeping the INR within the therapeutic range [195].

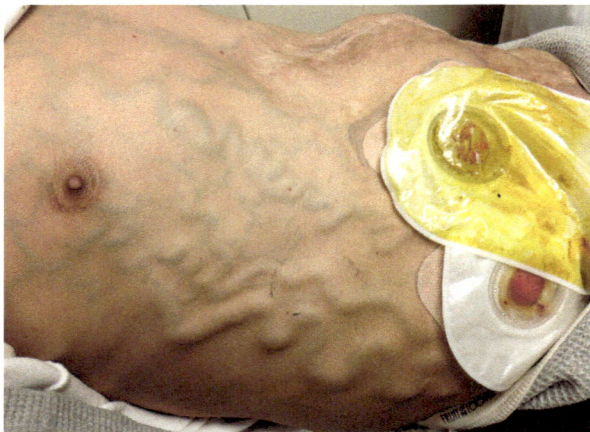

Fig. 10.6 Example of an HPN patient with "vanishing venous access," where extensive superior venacaval thrombosis resulting from long term and repeated SVC catheter placements. Figure 10.6 shows the clinical signs with gross distension of the collateral intercostal veins bypassing the obstruction

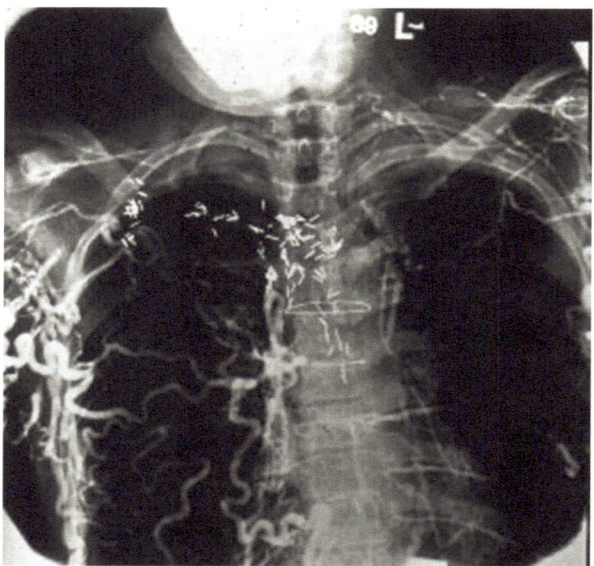

Fig. 10.7 X-ray demonstration with contrast injected into an arm vein finds its way through the collateral intercostal veins into the right atrium to the right atrium

TPN Liver Disease

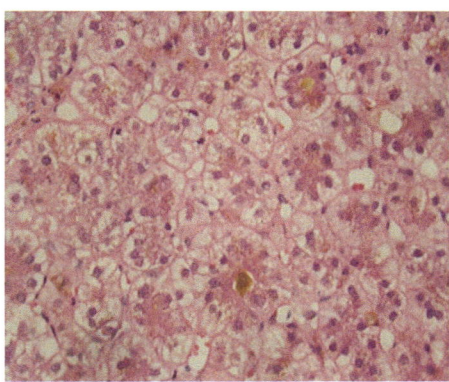

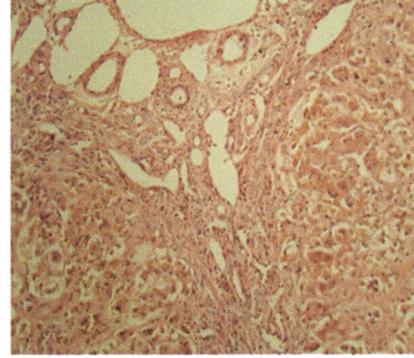

TPN Steatosis with early cholestasis   End stage liver disease demonstrating biliary cirrhosis without portal inflammation or fatty infiltration.

Fig. 10.8 Examples of advanced liver disease in patients dependent on long-term home TPN

Hepatic Complications: As with short term TPN, minor liver dysfunction, as indicated by abnormal plasma liver enzyme concentrations, is common, but the risk of severe progressive liver disease is considerably greater. The liver disease can be cholestatic or fibrotic, or a combination of the two. Most patients on HPN have some histological evidence of cholestasis or fatty liver on biopsy. The major types of TPN-associated liver disease are intrahepatic cholestasis, steatosis (microvesicular and macrovesicular), steatohepatitis, and cholecystitis (Fig. 10.8). Patients on HPN are at particular risk (10–15%) of progression to end-stage liver disease because, like alcohol abuse, the insult is perpetual and chronic [196].

The etiology and expression of the liver disease is complex as discussed in Chapter 9, p. 124, PN complications. Cholestasis with biliary sludge formation occurs most patients who have been on TPN and bowel rest for longer than a few weeks due to stagnation of biliary function and flow as a result of decreased vagal stimulation and cholecystokinin release. Many patients on HPN have short bowel and short bowel itself is associated with increased risk of gallstones. Intrahepatic disease is exacerbated by the low-grade chronic inflammatory state that exists in many HPN patients due to recurrent bacteremias, and due to bacterial overgrowth or dysbiosis. The other major risk factor is severity of loss of intestinal length, as risk of severe liver disease increases with increasing loss of absorptive function. Explanations include depletion of the portal flow of nutrients to the liver, disruption of the bile acid pool and small-bowel bacterial overgrowth resulting in chronic endotoxemia. There is good experimental evidence that compartmentation within the liver prevents IV nutrients being as efficiently utilized by the liver for protein synthesis as portal delivered nutrients as discussed in Chapter 5 "why is enteral feeding superior" [38].

The investigation and management of liver dysfunction is the same as that detailed above for short-term TPN. Excess calories from either glucose or fat contributes to the development of steatohepatitis (similar to non-alcoholic steatohepatitis (NASH)), much in the same way that French geese overfed with corn (carbohydrate) develop fatty livers from which "pate de foie" is harvested. Omega-6 fatty acids in excess of 1 g per kg per day in the absence of overfeeding has also increase the incidence of liver disease, and liver dysfunction is less commonly seen if total IV fat is kept below 40 g/day. In the USA we currently only have one form of IV lipid solution, derived from soyabean (Intralipid, Baxter, Chicago, IL), which contains predominantly n-6 fatty acids. Europeans are more advanced in this field with a variety of IV lipid emulsions derived from olive oil and fish oils (e.g., SMOF (Soy bean/Medium Chain Triglyceride/Olive Oil/Fish oil), Fresenius Kabi AG, Bad Homburg,—Germany) which, in uncontrolled studies, may reduce liver complications in pediatric HPN patients [197–199].

Treatment

1. Maintain oral or enteral feeding, even if the majority is malabsorbed and stomal output increases. Despite the fact that most is malabsorbed, the efficiency of digestion and absorption within the remaining proximal bowel (duodenum) is remarkably high and significant quantities will be absorbed into the portal system to maintain liver health and function. Eating also prevents gut stasis, bacterial overgrowth, and biliary stasis.
2. If possible, measure resting metabolic rate and match energy infusions, remembering that there might be significant residual food absorption that needs to enter the equation. Otherwise estimate energy requirements from 25 to 35 kcal/kg *ideal body weight*/day.
3. Cycle the TPN infusions rather than using continuous infusions, as this promotes physiological hepatic fat mobilization. Remember our physiological processes are not designed for constant feeding
4. Give a "TPN" holiday if remotely possible.
5. Suppress intestinal bacterial overgrowth with 2-week cycles of oral low dose broad spectrum antibiotics, such as metronidazole and/or Bactrim (trimethoprim and sulfamethoxazole). If ineffective, rifaximin (Salix, NY), a newer antimicrobial that is poorly absorbed and effective in controlling bacterial overgrowth, may be used.
6. Probiotics such as VSL#3 may be useful in patients with dysbiosis, and Lactobacillus plantarum may improve gut barrier and the absorption of hepatotoxins [200, 201].
7. TPN-induced cholestasis [202]

    (a) Ursodeoxycholic acid for restoring the bile salt pool balance [203].
    (b) Different lipid formulations (if available) containing medium-chain triglycerides or n-3 fish oils.

(c) Ultimately, however, patients with progressive jaundice and end-stage liver disease secondary to TPN-induced cholestasis require combined small-bowel-liver transplantation. Figure 10.9 well illustrates the dramatic resolution of progressive "end-stage" jaundice in a patient with "TPN failure" following combined small bowel and liver transplantation. This patient was very interesting as he developed progressive jaundice and weight loss, both of which were unresponsive to the above measures. Measurement of metabolic expenditure by indirect calorimetry showed that even if we matched expenditure with caloric infusion rates, he continued to lose weight down to a BMI of 14. This well illustrates the contention that the *liver is the heart of metabolism*, and liver failure results in breakdown of nutrient assimilation. Transplantation

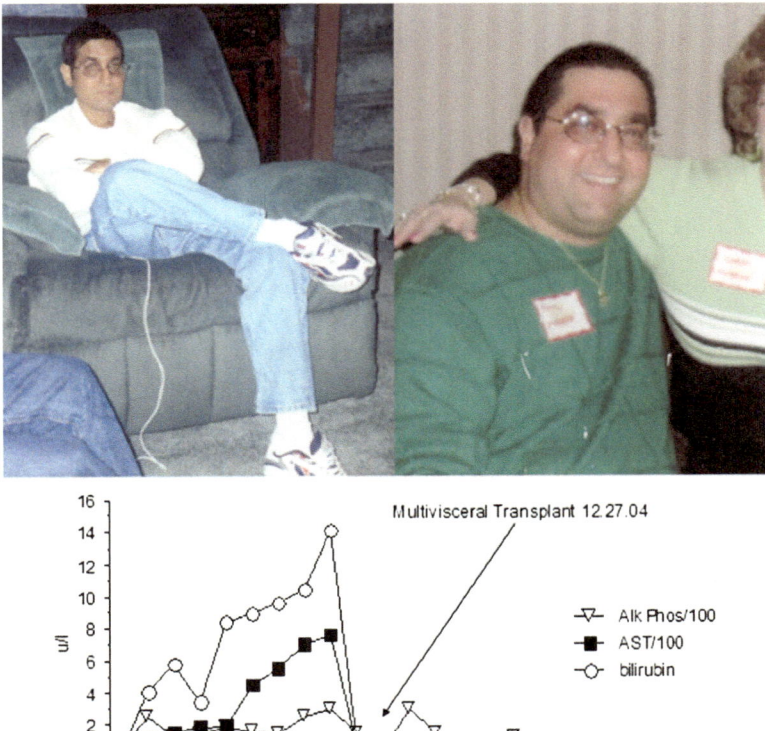

Fig. 10.9 Illustration of the effect of multivisceral transplantation on severe liver dysfunction and jaundice in a 40-year-old male with loss of his colon for familiar adenomatous polyposis and colon cancer, and his small intestine due to desmoid tumors, leaving him with an end-duodenostomy and permanent dependence on home TPN. Without combined liver and small bowel transplantation, this condition is uniformly fatal

was held because he was not quite 5 years out from his last resection for colon cancer, the arbitrary time that is used to determine "cancer cure." Following successful liver-small bowel transplantation, he made a remarkably full recovery, enabling him to return to work 6 months later. Today, 10 years later, he remains well, eating normally, and fully employed.

Home Enteral Feeding

Home enteral feeding (HEN) has now replaced home parenteral feeding for all those patients described above whose gut function can be restored by interventional feeding tube placement, as it is safer, cheaper, and allows for the discontinuation of all IVs and discharge from hospital, thus removing the risk of hospital acquired infections. HEN has also permitted earlier discharge from hospital those patients who have recovered from their critical illness, but are unable to eat normally, for example patients with necrotizing pancreatitis and fluid collections, further reducing healthcare costs and at the same time providing emotional support from the family. As with PN above, there is no need to keep patients dependent on tube feeding in hospital: it can be managed at home with (a) patient and family education and training, and (b) home care agency nursing. Alike HPN, HEN can be managed with the help of homecare agencies to provide the feeds, pumps, and associated equipment. These patients can be divided roughly into two groups, those with PEGs and those with nasoenteric feeding tubes. PEGs are more commonly used for patients with long-term need, with permanent disabilities, such as neurological disorders or events, while nasoenteric tubes are used for temporary disabilities, for example impaired gut function that is likely to recover with time, and in those at high surgical risk where time and nutrition is required to strengthen them sufficiently to withstand advanced or reconstructive surgery.

Home PEG and PEG-J Feeding: As discussed above, a common rule is to consider PEG placement in any patient likely to be dependent on tube feeding for longer than 4 weeks. Perhaps the best example is the stroke patient undergoing rehabilitation. Associated dysphagia, aspiration, and bulbar palsy can take months to resolve and such patients are best nursed in their home environment. PEGs are placed in patients with functional stomachs. Consequently, tolerance to feeding is generally good, permitting intermittent bolus feeding which the family unit can perform easily. Alternatively, home PEG feeding may be used to supplement normal eating in the chronically malnourished, anorexic patient. Here, it is often best to use the PEG feeding at night as a constant infusion by pump (e.g., 1–1.5 l over 8–10 h) and then to flush and clamp the tube by day and encourage the patient to participate in normal activities and eating. In the situation of patients with abnormal gastric emptying, a jejunal extension will be required (i.e., PEG-J). *It must be remembered that bolus feeding must not be used for jejunal feeding as the small intestine is designed to receive a slow continuous infusion from the stomach.* However, cyclical feeding can be effective where the total feed is delivered, like home PN, over a 10–18 h infusion infusion, depending on tolerance, by programmed pump. Another attribute to new pumps is that they can be programmed to provide regular free water flushes (up to 50 cc/4 h with gastric feeding, but not higher than 25 cc/4 h with jejunal feeding), to both assist hydration and prevent tube clogging.

Home Nasoenteric Feeding: If enteral feeding is needed for a limited time, e.g., 4–6 weeks, it is often preferable to continue the established nasoenteric feeding that was initiated in hospital, for example in patients recovering from critical illness. *Although a tube hanging out of your nostril is neither comfortable nor attractive, it is a safer alternative to home PN and allows delay in further interventions such as surgery, while maintaining or improving nutritional status.* Patients, their families, and unfortunately, sometimes even physicians are unaware of the relative risks of EN and PN, and time must be spent educating them on the pros and cons for both. An excellent example for HEN is the patient who has survived critical illness in the ICU due to severe acute pancreatitis, only to be left with a dysfunctional upper GI tract due to compression of the stomach and duodenum by the inflammatory pancreatic mass that has resolved into a chronic cystic fluid collection. Because of the gross disturbance of the anatomy of the upper GI tract (Chapter 8, Fig. 8.8), PEG placement is more difficult, risky, and will fail to function because of distal obstruction of the duodenum. The use of a J-tube extension (i.e., PEG-J) might work, but may also add further complications. For these reasons, we continue to use the NGJ tubes we place early on in the disease at the time of admission (for details of placement, see Chapter 8, p. 98 "Transnasal Endoscopy"). In our recently published experience, we commonly send patients home with their NGJ tubes for up to 6 weeks, waiting for resolution of their disease or improvement in their nutrition prior to elective surgery. In our recently published experience, we describe the outcome of 19 consecutive patients who were stable enough to be discharged home [116]. Feeding was delivered as cyclical infusions by pump at night over 14–18 h. Seven resolved spontaneously and were weaned back onto a normal diet, five continued to be obstructed and needed surgical decompression, and two were considered poor surgical risk and were given PEG/jejunostomy tubes for long-term feeding at home [116].

As mentioned above, jejunal feeding must NEVER be given in bolus form, as that is unphysiological. The feed is delivered by pump as cyclical infusions over 12–16 h over night, like HPN, and rates of <100 cc/h are best tolerated. Essential to success of long term home feeding is to prevent involuntary removal by securing the tube by the use of a nasal bridle (Fig. 8.3). If extra hydration is needed, it is best to add the water to the feed system so that it is delivered as a continuous infusion rather than intermittent boluses >30 cc, which might aggravate abdominal pain. Alternatively, the new pump mentioned above can be used and programmed to give small volume water flushes every 1–6 h.

Part III
Diseases that Affect Digestion, Absorption and Assimilation

Chapter 11
Permanent Intestinal Failure and the Short Bowel Syndrome

Permanent Intestinal Failure

Definitions: We have previously defined this as "Intestinal failure results from obstruction, dysmotility, surgical resection, congenital defect, or disease-associated loss of absorption and is characterized by the inability to maintain protein-energy, fluid, electrolyte, or micronutrient balance when on a conventionally accepted, normal diet" [173]. However, on reflection this is confusing, as conditions associated with obstruction and dysmotility prevent the intake of a conventionally accepted, normal diet, and it might be more accurate to use the definition of "any permanent condition that prevents the absorption of a normal diet." Intestinal failure due to obstruction is usually temporary until surgical reconstruction can be performed, but permanent failure can occur in patients who have undergone multiple surgical procedures with extensive adhesive disease, which cannot be released, or in those with "intestinal pseudo-obstruction," where the problem is not the length or absorptive area but the absence of motility and propulsive contractions. In Chapter 10, Table 10.1, we provided an illustration to the common makeup of permanent intestinal failure patients from our experience with 63 HPN patients at the Mayo Clinic in 1992, showing that the failure was roughly due to short bowel in 70% and obstruction in the remainder [183]. Note that today, a greater proportion of SBS patients have lost their bowel due to infarction than Crohn's disease due to the aging population.

Management of Intestinal Failure

This differs whether the cause is obstruction (O-IF) or short bowel (SB-IF). In general, the management principles are similar, aimed at maintaining fluid, electrolyte, and nutrient balances. However, the management of SB-IF is more complex because intestinal losses are considerably higher because of the additional losses of digestive

© Springer Science+Business Media New York 2015   149
S.J.D. O'Keefe, *The Principles and Practice of Nutritional Support*,
DOI 10.1007/978-1-4939-1779-2_11

secretions, which are high because these patients continue to eat and commonly eat excesses because of the hyperphagia, which is part of the "adaptive" response. It is ironic that patients with SB-IF would be easier to manage if they did not eat, because their PN volumes and electrolyte infusions would be lower. However, it is critical to understand a) that much of the nutrient digestion and absorption occurs in the duodenum and proximal jejunum and b) that the severe liver complications associated with SB-IF are related to the length of the remaining small bowel, probably because the shorter the bowel, the greater the depletion of portal nutrients. *Thus, patients must be encouraged to continue to eat, even if their stomal losses increase.* Because the management of SB-IF is more difficult than the management of O-IF, we will spend more time discussing its management below, but remember, the principles of conservation of body fluids, electrolytes, and nutrition remain common to both.

The Short Bowel Syndrome

The Principles

Loss of any amount of small intestinal length can result in short bowel syndrome (SBS). As with most of the other organs in the body, there is however a tremendous functional reserve capacity within the GI tract, such that segmental losses of the duodenum, jejunum, or ileum are well tolerated and do not have long-term effects, with the possible exception of impaired vitamin B12 and bile salt absorption if the terminal ileum is removed. *It must be emphasized that SBS has a spectrum of severity*, ranging from minimal loss of absorptive surface, such as the loss of the terminal ileum in patients with Crohn's disease, which can result in vitamin B12, bile acid, fat-soluble vitamin, and calcium deficiencies, all of which can be corrected by increased oral intake or supplementation, to moderate loss of the small intestine resulting in fluid, magnesium, sodium, and potassium deficiency, to severe loss of both the small intestine and colon resulting in the combination of fluid, electrolyte, vitamin, and protein, carbohydrate, and fat deficiency, resulting in what we term short bowel intestinal failure (SB-IF), where patients will die without total parenteral feeding.

   With progressive loss of intestinal length and mucosal absorptive surface, the first impairment is loss of fluid and electrolyte reabsorption, commonly presenting as dehydration evidenced by decreased urine flow, increasing BUN and creatinine, and electrolyte disturbance, most commonly hypokalemia and hypomagnesemia. To understand this, you have to understand gut physiology and the process of digestion and absorption. For food to be digested, it has to be broken down into small particles and emulsified so that the surface area is increased to allow the efficient attachment and activation of digestive enzymes. This requires an outpouring of ~7 l of fluid per day in the form of secretions from the salivary glands, the stomach, the pancreas, and the liver. Further fluid is drawn across the upper small intestine by osmotic forces, as the proximal mucosa is freely permeable to water. Under these conditions, enzymatic food digestion and active nutrient absorption is so efficient that the process is virtually complete by the proximal jejunum. However, not all nutrients have active transport mechanisms and as pointed out above, the mucosa is leaky. Consequently, large volumes of fluid and electrolytes remain in the jejunum and it is the job of the remaing distal small intestine to reabsorb what remains. As the fluid makes its way down to the ileum, the mucosa becomes progressively less permeable, allowing efficient reabsorption of fluids and electrolytes against a concentration gradient. *This makes it understandable that the first clinical sign of short bowel intestinal failure, particularly due to distal bowel, is dehydration and electrolyte deficiency.* The electrolytes most affected are the polyvalent cations magnesium and calcium, but because body stores of calcium are vast, plasma levels are maintained at the expense of bone mineral losses. Thus, remember to measure bone mineral density with DEXA scans to detect chronic body calcium deficiency in established patients. The body pool of magnesium is, by contrast, small, accounting for the high frequency of hypomagnesemia, which can become so severe as to present as clinical tetany—spontaneous curling up of the fingers, wrists, and toes. In evidence, studies have shown that there are critical lengths of the small intestine that are needed before nutrient malabsorption becomes significant but that the length has to take into consideration the health of the remaining mucosa and whether the colon remains in continuity. Thus, the functionality of the remaining bowel in a patient with SBS due to Crohn's disease may not be the same as that from a patient who developed SBS from trauma or infarction.

The remarkable absorptive capacity of the colon is becoming increasingly recognized. Despite the fact that it does not secrete digestive enzymes, its microbiota does, first ingesting and metabolizing dietary residues for its own metabolic demands and then releasing partly degraded nutrients, such as short-chain fatty acids derived from carbohydrate or protein residues, which can be used by the mucosa to maintain colonic health, e.g., butyrate, or absorbed into the systemic circulation for hepatic and general body health, e.g., propionate and acetate. Furthermore, the microbiota play an important role in the maintenance of essential micronutrient sufficiency as fermentation releases phytochemicals and minerals from vegetable cell walls and synthesize folate, B12, biotin, and niacin [46]. As discussed earlier, studies in patients with adapted SBS have shown that energy salvage can reach 1,000 kcal/day and account for the survival of patients with only 6 in. of small bowel plus colon in the days prior to TPN [204].

Short Bowel Intestinal Failure

This extreme condition is associated with major morbidity and mortality, consuming considerable health-care resources. It occurs only when the considerable reserves of the intestines are exceeded resulting in rapid and progressive losses of body stores and death. Some working guidelines, based on clinical experience [173, 205, 206] are that nutritional autonomy usually begins to be compromised when you lose >80% of the small intestine but retain the colon or lose >70% of the small intestine PLUS the colon. In practice [206], it is likely that a state of **permanent intestinal failure** will exist if you have:

- *<60 cm of small intestine, plus the colon.*
- *<120 cm of small intestine, without a colon.*

It has been estimated from this that the salvage capacity of the colon is roughly equivalent to 60–100 cm of small intestine. It must, however, be remembered that these measurements assume that the remaining small bowel mucosa and motility are normal and the presence of residual disease, or the presence of rapid transit, will exacerbate losses.

Intestinal Adaptation

The ability of the body to adapt and survive in a hostile environment is remarkable. Vital organ function is preserved by there being duplicate organs, in which case loss of one is covered by increased function of the other, for example, the kidneys, or as in the case of single organs such as the liver, pancreas, and gut, by increasing the function of the remaining tissue, a process termed "adaptation." With regard to the gut, the loss of the colon is compatible with life as the intestine progressively holds on to fluid, reducing ileostomy losses. Similarly, the small intestine can afford to lose 50% of its length by compensatory increases in digestion and absorptive capacity in the remaining bowel. *The process of adaptation commences within 48 h, is maximal in the first 6 months, but continues up to or even beyond 2 years.* The mechanisms have been extensively studied in animal models and short bowel patients (Fig. 11.1) and have been shown to involve:

- Villus hyperplasia.
- Muscular hypertrophy.
- Increased nutrient transport.
- Increased digestion.
- Changes in motility.
- Secretion and blood flow.

However, the dramatic increases in villus size and thus absorptive area (4×) shown in rodents are not seen in humans [205, 207, 215, 216], suggesting that the major explanations involve changes in motility, secretion, and blood flow. The initiating factors and control mechanisms are unclear but probably involve hyperphagia and increased topical nutrient stimulation resulting from the loss of negative feedback control of appetite from loss of the distal bowel. In normal digestive physiology, the failure to absorb food in the proximal bowel and delivery of undigested nutrients into the distal ileum and colon triggers what has been termed *the ileal brake*. There are specific L cells in the mucosa which synthesize and release a battery of peptide hormones, including peptide YY (PYY), glucagon-like peptide-1 (GLP-1), and GLP-2 into the circulation which suppress appetite and food intake, delay gastric emptying, and inhibit pancreatic secretion, and thus stem the rate of flow of undigested food into the distal bowel. *GLP-2 is perhaps the most intriguing of these peptides as it is strongly trophic to the mucosa, resulting in remark-*

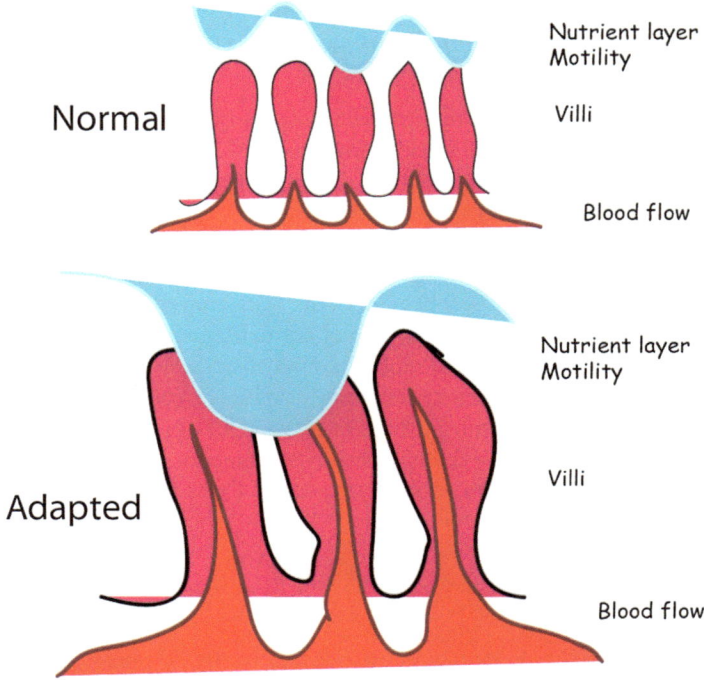

Fig. 11.1 Illustration of the basic changes after adaptation in short bowel patients. The blue represents the luminal flow of nutrients which increases with hyperphagia, which stimulates villus growth and blood flow

able villous hyperplasia and increases in mucosal blood flow—factors that suggest it plays a key role in the adaptation process when the proximal intestine is lost [219–225]. However, GLP-2 cannot provide the whole explanation for adaptation as adaptation still occurs when the GLP-2-producing distal small intestine and colon are lost. When the distal bowel is lost, negative feedback ceases and hunger continues, explaining the observation that patients with severe short bowel commonly are hyperphagic, consuming roughly twice normal dietary intake levels [213]. Colonic adaptation is characterized by massive dilatation and sometimes excessive gas production from increased fermentation. Patients need to be advised that this is an *appropriate* change, albeit antisocial! In normal health, colonic fermentation salvages about 200–400 kcal of energy from dietary residues per day, but, as mentioned above, in SB-IF patients, this quantity quadruples [187].

Assessment of Degree of Severity

From the above, it can be understood that treatment and management will depend upon the severity. First, patients have to be stabilized, with correction of hydrational status (i.e., normalization of plasma creatinine) and blood levels (e.g., potassium, magnesium), and established on a normal diet. IV supplements are then held, while carefully monitoring plasma creatinine and magnesium and 24-h urine volumes and sodium content.

- *Mild*: If plasma creatinine remains within the normal range and urine output is >1,000 ml/day, the SBS will be categorized as mild. These patients can be managed by dietary, oral fluid, and anti-motility drug management alone.
- *Moderate*: If the plasma creatinine increases above the normal range and urine output is <1,000 ml/day and urine sodium content is <20 mmol per day, a state of moderate SBS will exist. These patients are at risk for readmission for dehydration and prerenal failure and may need periodic "customized" IV infusions at home, one to three times per week, consisting of normal saline supplemented with potassium and magnesium salts and multivitamins.
- *Severe*: Finally, if body weight decreases despite correction of fluid and electrolyte losses with IV infusions, a state of severe SBS, or SB-IF, will exist. These patients need HPN, i.e., IV fluids, electrolytes, minerals, vitamins, trace elements, plus macronutrients, amino acids, dextrose, and lipids for survival.

Composition of PN

Ideally, absorption should be measured, conventionally by placing the patient on a normal diet containing 100 g fat/day for 72 h and measuring stool or stomal fat content. If the coefficient of fat absorption is <50%, PN will be necessary to prevent weight loss. In practice, absorption is rarely measured because of time and expense. Instead, most patients with massive intestinal loss, who are likely to develop SB-IF from the definitions above, are initially started on PN, and body weight is monitored closely to detect change. It is extremely important to allow these patients to continue to eat in order to stimulate the adaptation process, but feeding style must be modified to small frequent meals and snacks, as described below. Caloric IV infusions are then modified to maintain a BMI within the normal range ($18.5–24$ kg/m^2), and amino acid infusions are tailored to keep the BUN within normal limits (assuming plasma creatinine is also within normal range). In the obese, caloric infusions are reduced to 400 kcal/day until weight normalizes. Patients with SB-IF are stable once these issues have been addressed, and there is no need to keep them in the hospital, so training for home parenteral nutrition should be commenced to allow discharge, as described in the previous section.

Principles of Management

The essential management principle for SBS is *to overcome malabsorption by making the remaining bowel work harder*. Our GI tract is designed to allow us to eat intermittently, allowing more time for other essential activities: hunting in our predecessors and going to work for us. With SBS, this capacity is lost, and we have to *behave more like rabbits, nibbling throughout the day.* This provides the absorptive mucosa with a continuous flow of nutrients, maximizing daily absorption. It is also important to note that digestive function is preserved; indeed pancreatic secretion increases in compensation [207, 209] (Fig. 11.2), so elemental diets are not needed as the digestive process is almost complete by the proximal jejunum. More important is to keep the digesta in contact with the mucosal surface for as long as possible with the use of anti-motility agents. Finally, dietary restriction should *not* be stringent [210]. In previous years, low-fat diets were mandated to reduce steatorrhea, but it soon became recognized that as soon as patients got home, they eat whatever they wanted, when they wanted [204], because SBS causes hyperphagia and low-fat diets are unpalatable. Studies were performed and showed that more fat was absorbed from a high-fat diet, despite the exacerbation of steatorrhea [212], and we now recommend a normal fat diet. Protein is highly digestible and generous intakes are acceptable. Finally, carbohydrate is best given in complex form to increase tolerance and stimulate colonic fermentation and thus energy salvage in those with colonic conservation [211]. All these points need to be discussed with the patient and their family, as they have to realize that although the long-term prognosis of SB-IF is good, their GI anatomy has forever changed and will not tolerate the consumption of large irregular meals.

- *Mild:* Nutritional status should remain stable with a normal balanced diet plus oral supplements of vitamins and minerals (e.g., "once-a-day" preparations) to overcome exaggerated losses. It must be remembered that B12 absorption continues even after the loss of the terminal ileum, but it is much less efficient and high oral doses will be required to prevent deficiency. In the long term, plasma magnesium, vitamin D and bone mineral density, and vitamin B12 should be monitored.
- *Moderate:* Here, the prevention of dehydration and electrolyte deficiency is key. Plasma creatinine should be monitored closely and kept within the normal range by adopting the following preventative measures: Diarrhea or high stomal losses should be suppressed by dietary modification in the form of small frequent meals, together with the avoidance of water, the use of WHO-type solutions, and anti-motility therapeutic agents, such as Imodium, typically in high does (e.g., 2–4 tabs 3–4× per day ½–1 h before meals). *Urine volume must be monitored*; the patient must be taught how to measure total 24-h urine volumes at home, daily for the first week, then dropping to weekly if volumes are greater than one liter per day. He/she must be informed that daily urine output must *never* be allowed to drop below one liter per day. If this is noted, he/she must report this to the HPN team and/or self-administrate IV rehydration in the form of one liter normal saline, if feasible. Chronic dehydration will result in progressive rises in serum creatinine concentrations, and if levels are left >2 for any length of time, irreversible chronic renal failure will complicate management and outcome severely. Chronic hypomagnesemia, with or without carpopedal spasm (tetany), characterizes untreated moderate SBS. Again, oral supplements should first be tried in divided doses, added to food, throughout the day. However, high oral doses are not recommended long term as they will exacerbate diarrhea and create a vicious cycle. Rather, weekly IV supplements

should be started in the form of 30–50 mEq added to their hydration fluids or 1 l saline given at least once a week. We have used weekly intramuscular injections of magnesium, but it is painful and not commonly used.

The indications for commencement of IV supplementation in patients established on dietary and oral fluid modification are:

1. Urine volumes remaining below one liter per day, with sodium content <20 mmol/day.
2. Plasma creatinines remaining above the normal range.
3. Serum magnesiums remaining low, associated with symptoms suggestive of tetany (hand–foot muscle spasms).

   Some patients need daily IV infusions of 1 l of saline together with the appropriate quantities of potassium and magnesium to maintain normal renal function and electrolyte balance; others, particularly those with chronic magnesium deficiency, may only need a single infusion weekly as described above. This also determines the type of IV catheter they will need: those with daily infusions will need a central line, or PICC line; those with once weekly will only require an intermittent peripheral IV catheters. Try to avoid central lines as long as possible to avoid long-term access problems and infections.

• *Severe:* This is the group with *short bowel intestinal failure (SB-IF)*, and they will be home TPN dependent (HPN, see p. 127) to maintain not only fluid and electrolyte balance but also nutrient balance.

Practice

Initial Management

Stimulation of Adaptation

Food: The most powerful stimulatory factor is complex food. Patients should be encouraged to start eating *normal* food as soon as possible after the loss of intestine as the topical effect of complex nutrients on the mucosa triggers the release of the endocrine and paracrine factors that are responsible for adaptation. Often, however, patients are critically ill and recovering from surgery or polytrauma, and so food has to be delivered by feeding tube as a liquid formula diet. Although elemental formulae may be better absorbed in patients with compromised bowel function, they are less stimulatory, and so it is better to commence with a standard polymeric diet, and one containing fiber to maintain the microbiota if the colon is intact, and to make up for the likely malabsorption with IV fluids and electrolytes or parenteral nutrition. It should also be noted that pancreatic enzyme secretion is raised in adapted SB-IF patients as mentioned above [207, 209] (Fig. 11.2), and so digestion is not the rate-limiting factor in absorption. An estimate of the length of the remaining bowel should be obtained from the operative records, or from small bowel imaging (barium) studies, to predict the likelihood of permanent intestinal failure from the information given above, i.e., *<60 cm of small intestine plus the colon or <120 cm of intestine without a colon.*

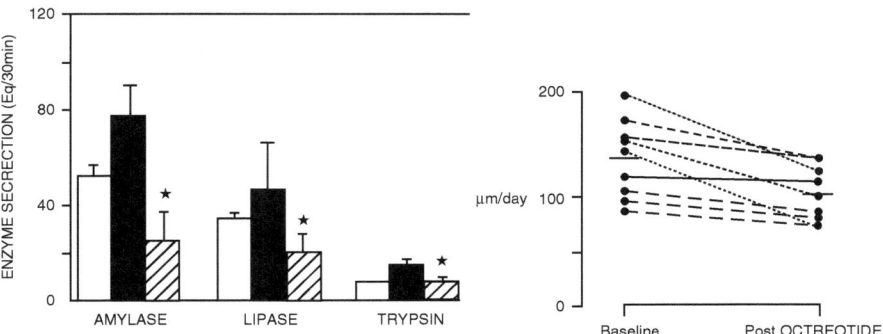

Fig. 11.2 *Left panel*: Summary of the changes in amylase, lipase, and trypsin secretion in response to CCK in SBS-IF patients before (black bars) and after 10 days of treatment with octreotide (striped bars), compared to normal controls (white bars), showing significant ($P < 0.05$) decreases in all three. Values represent the mean enzyme secretion during the 30-min collection periods during the 4-h study. *Right panel*: Individual changes in villus growth rates calculated from isotope incorporation and morphological measurements in patients before and after 10-day octreotide treatment, showing significant ($P < 0.05$) suppression of the pancreatic hypersecretion and suppression of villus growth rates [209]

With time and in the absence of chronic obstruction, SB-IF patients will develop hyperphagia as part of the natural adaptation response. This develops, as discussed above, because the ileal brake is missing, and satiation does not last long after a meal because most of what is eaten, plus secretions, are lost in the bag or toilet. In the old days, patients were given strict instructions to restrict the intake of food and, in particular, fat, as this would help suppress stomal or stool losses. However, as described above, this also reduces absolute nutrient absorption. The importance of preserving some degree of intestinal absorption is that portal nutrients are essential for maintain hepatic function, even if TPN is given, as IV nutrients are not used as efficiently as enteral nutrients for hepatic protein synthesis [39]. Consequently, we now allow patients to eat a balanced diet in small portions split up throughout the day, bearing in mind that patients tend to eat "what they want, when they want" when they get home. As a consequence, actual intakes end up being about twice the normal [213].

Enhance Absorption

Avoid Water: In addition to hyperphagia, adapted patients often also develop insatiable thirst and crave water, often iced water. It is a simple physiological fact that if SB-IF patients drink water alone, endogenous fluid and electrolyte losses will worsen. *This can set up a vicious circle, as the more you drink, the more fluid and electrolytes you lose from the body, the thirstier you get, eventually creating "the wash-out syndrome"* [207, 209]. This was explained above and is related to the porous nature of the proximal gut and lack of intestinal length. In order to prevent these losses, SB patients need to be advised to add carbohydrate source (it can be

Oral Rehydration Solutions

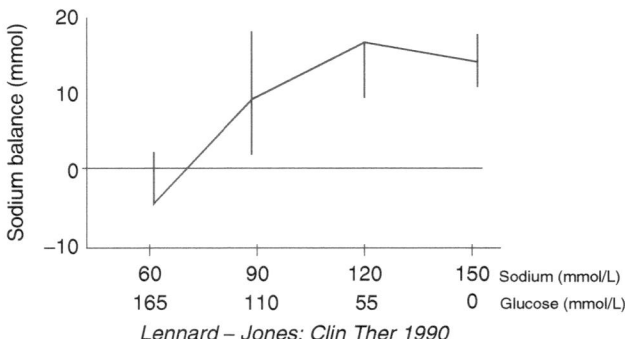

Lennard – Jones: Clin Ther 1990

Fig. 11.3 The physiological basis for WHO rehydration fluids. Sodium balance is only achieved when luminal concentrations exceed 70 mmol/l with glucose concentrations of 140 mmol/l

Table 11.1 Examples of scientifically based oral rehydration solutions (WHO-ORS) and more commonly used fluids for comparison to ideal*

	Sodium (mmol/l)	Carbohydrate (g/l)	Osmolality (mOsm/kg)
WHO-ORS	90	20 (111 mmol/l)	310
Pediatric solution	50	20	270
Gatorade-type	20	60 (333 mmol/l)	380
Ginger ale	3*	90	540
Apple juice	3*	124	730
Chicken broth	250	0	450
Chicken noodle soup	150	50	400

* need to add salt

sugar, polycose, or starch) and salt to their water (a) to maintain isotonicity and (b) to activate active transport of glucose and sodium in the proximal gut. Note glucose co-transporters cannot function without sodium. This is the foundation of the WHO oral rehydration solutions (see below) used extensively in the developing world to counteract dehydration from acute enteric infections, such as cholera, which increase the permeability of the mucosa throughout the GI tract. Classic studies of Lennard-Jones demonstrated that you need more than 90 mEq/l of sodium to achieve net sodium absorption (Fig. 11.3) [214].

Perhaps the most common oversight in SBS management is the failure of the managing team to instruct the patient to NEVER drink straight tap or bottled water. WHO solutions can be made up at home from a simple recipe: 6 level teaspoons of sugar, 1/2 level teaspoon salt, 1 liter water. Unfortunately, patients generally tire of WHO-type solutions, and the best compliance is gained by using sports drinks, such as "Gatorade," which is better than water but lower in salt and higher in sugar than a WHO solution (Table 11.1). *In practical terms, advise patients to drink fluids that contain a carbohydrate source and salt, such as soups.* My favorite suggestion is soups containing pasta, potato, or rice, with lots of added salt!

Prolong Food: Mucosal Contact Time

This is the cornerstone of the management of patients with short bowel as malabsorption primarily occurs due to insufficient contact between the digested food and the absorptive surface, rather than incomplete digestion. The prolonged dwell time, however, also increases digestion. We have shown that pancreatic enzyme secretion is increased in SBS, and the digestive process is virtually complete by the proximal jejunum [207]. Thus, as discussed above, the need for a long intestine is to enable reabsorption of the secretions needed to efficiently support the digestive process, rather than support digestion. Motility changes, becoming less coordinated, with adaptation in an attempt to hold everything in for as long as possible. In general, solid food remains in the gut longer, and it is best to avoid drinking large quantities of fluid with meals or snacks to avoid "washout." Perhaps the most effective means of prolonging mucosal contact time is to use anti-motility drugs.

Imodium: The cheapest and most effective is loperamide (Imodium). It is an opioid derivative, which, like morphine, suppresses the contraction of longitudinal smooth muscles and enhances the contraction of the circular muscles of the gut but, unlike morphine, is poorly transported across the blood–brain barrier making it more bowel specific. Because Imodium has a wide therapeutic range and because its absorption may be impaired in SBS, it should be used in high doses, up to 18×2 mg tabs per day spread out to cover dietary intakes. It is best given 1 h before meals and with meals, e.g., 2 1 h before and 2 with meals and 1–2 with snacks. Often confused with Imodium is Lomotil, a drug with similar properties. However, it is important to understand that in addition to the active ingredient, the opioid derivative diphenoxylate, it contains atropine, which can produce significant anticholinergic side effects (dry mouth, vision), which prevents its use in the large quantities suggested for Imodium above. Other opioids are equally effective, such as codeine phosphate and tincture of opium, but they have strong central effects. We prefer to use Imodium alone in high doses.

Antisecretory Agents: Antisecretory agents are attractive because secretion rates are often high in SB-IF patients because of the continued gut stimulation due to hyperphagia, and as I have mentioned earlier, dehydration is often the earliest sign of intestinal failure because the reason we have many meters of the small intestine is to reabsorb the secretions that are needed for efficient digestion and absorption. Clearly, however, this is a balancing trick, as too effective suppression will impair digestion and absorption. As in most chronic GI disorders, proton pump inhibitors are overused. Their initial use after bowel resection can be justified by the reports of peptic ulcers in association with hypersecretion [215, 216]. However, our measurements of gastric acid secretion in adapted patients were normal [207, 209], and therefore, I discourage the use of PPIs in adapted patients, particularly because they encourage bacterial overgrowth in the remnant gut, which interferes with digestion and absorption, thus exacerbating stomal or diarrhea losses. Furthermore, it must be remembered that gastric acid forms the first line of defense against environmental pathogens.

Somatostatin Analogues: Somatostatin has glibly been termed "intestinal cyanide" as it suppresses most functions of the bowel, including motility, as well as pancreatic endocrine and exocrine function, thus removing the additional problem of secretory losses associated with SB-IF and effectively reducing high stomal and fistula losses. Studies of ours in adapted hyperphagic end-jejunostomy HPN-dependent patients showed that stomal losses were reduced by half (see below) [207], while octreotide is very effective in the short term and can initially precipitate heart failure in patients with severe SB-IF due to the dramatic effects on suppressing secretory losses in patients receiving high IV infusion rates to maintain renal function [207]. Furthermore, there is concern that its long-term use is counter-adaptive, as it suppresses not only pancreatic secretion, and therefore potentially digestion and absorption, but also mucosal blood flow and villus growth [207] (Fig. 11.2). To show this, we infused stable isotope-labeled amino acids (^{13}C-leucine tracer) in nine adapted SB-IF patients dependent on home TPN and matched healthy controls. With our 4-h IV infusions, where gastric juice and pancreatic enzymes were sampled continuously by intubation, we were able to simultaneously measure nitrogen balance, gastric and pancreatic secretion, and the rates of pancreatic enzyme and gastric and duodenal mucosal turnover before and after subcutaneous octreotide (100 μg) injections. Interestingly, rates of gastric and duodenal mucosal turnover and their morphology were normal, but rates of pancreatic amylase and trypsin secretion and synthesis were significantly higher in patients (Fig. 11.2). Octreotide treatment significantly suppressed not only stomal fluid losses from 8.1 ± 1.8 to 4.8 ± 0.7 l/day ($P < 0.001$) but also gut hormones and mucosal and pancreatic synthesis rates and calculations of villous growth rates based on isotope incorporation and measurements of villous heights and widths (Fig. 11.2). Although stomal nitrogen losses were also reduced, this was at the expense of increases in urine nitrogen losses such that overall nitrogen balance remained unchanged. Another concern is that octreotide also reduced insulin levels, which, in conjunction with IV glucose infusions in TPN-dependent patients, will result in the unwelcome complication of hyperglycemia.

Therapy to Increase Adaptation

Growth Hormone and Glutamine

Recognizing the facts that glutamine is the preferred fuel for enterocytes and that, in experimental models, it is trophic to the small bowel mucosa and, secondly, that growth hormone was also trophic to the mucosa, Wilmore and colleagues investigated the possibility of enhancing adaptation in SB-IF patients in order to wean them off HPN. Their initial uncontrolled studies in 8 PN-dependent patients showed that the combination of a modified diet (low-fat, high-complex carbohydrate), oral glutamine supplements, and daily injections of recombinant growth hormone for 3 weeks indeed increased fluid, electrolyte, and carbohydrate absorption, leading them to conclude that this therapy may offer an alternative to long-term dependence on total parenteral nutrition for patients with severe short bowel syndrome. Because of criticisms that this study was not randomized and controlled, the same group published a follow-up study 10 years later where 41 SB-IF patients were randomized to one of 3 treatment arms (1:2:2 ratio): oral glutamine (30 g/day)+GH placebo (control group, $n=9$), glutamine placebo + GH (0.1 mg/kg per day, $n=16$), or glutamine + GH ($n=16$) for 6 weeks [217]. Patients who received GH + Gln + diet showed the greatest reductions (7.7 ± 3.2 l/week; $5,751\pm2,082$ cal/week; 4 ± 1 infusions/week, $P<0.001$ vs. Gln + diet) [217]. At 3-month follow-up, only patients who had received GH + Gln + diet maintained significant reductions in PN ($P<0.005$) compared with the Gln + diet group. Furthermore, continuation of the treatment for 1 year was associated with a reduction in PN volumes in 40% of patients. These were exciting results as they suggested we could "superadapt" SBS patients with hormonal therapy. Unfortunately, a series of subsequent studies gave mixed results and raised concerns about side effects. The chief concern is that GH promotes growth in organs throughout the body, not just the gut, as illustrated by its natural overproduction in acromegaly. Finally, in a Cochrane analysis of the five RCTs, the authors concluded that "the results suggest a positive effect of human growth hormone on weight gain and energy absorption. However, in the majority of trials, the effects are short-lived returning to baseline shortly after cessation of therapy. The temporary benefit calls into question the clinical utility of this treatment" [218]. One can safely say that oral glutamine is a waste of money as it is an inessential amino acid and excess will simply increase urine nitrogen. What the residual gut needs is exposure to *complete, complex, food* as studies have shown that although glutamine increases villus growth in TPN-fed rats, rat chow, which contains a wide spectrum of essential nutrients, is, not surprisingly, far superior (Chapter 3, Fig. 3.4).

Gut Peptides: The search for the mechanism behind natural adaptation switched next to gut-specific hormones. Interest in the potential role of glucagon was aroused when patients with endocrine tumors producing glucagon were shown to have mucosal hypertrophy. For example, a patient with a glucagon-producing endocrine tumor of the kidney was found, on laparotomy, to have marked hypertrophy and enlargement of the whole intestine, especially the jejunum [219]. The villus hypertrophy was evident on visual inspection (Fig. 11.4), and histological measurement confirmed

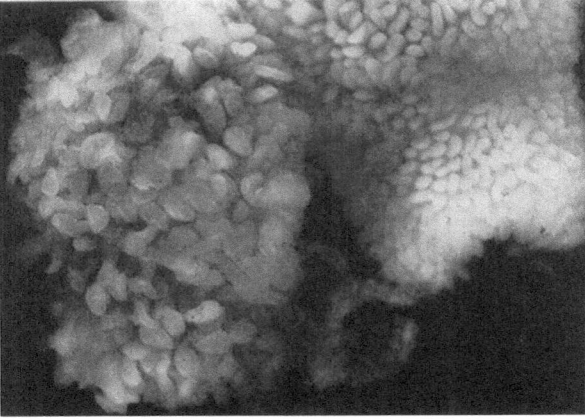

Fig. 11.4 Dissecting microscopic appearances of the jejunum of a patient with a glucagonoma of the kidney on the left illustrating villous hyperlasia (left). On the right is a jejunal biopsy from a normal healthy person (Gleeson et al. [219])

that villus length was on average 1,350 μm, compared to control of 350–800 μm. The diagnosis of a functional endocrine a-cell tumor was made on histochemistry and the detection of ten times normal blood levels of glucagon. At that time, GLP-2 was unknown, but interestingly the authors speculated that there might exist "a second hormone that stimulates villous growth...."

Since then, it has been recognized that proglucagon undergoes posttranslational modification to a variety of peptide hormones, including glucagon, GLP-2, and GLP-1. Together with peptide YY (PYY), it functions as the "ileal brake," turning off pancreatic secretion and slowing gastric emptying and intestinal motility if nutrients arrive unabsorbed in the ileum. However, experimental studies have shown that *GLP-2* has multiple other effects on gut function through the activation of its receptor in the intestinal mucosa with the release of insulin-like growth factor-1, keratinocyte growth factor, nitric oxide, and vasoactive intestinal polypeptide and the promotion of ErbB signaling, all of which participate in the observed increases in intestinal growth through enhancement of proliferation, suppression of apoptosis, increased blood flow, and absorption following experimental injection of the peptide [220, 221].

GLP-2 Analogues (Teduglutide, "Gattex")

Teduglutide: As with peptide hormones in general, GLP-2's biological half-life is short, and so, based on the positive results of pilot IV infusion studies, a long-acting analogue, teduglutide, was synthesized with one amino acid substitution (glycine for alanine, Fig. 11.5) that was resistant to protease degradation, extending its

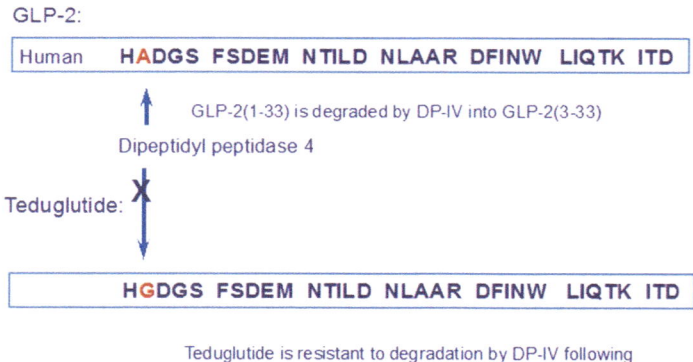

Fig. 11.5 Modification of the natural structure of GLP-2 with a single amino acid substitution makes it resistant to proteolytic degradation and therefore extends its half-life from minutes to hours, making it suitable for a single daily injection

half-life from minutes to hours so that it could be administered as a single daily subcutaneous injection.

Two multicenter, multinational, randomized controlled studies have now been completed which show that the drug at a dose level of 0.05 mg/kg/day is effective in reducing IV fluid requirements in patients with adapted SB-IF. In the first, 83 patients were randomized to two dose levels of teduglutide or placebo for 6 months [222]. Using a 20% or greater reduction in PN volume requirements to maintain normal renal function (i.e., a urine output of 1–2 l/day) as "clinically significant" (note, this level of reduction would allow the average HPN patient to drop one night of IV infusions), the low dose (0.05 mg/kg/day) was significantly more effective than the placebo (6% vs. 46%, $P=0.007$). This was accompanied by significant increases in villous height and citrulline synthesis (citrulline can only be synthesized by enterocytes, so fasting blood levels have been proposed as a measure of enterocyte mass) thus suggesting a potentiation of the normal adaptive response. At the end of the study, patients continued on taking drug for an additional 6 months to assess sustainability and safety [223]. Figures 11.6 and 11.7 illustrates that the potency of the drug was preserved; in fact, PN requirements continued to drop, and, at the end of 12 months, 68% of patients had achieved >20% PN reductions and four subjects had been weaned off PN completely.

Because of concern about the apparent lack of efficacy of the higher dose level, 0.1 mg/kg/d (note this dose reduced PN requirement (25 % reduced PN by >20 %), but not significantly, for a variety of reasons probably unrelated to the drug), a confir-

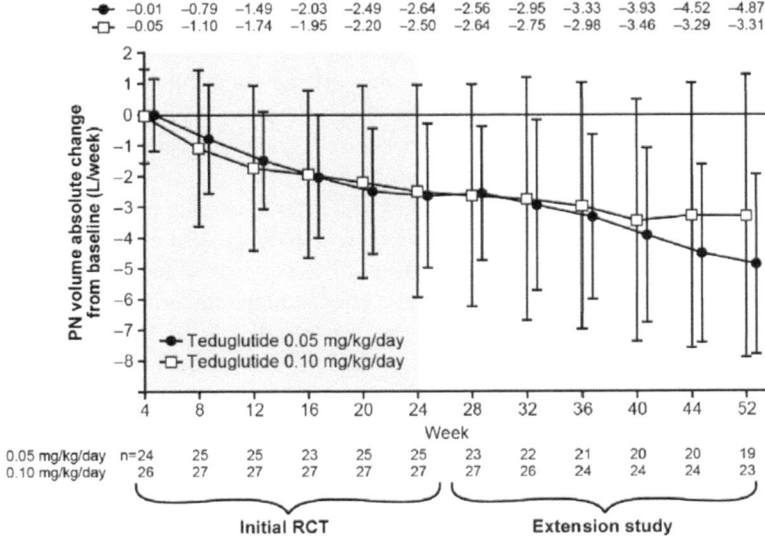

Fig. 11.6 Mean reduction in parenteral support over 52 weeks for the two dose levels of teduglutide. Patients enrolled in the extension study were continued on teduglutide at the same dose as they were given during the RCT (*O'Keefe et al.* [223])

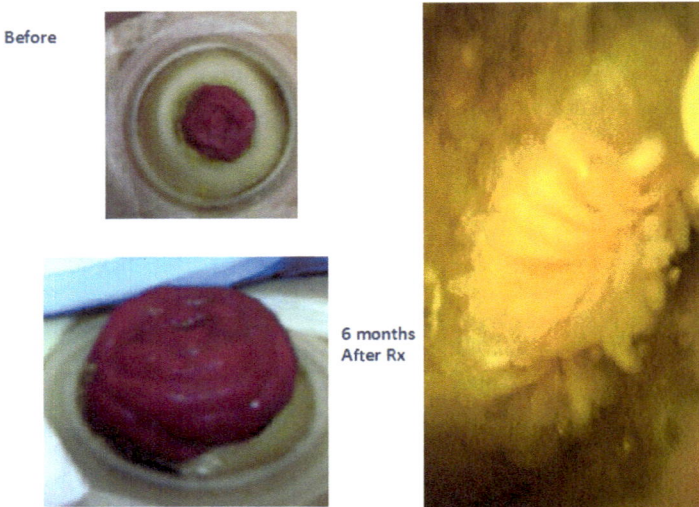

Fig. 11.7 Illustration of the macroscopic proliferative effects of teduglutide in a patient with SB-IF with an end jejunostomy. Note the enlargement of the stoma (*lower left*), and hypertrophy of the villi seen via jejunoscopy using a regular endoscope (*right*)

matory study was demanded by the FDA before release of the drug for clinical use, based on the low dose alone vs. placebo. In this, 86 SB-IF patients were randomized and treated for 6 months [224]. Sixty-three percent of patients achieved a clinically significant reduction in PN requirements as compared to 30% on placebo ($P = 0.002$). Again, participants were invited to continue on a 2-year extension open-label study. The preliminary results indicate continuing efficacy with further reductions in PN requirements and complete weaning in seven patients. With all the studies combined, 11 of the 173 SB-IF patients have been completely weaned from PN (*O'Keefe et al. ESPEN proceedings, Clinical Nutrition 2012*).

In summary, these studies are exciting and offer a novel approach to the clinical management of SB-IF, but the true efficacy and safety of the drug has still to be revealed in clinical practice; now, the drug is FDA approved and marketed. There is no doubt that this drug has potent trophic effects on the remaining intestine as they can be observed by looking at the increase in stoma size and villi with a normal endoscope (Fig. 11.7). As with any potent therapy, there could be potent side effects, and although the incidence of side effects so far is low, there is particular concern about the long-term use of a proliferative agent, particularly in an aging population. Careful surveillance with regular colonoscopy will be mandatory.

Other "Ileal Brake" Peptides: It is likely that other ileal brake peptides will also have beneficial effects in the management of SB-IF by helping regulate dietary intake and gut motility. For example, in a recent uncontrolled study, *GLP-1* infusions helped wean three patients from IV infusions by suppressing hyperphagia and gut motility [225]. Peptide YY may have similar effects. The results of RCTs are eagerly awaited.

Chapter 12
Small Bowel Transplantation

The Principles

The ultimate treatment of short bowel intestinal failure is small bowel transplantation (SBTx). While many remedies, such as those described above, can reduce the severity of intestinal failure due to SBS, e.g., GH and GLP-2 treatment was associated with an increase in caloric absorption by 400–800 kcal/day [222, 224, 226], only SBTx can predictably restore normal digestive and absorptive function, making patients with extreme intestinal failure nutritionally autonomous. Indeed, successful transplantation is remarkable in allowing young patients with chronic obstruction to eat normal food for the first time in their lives. Current Medicare guidelines restrict the use of small bowel transplantation to those with "TPN failure," as defined below:

Indications: "TPN Failure"

TPN failure results chiefly from 3 conditions associated with HPN, namely:

1. *Recurrent life-threatening bacterial infections or fungal septicemias.*
2. *Loss of venous access due to extensive central vein thrombosis.*
3. *Liver failure and cirrhosis.*

"TPN failure" constitutes a condition recognized by Medicare as the prime indication for small bowel transplantation, as patients would likely die without transplantation [227, 228]. However, some private insurance coverages allow patients with *high risk of* developing TPN failure to advance to early transplantation [227]. This is particularly relevant to patients with extreme SBS with end jejunostomies <50 cm, as prospective studies have shown that they are at extreme risk of developing liver failure—which, if waited for, will necessitate not only intestinal transplantation but also liver transplantation [227]. The likely explanation for the

© Springer Science+Business Media New York 2015
S.J.D. O'Keefe, *The Principles and Practice of Nutritional Support*,
DOI 10.1007/978-1-4939-1779-2_12

higher risk of liver problems with shorter remnant bowel is that the shorter the bowel, the lower the rate of residual absorption and the lower the delivery of portal nutrients to the liver. This would explain the resolution of liver dysfunction after small bowel transplantation [192].

Success has improved dramatically over the past decade, such that current 1-year survival rates equal those for liver and renal transplantation. In their paper entitled *A New Era Has Dawned*, the International Intestine Transplant Registry, which has a database of 989 grafts in 923 patients from 61 programs in 19 different countries, presented their cumulative results that 1-year survival in the USA ranges from 78 to 84% and 5–10-year survival from 56 to 61% [228]. They concluded that survival can be expected to improve further with earlier referral, as the procedure is more successful when patients are transplanted from home. However, survival is not the only outcome parameter that should be examined. One of the most concerning aspects of HPN management is the poor quality of life. Consequently, we examined outcome and QoL, measured by a validated self-administered questionnaire containing 26 domains and 130 questions, for a minimum of 12 months in a cohort of 46 consecutively transplanted adult patients in Pittsburgh between June 2003 and July 2004 [192]. The majority of the patients (76%) had intestinal failure because of extreme short bowel, mostly due to mesenteric infarction, the remainder having either chronic pseudo-obstruction or porto-mesenteric vein thrombosis. All but the latter group were dependent on home HPN (median 2, range 0–25 years) and had developed serious recurrent infective complications with or without central vein thrombosis and liver failure. Two thirds received a liver in addition to a small intestine. All were weaned from PN at a median of 12 days posttransplant and were independent of tube feeding by 69 days, eating normally. Five patients died, two with acute rejection and the remainder with sepsis or surgery. The remaining patients were followed for a median of 21 months, range 12–36 months, experiencing an average of 1.2 episodes of acute reversible rejection detected by surveillance ileoscopy and biopsy as described below. As there has been much debate about the relative QoL between transplanted and HPN-managed patients, we included a "control" group of our HPN patients who chose not to pursue the transplant track. Although their underlying diseases and PN requirements were similar, global assessment of their QoL was significantly higher, indicating that the patients going to transplant were in general sicker. Following transplantation, global QoL improved in all subjects to a level higher than the HPN patients, and there was a significant improvement in 13 of the 26 specific domains examined. We concluded that with continued progress, small bowel transplantation could potentially become an alternative to HPN for the management of permanent intestinal failure, rather than a last-chance treatment for "TPN failure." The success of this procedure can be remarkable allowing patients to eat normally after years of PN dependency (e.g., we had one patient who had never learned to eat normally because of intestinal pseudo-obstruction who had to be taught how to eat after successful transplantation!) and, combined with a liver, can allow for the first time good quality survival in patients with extreme jaundice, metabolic failure and marasmus due to end-stage liver disease due to ultrashort bowel, as illustrated on Chapter 10, Fig. 10.9.

Ileoscopy & Biopsy

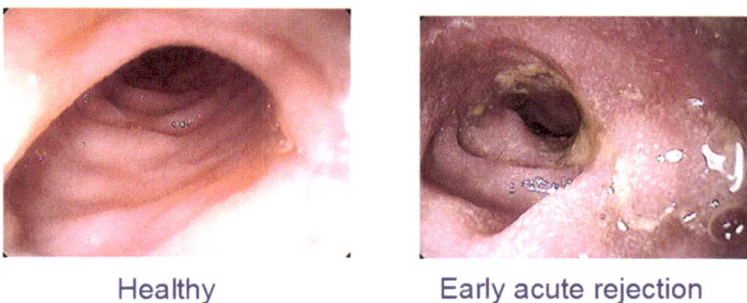

Healthy   Early acute rejection

Fig. 12.1 Endoscopic appearances of small bowel transplant grafts via the ileal 'chimney'. View on left shows healthy ileal graft mucosa while photo on right illustrates early, reversible, acute rejection

The downside is the need for lifelong immunosuppression and graft surveillance by endoscopy, and some patients develop acute recurrent or chronic rejection requiring considerable lengths of hospitalization (Fig. 12.1). The management of acute rejection is, however, easier that in other forms of solid organ transplantation as the graft can be biopsied relatively noninvasively, through the creation of an ileal graft "chimney" for the first year of surveillance. In our recent review of our experience with ileoscopies, we showed that severe rejection is easy to identify by visualization alone, but more moderate forms—which are rapidly reversible with specific therapy—can be missed, necessitating histological examination of endoscopic biopsies [229].

The Practice

Small bowel transplantation has not "taken off" in the USA and Europe as liver transplantation did in the 1980s. For example, in a European survey, only 15% of HPN patients with Medicaid criteria for "TPN failure" and small bowel transplant were referred to a center for transplantation, and only 36% of adults and 43% of children with HPN-liver failure were described as needing immediate transplantation [230]. The explanation for the reticence is unclear, particularly since SB-IF-associated liver failure is generally a fatal condition and also because late referral is associated with poor outcomes. The most likely explanation is the unfamiliarity with transplant outcomes and the fact that few centers around the country—or the world—offer small intestine transplantation, because the volume is small and the specific skills needed to perform the surgery, and manage the problems, are scarce.

Chapter 13
Acute and Chronic Pancreatitis

The pancreas plays the major, arguably the central, role in nutrition of the body. Through its exocrine function, it converts complex food into simple "elemental" nutrients that can be absorbed by active or passive mechanisms across epithelial membranes into body fluids for distribution to all organs of the body for respiration, anabolism, or storage. It also controls the utilization of absorbed nutrients through its endocrine functions: absorbed nutrients are sensed, and hormones such as insulin, glucagon, and somatostatin are released in concert with the flow of nutrients to maintain blood levels and stimulate anabolism or catabolism. This explains the extremely poor nutritional state of patients with end-stage chronic pancreatitis where exocrine failure results in maldigestion and endocrine failure results in the failure to utilize the small amount of nutrients that are absorbed. It also explains why diabetes associated with chronic pancreatitis is "brittle." The encouragement of increased food consumption, coupled with adequate pancreatic enzyme supplementation, will increase the flow of digested nutrients into the portal vein. The inability of the pancreas to sense the increase in absorbed nutrients and secrete insulin will result in reduced liver and tissue uptake resulting in hyperglycemia, hyperaminoacidemia, and hyperlipidemia in the systemic circulation. Even more dangerous is the other side of the coin, where dietary intake is interrupted and the portal flow of glucose ebbs. This normally stimulates the pancreas to secrete glucagon and somatostatin to generate gluconeogenesis, but in their absence, the regular insulin injections are unopposed, resulting in progressive systemic hypoglycemia and ultimately life-threatening neuroglycopenia. Nutritional management of acute pancreatitis is equally challenging as food increases the synthesis of trypsinogen, and trypsinogen pre-activation within the pancreas is the initiating and perpetuating factor in the acute inflammatory process [231].

© Springer Science+Business Media New York 2015
S.J.D. O'Keefe, *The Principles and Practice of Nutritional Support*,
DOI 10.1007/978-1-4939-1779-2_13

Severe Acute Pancreatitis (SAP)

It is important to understand that acute pancreatitis varies considerably in severity and that >75% of patients admitted with the disease have the mild form which recovers within a few days, allowing resumption of normal eating without the need for nutritional support. Our prospective study on nutrition and outcome in 156 consecutive patients admitted with acute pancreatitis showed that conservative treatment with IV fluids and analgesics resulted in the remission and discharge on normal food in 75% within 4 days (Fig. 13.1) [62]. On the other hand, the severe form of the disease is associated with high mortality rates, multiple organ failure, high demands for ICU management, and lengthy ICU and hospital stays and is one of the most catabolic of critical illnesses. Put together, this translates to one of the most challenging of hospital nutritional managements, which consumes much of our clinical time as nutritional gastroenterologists working in tertiary referral centers [161].

Percentages of Admissions in Each of the Three Groups

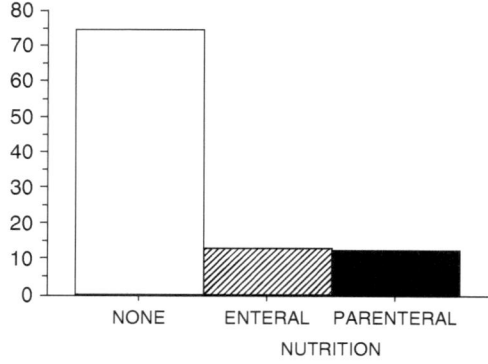

Fig. 13.1 Breakdown of admissions for acute pancreatitis into the following three groups: group O ("none") needed no nutritional support, group EN ("enteral") received jejunal tube feeding, and group PN ("parenteral") received IV nutrition (Abou-Assi et al. [62])

Management Principles

Management of SAP is particularly difficult because of:

- *Feeding may exacerbate the disease.*
- *Enteral feeding is difficult because of compression of the upper GI tract by the swollen pancreas and inflammatory mass.*
- *TPN will exacerbate the inflammatory response and hyperglycemia.*

In order to understand how best to treat the disease, we need to understand the pathophysiology.

The Pathophysiology

The excess mortality of severe acute pancreatitis is associated with the consequences of pancreatic injury rather than the pancreatic damage itself. In contrast to patients with mild disease, those with severe pancreatitis develop a systemic inflammatory response characterized by a flood of pro-inflammatory cytokines [232], which impair respiratory, renal, and intestinal function, resulting in multiple organ failure [232, 233]. This process has been extensively studied in animal models. The initiating factor in the inflammatory cascade is accepted to be an increase in intracellular calcium flux with premature activation of trypsinogen within the pancreas, leading to intracellular proteolysis or "autophagia" [43, 234, 235]. Figure 13.2 helps illustrate some of what is known to happen in the evolution of multiple organ failure and emphasizes the key role of the intestine in its genesis and the potential for enteral feeding to break the vicious cycle of events. Intracellular injury results in the generation of a cascade of pro-inflammatory cytokines such as IL-1b, TNF-alpha, IL-17,

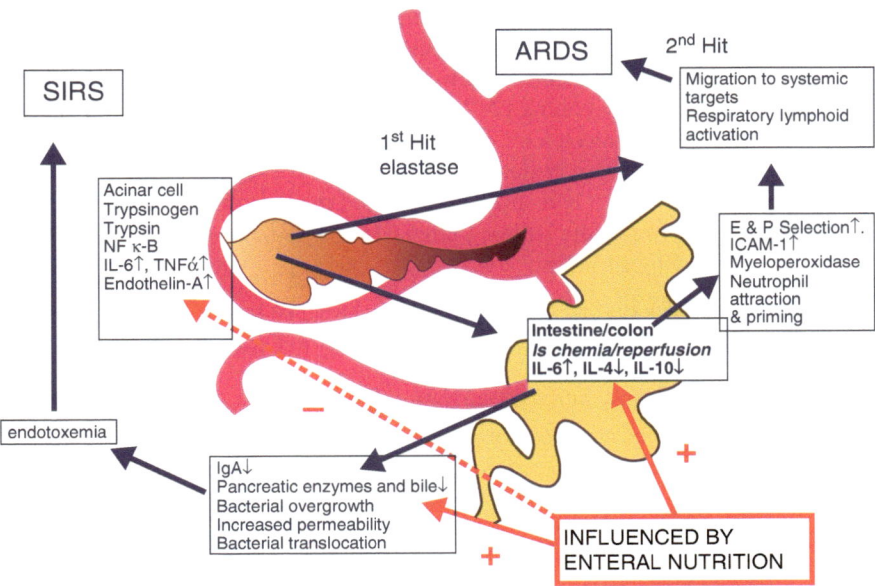

Fig. 13.2 An explanation for the frequent progression of acute pancreatitis to multiple organ failure and how early enteral feeding may suppress the progression. The initial pro-inflammatory cytokine generation from the autophagic pancreatic acinar cell injury sets up secondary ischemic injury in the bowel which amplifies the "cytokine flood" which provides a second hit on the lung injury induced by circulating pancreatic proteases and activated neutrophils producing ARDS. Reduced luminal secretion of pancreobiliary secretions plus ileus allows small bowel bacterial overgrowth with consequent endotoxemia, amplifying the systemic inflammatory response. Early (low volume) enteral feeding promotes mucosal blood flow and prevents ileus and stagnation, suppressing the cytokine response

and IL-18 via activation of periacinar myofibrocytic NF kappa B and MAP kinase [236–239]. This in turn stimulates the release of IL-6 and the cytoattraction of neutrophils, which in turn leads to further cytokine generation which spills into the systemic circulation, and a secondary response commences, approximately 48 h later, which leads to the further generation of PG-2, thromboxane, LTB-4, and oxygen-derived free radicals within the bronchial and intestinal mucosa leading to cytotoxic injury in distant organs. Arterial constriction induced by endothelin-A activation can lead to necrosis of the pancreas and gangrene of the intestine [239]. Splanchnic and whole body protein catabolism is accelerated by inflammatory cytokines [240]. The situation is compounded further by the release of proteolytic enzymes such as trypsin, elastase, phospholipase, and caspase 1 from the injured pancreas into the circulation which leads to amplification of cell injury within the lung and GI tract leading to ARDS, intestinal ischemia, bacterial translocation, and the well-recognized systemic inflammatory response syndrome (SIRS) (Fig. 13.2) [241].

It is these complications that account for the high mortality rates, which can approach 30–50%, in severe necrotizing pancreatitis. Despite the accumulating knowledge of the mechanisms involved, there have unfortunately been no major breakthroughs in treatment—other than enteral feeding. The use of antiprotease therapy has been disappointing, and the initial excitement that specific anti-cytokine therapy might prevent the cytokine activation cascade has not been realized on formal testing in the clinical arena [240]. This is reminiscent of the attempts to use corticosteroids for the management of overwhelming sepsis in the ICU. Inflammation is the way we recover from critical injury, it is the *appropriate* response, and suppression may well worsen outcome. As discussed in Chapter 4, we need to support the response and provide the building blocks for tissue repair and recovery. This is where enteral feeding comes in:

1. Promotes intestinal blood flow, reducing intestinal ischemia.
2. Suppresses the additional inflow of inflammatory cytokines from the gut into the circulation.
3. Maintains intestinal motility and "housekeeping," preventing bacterial overgrowth, endotoxemia, and bacterial translocation.
4. *But* proximal enteral feeding stimulates the pancreas to produce more trypsinogen and thus might exacerbate the intrinsic disease process.

These points explain why the use of TPN and bowel rest actually worsens outcome. While TPN is the best way of providing feeding without can stimulating the pancreas, i.e., providing "pancreatic rest" (Fig. 13.3) [30], it negates points 1, 2, and 3. Bacterial translocation may be of critical importance, as the organisms most commonly responsible for pancreatic infections are of colonic origin [80], and endotoxemia commonly accompanies severe disease [77]. Second, the presence of a central vein catheter in TPN-fed patients provides an open conduit for nosocomial infection. Third, intravenous feeding invariably results in hyperglycemia in patients with severe acute pancreatitis because (a) the glycemic effect of glucose administered parenterally is greater than if it is given enterally [30], (b) acute pancreatitis impairs pancreatic endocrine function resulting in a relative insulin deficiency [243], and (c) the acute inflammatory response and secretion of counter-regulatory hormones

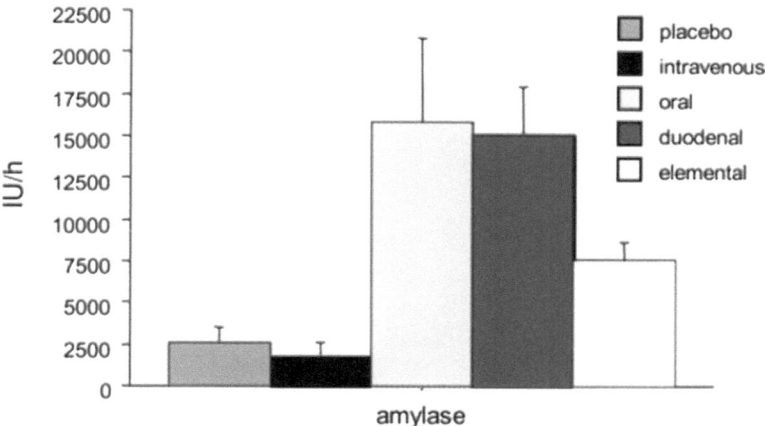

Fig. 13.3 Amylase secretion in response to enteral and parenteral nutrition. Relative amylase secretory responses to enteral and parenteral feeding, illustrating no difference between oral and duodenal feeding of a complex diet, an intermediate response to duodenal elemental diet feeding, and no stimulatory effect of intravenous feeding compared with placebo saline (*O'Keefe et al.* [30])

increase endogenous glucose production and create insulin resistance [50]. Recent studies have clearly demonstrated that hyperglycemia worsens outcome in any form of critical illness [59]. In hyperglycemia, leukocyte function is impaired and intestinal motility reduced leading to increased infection risk from enteric pathogens [55]. *Consequently, it is likely that the potential benefits of TPN on "resting" the pancreas are overshadowed by its detrimental effects on intestinal function and mucosal integrity and by its septic and metabolic complications.*

These considerations stimulated us to develop an "ideal" form of nutritional support, based on adequate access for enteral feeding, plus avoidance of pancreatic stimulation—*distal jejunal feeding*.

Enteral Feeding Without Pancreatic Stimulation, Distal Jejunal Feeding

Classically, the stimulatory effect of feeding has been divided into three phases: the cephalic phase, the gastric phase, and the intestinal phase (Chapter 3, Fig. 3.1). Cholinergic (vagal) stimulation induced by ingestion of food in the mouth and luminal transit in the esophagus, stomach, and duodenum provides the chief stimulus, but in the duodenum, CCK release by food contact augments secretion. Our physiological studies in healthy volunteers showed that avoidance of the cephalic phase had little effect, but conversion of a polymeric to an elemental diet reduced secretion by 50% (Fig. 13.3) [30].

As undigested food moves further down the intestine, the stimulatory effect tapers, and if it gets to the end of the ileum, it activates the ileal brake to secrete peptide hormones, PYY and GLP-1, that actively inhibit pancreatic secretion [244].

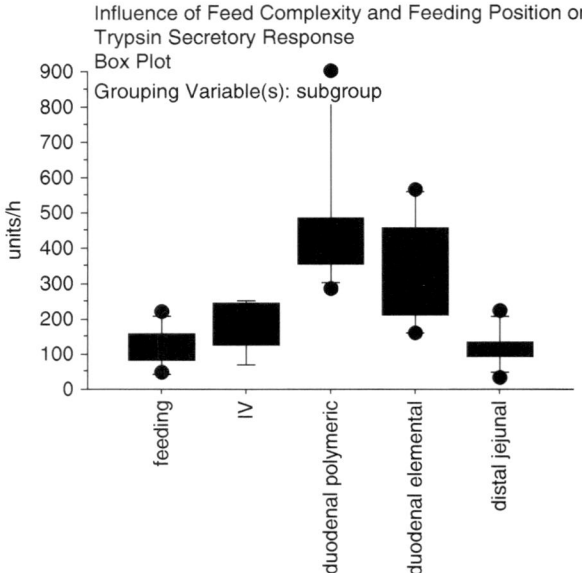

Fig. 13.4 The relative pancreatic stimulatory effects of enteral and parenteral (IV) feeding on pancreatic secretion in normal healthy volunteers showing that distal jejunal (i.e., >40 cm past the ligament of Treitz) feeding had no stimulatory response (Kaushik et al. [159])

Consequently, there must be a point between the duodenum and the ileum where infusion of a liquid formula diet would neither stimulate nor inhibit pancreatic enzyme secretion. To determine this level, we placed feeding tubes at progressive distances past the ligament of Treitz, namely, 20, 40, 80, 105, and 120 cm. The pattern of the secretory responses during 360 min of feeding is shown on Fig. 13.4 demonstrating that there was no significant secretory response to mid-distal jejunal feeding, as secretion rates were no different from those measured during fasting or IV feeding [159]. Examination of the gut peptide responses supported the suggestion that pancreatic secretion might have been suppressed by induction of the ileal brake, with substantial increases in plasma GLP-1 and PYY but not CCK. Our results are consistent with those of Vu et al., who showed that the infusion of a mixed polymeric liquid diet at normal tube feeding rates (i.e., 1.6 kcal/min) into the proximal jejunum stimulated basal trypsin secretion fourfold whereas infusion 60 cm below the ligament of Treitz had no stimulatory effect over 3 h [245].

Pancreatic Stimulation by Enteral Feeding in Severe Acute Pancreatitis

Of course, all of this would be meaningless if pancreatic secretion is arrested by acute pancreatitis. To investigate this, we first examined the pancreatic secretory response to feeding in 12 patients with moderate and severe (four necrotizing) pancreatitis and noted that secretion into the duodenum was indeed suppressed approximately 90% (Fig. 13.5 upper panel [128]), which is at the level where fat malabsorption commences [42]. However, a reduction in luminal secretion does not necessarily equate with the arrest of synthesis, as we know that a large proportion of synthesized enzymes leak from the pancreas into the systemic circulation, where they are used as biomarkers for the diagnosis of acute pancreatitis, e.g., serum amylase and lipase. In order to examine this, we next studied the kinetics of trypsin production by labeling trypsin with stable isotope-labeled amino acids (^{13}C-leucine) and showed that the synthesis time for secreted enzymes was no different to that measured in healthy subjects (Fig. 13.5 lower panel [128]). Thus, we concluded that it was still possible for proximal enteral feeding to stimulate pancreatic trypsinogen synthesis even in patients with pancreatic necrosis, and consequently the ideal feeding method should avoid pancreatic stimulation.

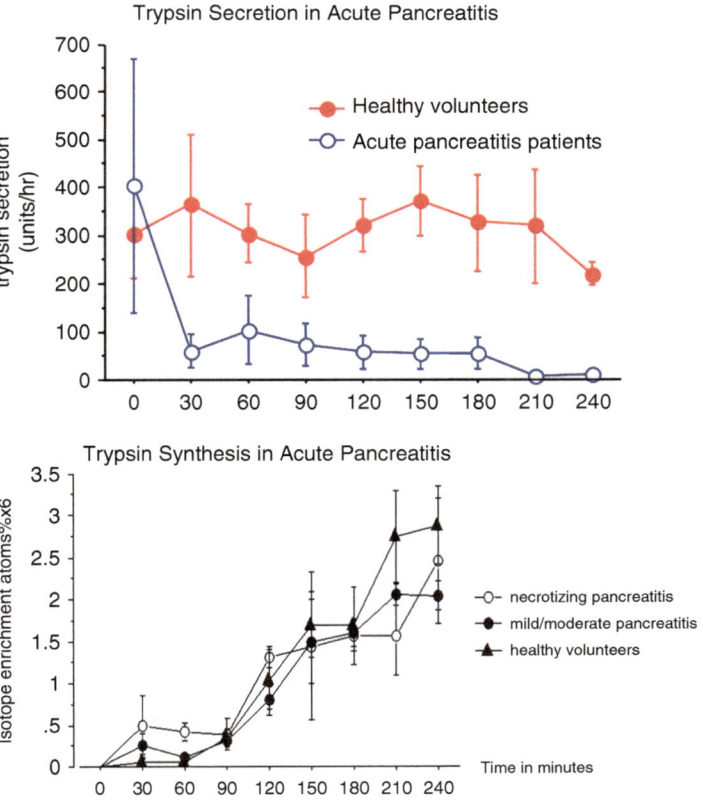

Fig. 13.5 Upper panel shows that luminal secretion of pancreatic enzymes is dramatically reduced in severe acute pancreatitis but, as shown in the lower panel, the pancreas retains its ability to synthesize new enzymes (lower panel, incorporation of labeled amino acids into trypsin protein) (*O'Keefe et al.* [128])

The "Ideal" Feeding Method

Based on the above discussion, in Pittsburgh we have championed the use of transnasal endoscopic placement of double-lumen gastric decompression, mid-jejunal feeding tubes (Chapter 8, p. 98 "Transnasal Endoscopic Placement of Feeding Tubes"), to deliver semi-elemental diets, in order to:

1. *Bypass the obstructed and dysfunctional upper GI tract.*
2. *Avoid the use of TPN and to maintain gut function distal to the stomach.*
3. *Provide enteral feeding without pancreatic stimulation.*
4. *Provide feeding in the form of a semi-elemental diet because enzyme secretion and therefore digestion can be compromised.*
5. *Decompress the obstructed stomach and reduce aspiration risk.*

The Europeans, however, favor the use of simple nasogastric feeding as NG tubes are placed routinely on arrival to the hospital in patients with acute abdominal conditions, providing enteral access for rapid commencement of early feeding. Several studies, including one of our own on 17 severely ill patients with APACHE II score of 14 (range 9–24), suggest that the earlier you start enteral feeding, the better the outcome [246], and an alternative approach may be to attempt to use the routinely placed NG tube for feeding on admission and to only convert to distal jejunal feeding if it is not tolerated. We conducted an NIH-supported clinical trial to determine the value of pancreatic rest in the final outcome, but only recruited 25 of the proposed 140 patients because the entry criteria were too tight. The preliminary results showed that "feeding failure" defined as failure to achieve a feeding rate of >10% of goal for a 48-h period occurred in 0/14 patients randomized to distal jejunal feeding and in 6/11 patients randomized to NG feeding (primarily due to nausea, vomiting, or GRVs >500 ml/4 h), necessitating cross-over to distal jejunal feeding. As a consequence, the quantity of feed delivered was significantly higher in distally fed patients. Taken together with our clinical experience, these results indicate that if you have the expertise to place double-lumen gastric decompression, distal jejunal (NGJ) feeding tubes (for instructions see Chapter 8, "Transnasal Endoscopic Placement of Feeding Tubes"), these tubes should be placed as soon as the patient has been resuscitated in the ICU.

How 'Early' is Early? The Dutch Pancreatitis Study Group have just published the first large scale RCT comparing early enteral feeding (n=101; a jejunal feeding tube placed a median of 23 hours after presentation at the emergency room, feeds started at 20cc/h for 24 hours, then increased gradually) to an offered oral diet (n=104) initiated 72 hours after admission [247]. If the oral diet was not tolerated, jejunal feeding was commenced (32% of patients). From what we have discussed in Chapter 5, it was not surprising that their 'composite' end point based on the development of major infection or death, was no different at the 6-month follow-up (Fig. 13.6). It is unlikely that the additional 48 hours of bowel rest that occurred in the orally-offered group would significantly affect outcome in a disease process that was already established. Furthermore, malnutrition was not the indication for nutritional intervention and so body stores were never seriously threatened. In addition, 'fucolysation' may well maintain luminal nutrition in this situation obviating the need for immediate enteral feeding (see Chapter 5,

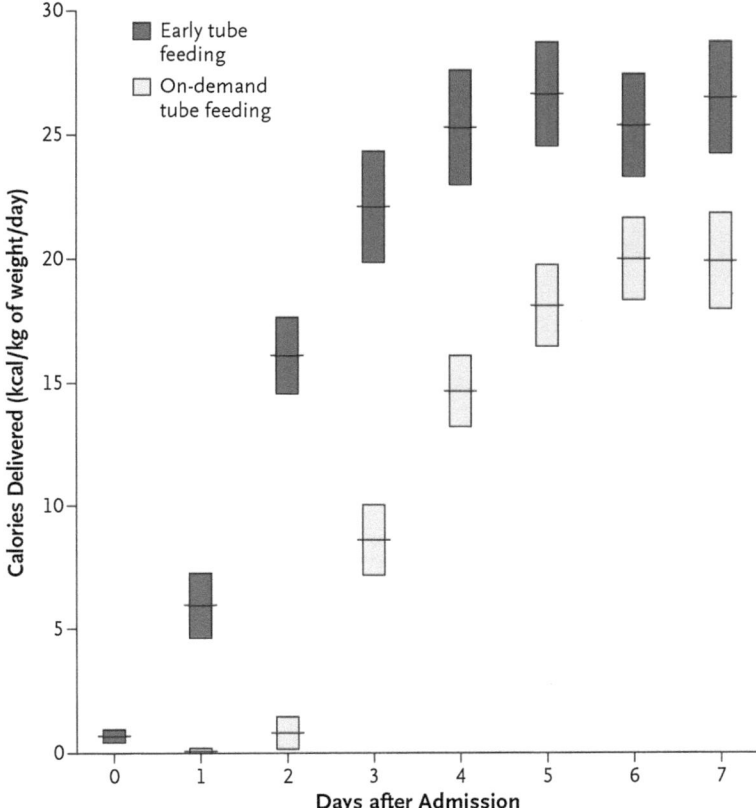

Fig. 13.6 Calories delivered with the use of early versus on-demand nasoenteric tube feeding in the management of acute pancreatitis [247]

[101]). Perhaps the most important thing to be illustrated by this study was the fact that nobody needed PN, and thus PN complications did not worsen outcome in either group!

The Practice

Prediction of Severity and Outcome

As discussed earlier, most patients (80%) admitted with acute pancreatitis recover rapidly and do not need nutritional support. The diagnosis is usually made by the combination of acute abdominal pain and >3× elevation of serum amylase and lipase. However, initial enzyme levels do not predict the severity or outcome. This has led to the search for predictors of severity on admission, because early aggressive management, including fluid resuscitation and commencement of enteral nutrition, reduces the systemic inflammatory response and organ failure and thus will

Table 13.1 Ranson's score for the prediction of severity of acute pancreatitis. A score >3 predicts poor outcome

Upon admission	48 h later
Age >55 years	Hematocrit fall >10%
WBC >16,000/mm^3	BUN rise >5 mg/dl
LDH >350 IU/l	Serum calcium <8 mg/dl
AST >250 IU/l	PaO$_2$ <60 mmHg
Glucose >200 mg/dl	Base deficit >4 mEq/l
	Fluid sequestration >6 l

Table 13.2 The systemic inflammatory response syndrome (SIRS)

The incidence and severity (*mild 2, moderate 3, severe 4* of the following criteria) defined by:
1. Temperature >38 °C or <36 °C
2. Pulse >90/min
3. Respiratory rate >20/min or PaCO$_2$ <32 mmHg (<4.3 kPa)
4. WBC >12,000 or <4,000 cells/mm^3 or >10% immature (band) forms

improve outcome from severe disease. The classic categorization is the Ranson's score (Table 13.1), which is based on commonly measured parameters such as hematocrit, WBC, blood gases, glucose, LFTs, BUN, calcium, and age [248]. Other indicators of disease severity such as C-reactive protein and the APACHE II score [249], based on multiple physiological parameters, are also useful but less commonly available. A recent study from the UK provided evidence that the simple systemic inflammatory score (SIRS) [250] (Table 13.2) based on temperature, pulse, respiratory rate, and WBC is predictive of the development of organ failure and mortality, particularly if it is resistant to treatment [250, 252]. These considerations have led to our use of the following criteria to predict who is likely to progress to the severe form of the disease, or who already has the severe form of the disease, and who will benefit from urgent establishment of enteral feeding:

Predictive

(a) The systemic inflammatory (SIRS) score >2.
(b) Ranson's criteria equal or >3.
(c) APACHE score equal or >8.

Established

(a) The presence of organ failure resistant to early aggressive IV fluid resuscitation as defined by a Marshall score [81] of 2 or more, excluding the liver component as the abnormality, may be due to gallstones rather than the systemic inflammatory response.
(b) Pancreatic necrosis >30% on CT scan or a CT severity index +/>5 [251].

In summary, recent studies have shown that early organ failure is possibly the best indicator of severity of illness as it correlates strongly with mortality. A CTSI of 5 or more was recently shown to be associated with an eightfold increase in mortality rate and a 17× increased chance of prolonged hospital stay and a 10× need for surgery [252]. The APACHE II score is probably the best *early* indicator of severity, as a score of >7 has an accuracy of predicting severe disease in 53–68% on admission, while a Ranson's score becomes maximally useful only at 48 h when a score >2 has a reported accuracy of 62–75%.

The need for a protocol for prediction of severity is important in practice, as it is important to start enteral feeding during the first week in patients with predicted severe disease, as the condition is invariably associated with ileus, *and ileus is more difficult to reverse once it becomes established.*

Feeding Protocol

1. *Use a semi-elemental formula* because it is less stimulatory and overcomes maldigestion. We have shown, as discussed above, that luminal enzyme secretion is often reduced >80% in acute pancreatitis—the level at which fat malabsorption commences—and so it is logical to use a semi-elemental formula, which also evokes less pancreatic stimulation [30].

2. *Start slowly, progress slowly.* It is of critical importance not to overburden the fragile gut with overfeeding, more than any other disease because of the pathophysiology described above. It is likely that the high complication rate of intestinal ischemia and mortality reported in the Dutch study on feeding and prebiotics was a result of the combination of high early feeding rates plus the injection of massive quantities of viable organisms [253]. Some have recommended that critically ill patients in the ICU needing pressors for poor cardiac outputs should not be given enteral feeding as it will precipitate gut ischemia. This doesn't make sense, as nutrients promote mucosal blood flow, but clearly mucosal function will be impaired, and feeding rates must be slow until overall perfusion improves. Most patients with this disease were previously well nourished; in fact, 60% of our patients are obese (particularly those with gallstone-induced disease), and so there is no rush to meet full nutritional requirements as supported by the second recent study from the Dutch group [247]. Enteral feeding is used chiefly to preserve mucosal and gut function; so "trophic" rates are appropriate. Fluids and electrolytes are maintained by IV infusions, watching renal and respiratory function closely.

   Start jejunal feeding at 20–25 cc/h for the first 24 h while maintaining low intermittent (50 mmHg) gastric suction. If tolerated and if the patient's general condition is stable, advance feeding to 50 cc/h for 24 h and then to goal (to provide 1.5 g of protein/kg ideal body weight/day) by day 3, maintaining gastric decompression. If gastric volumes are >500 cc/24 h, continue low intermittent suction. If less, clamp and check gastric residual 4–6 hourly as described in Chapter 8, "Transnasal Endoscopic Placement of Feeding Tubes".

3. *Avoid prophylactic antibiotics and PPIs*. Patients with SAP have all the signs of severe sepsis, with fever, very high white cell counts, and high C-reactive proteins, and the urge to start broad-spectrum IV antibiotics (e.g., meropenem) and even antifungal (e.g., caspofungin) is high. However, this is often a consequence of pancreatic necrosis and not infection, and controlled studies, and their meta-analysis, do not show that they improve outcome [254, 255]. In fact, they might impair outcome by their detrimental effect on the gut microbiota, and studies of ours have shown that the combination of IV PPIs and antibiotics is commonly associated with diarrhea and dysbiosis, raising the risk of *C. difficile* infections [34].

4. *Avoid early surgery and home enteral feeding*. Another urge that needs to be suppressed is the urge to perform surgery. In the early stages, weeks 1–2, of SAP, the patient has an "acute abdomen," with severe pain, distension, rebound tenderness, and high white cell counts: a constellation of signs that normally indicate the need for a laparotomy. Surgery under these conditions is hazardous producing more harm than good, as the pancreatic inflammatory mass usually involves all local organs, and a demarcation plane is absent. Indeed, outcome studies have indicated that mortality is reduced if surgery can be delayed 4–6 weeks, or avoided, by conservative management [256]. Since the gut is obstructed, interventional feeding is essential to allow conservative management to work. Previously, TPN was used, but the risk of sepsis from central vein catheters, plus the inevitable hyperglycemia discussed above, precludes its use, and NGJ feeding is the best supportive management. Our experience shows that patients commonly recover almost completely with the exception of a blocked upper GI tract because of the cystic mass. Withdrawal of the tube and oral feeding will result in persistent vomiting and aspiration risk. So, in such patients, we discharge them home on home NGJ enteral feeding (14–18 h cyclical nocturnal infusions with a fiber-supplemented semi-elemental formula, not exceeding 100 cc/h). Despite the gastric outlet obstruction, vomiting is not usually a problem if the patient remains NPO, but if it is, they are taught how to decompress their stomachs through the G-port on the NGJ tube. In this way, they are safely managed at home until (a) spontaneous resolution of the cystic collection, manifested by oral tolerance to fluids, with subsequent weaning back onto normal food, or (b) elective surgical, endoscopic, or radiological cyst decompression at 4–6 weeks [116].

5. *Add soluble fiber* to the formula after day 7, e.g., 4–8 g three times a day, to ameliorate the problem outlined in 3 above [34]. The most physiological way of doing this is to dissolve the fiber in a minimum volume of water and add to the feed so that it can be given together as a constant jejunal infusion. As mentioned in Chapter 9, it is best to avoid boluses >30 cc down the J-tube.

6. *Wean as soon as upper GI function returns*. In patients with mild and moderate disease, gastric emptying is usually adequate as patients can be slowly weaned back on to normal feeding as soon as symptoms, notable abdominal pain,

resolve. However, patients with SAP have a bimodal course with regard to feeding. Initially, interventional enteral feeding is required to overcome upper GI dysfunction, with poor gastric emptying and poor motility, and to feed without stimulating the pancreas. However, in the second week, the inflammatory response settles, and the disease begins to resolve with lysis of the necrosis and the formation of cystic fluid collections. Unfortunately, these collections prevent the resumption of normal eating, as they exacerbate the outlet obstruction problems. Hence, deep jejunal feeding and gastric decompression are still needed to maintain enteral feeding. Pancreatic rest becomes less important, unless the disease is complicated by pancreatic duct rupture and pseudocyst formation (Fig. 13.8). Resolution of the obstruction can be identified by a drop in gastric residual volumes and the absence of nausea and vomiting. A trial of oral fluids is then appropriate, and if tolerated, feeding can be progressed through full liquids to a soft and then low-fat (20 g/day) diet. Remarkably, digestive function usually returns to normal, even in patients who have lost much of their pancreas to necrosis, but exogenous enzyme supplements may be helpful during the weaning–recovery stage.

The Nutritional Management of Pancreatic Fluid Collections

As illustrated in Figs. 13.7 and 13.8, there are multiple reasons for upper GI dysfunction in patients with pancreatic diseases. First, there is the scenario in SAP, as described above, where the pancreas and surrounding tissues become massively inflamed and swollen, producing what has been termed a "phlegmon." This distorts and compresses the stomach and duodenum producing gastric outlet and duodenal obstruction. Failure of the upper GI tract is exacerbated by the reductions in motility associated with the cytokine storm and systemic inflammatory response. Here, the use of the NGJ tube is essential (a) to overcome the obstruction and feed into the open jejunum and (b) to place the tip of the jejunal feeding tube approximately 40 cm past the ligament of Treitz in order to maintain pancreatic rest to allow the disease process and inflammation to resolve. Second, gastroduodenal obstruction can occur from pancreatic cystic fluid collections resulting from pancreatic duct injury with leakage of secretions in more established post-acute or acute-on-chronic or chronic pancreatitis. Here, an NGJ tube is useful (a) to overcome the obstruction and feed into the open jejunum and (b) to maintain pancreatic rest to allow the leak to heal. Unfortunately, in patients with chronic disease, pancreatic rest will reduce the size of the cyst, but when normal feeding is resumed, the cyst will recur. Consequently, NGJ feeding is more successful in obtaining spontaneous resolutions in the acute than chronic situation, and recurrence in chronic patients should be treated with endoscopic stenting.

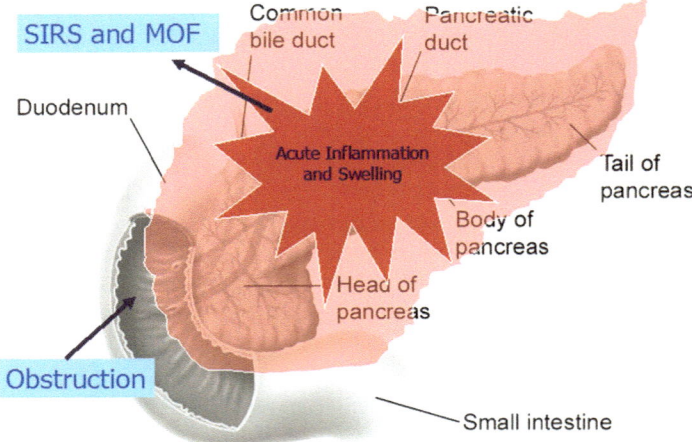

Fig. 13.7 Severe acute pancreatitis: dysfunction of the upper GI tract due to inflammatory swelling of the pancreas with gastroduodenal compression and impaired motility

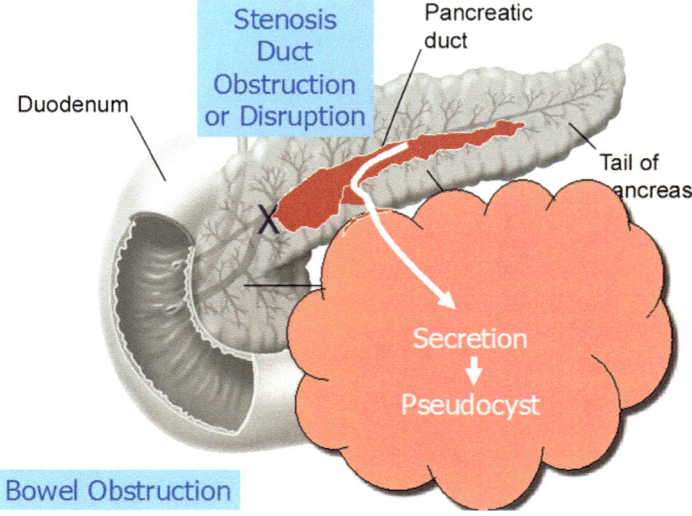

Fig. 13.8 Post-acute, acute-on-chronic, or chronic pancreatitis resulting in pancreatic duct rupture, stenosis or obstruction, pancreatic juice leakage, and pseudocyst formation

Chronic Pancreatitis

Principles

As with the small intestine and the liver, there is tremendous functional reserve in pancreatic exocrine function, and malabsorption due to maldigestion only develops after >90% of the enzyme secretion is lost [42]. Despite the commercial development of potent pancreatic enzyme supplements, it is currently rarely possible to restore normal digestion once pancreatic steatorrhea has developed [257, 258]. This well illustrates the fine orchestration of pancreatic secretion in response to feeding, as it is impossible to mimic the timing and quantitative release of enzymes from the pancreas into the digesta by giving them by mouth. For example, it has been estimated that the normal pancreas releases 60,000 U of lipase per day. Consequently, a daily supplementation of 60,000 U should prevent steatorrhea. However, when we performed a controlled study in 29 patients with pancreatic insufficiency and gave the active therapy group supplements amounting to 160,000 U per day (given as four capsules containing 10,000 lipase units per capsule with meals and two with snacks), steatorrhea remained in 70% [261]. Explanations probably include the incomplete release and mixing of enzymes with the digesta and the presence of secondary mucosal abnormalities due to pancreatic endocrine insufficiency, malnutrition, and/or bacterial overgrowth.

The Vicious Cycle

End Stage Pancreatitis or Pancreatic Failure

In advanced chronic pancreatitis, the progressive deterioration of pancreatic exocrine and endocrine function converges to have a massive impact on gut function and nutrition. Exocrine deficiency alone will impair the digestion and thus absorption of food, resulting in progressive loss of body stores and malnutrition. Malnutrition will exacerbate the situation, as the pancreas has one of the highest demands for amino acids within the body, and a reduction in their supply will suppress enzyme synthesis, culminating in further reductions in enzyme secretion and digestive capacity. Malnutrition also impairs mucosal growth and repair, reduces acid secretion, promotes bacterial overgrowth, and can be a primary cause of malabsorption as discussed in Chapter 3. The supply of pancreatic enzyme supplements may initially help break the cycle, but as pancreatic endocrine failure develops, the cycle can develop momentum again. First, the development of hyperglycemia will lead to disturbance of gastrointestinal motility, leading to stasis, bacterial overgrowth, interference with nutrient–enzyme interaction, diarrhea, and malabsorption. Secondly, it must be remembered that insulin is one of the most powerful anabolic hormones of the body, and deficiency will impair the utilization of absorbed nutrients for all body functions. We tend to focus on the importance of insulin in glucose metabolism, but insulin is also essential for protein and fat storage and utilization. So, even if digestion and absorption can be increased with enzyme supplements, insulin deficiency will impair the utilization of the absorbed amino acids for pancreatic enzyme synthesis, as well as for mucosal regeneration and villus function. Thus, the whole process of digestion, absorption, and regeneration will be impaired – unless the provision of pancreatic enzyme supplements is covered by a regular supply of insulin.

Pancreatic Diabetes Is "Brittle" Diabetes

Perhaps the most important clinical observation in the controlled study in 29 patients with pancreatic insufficiency mentioned above was the ability for potent enzyme supplements to produce potentially life-threatening disturbances in glucose control of insulin-dependent patients with diabetes. On restarting pancreatic mini-microspheres, one patient developed hyperglycemic ketoacidosis due to increased glucose absorption, and on discontinuing, two developed symptomatic hypoglycemia due to overtreatment with insulin, necessitating hospitalization. As illustrated in Fig. 13.9, the management of exocrine failure can be fraught with difficulty because of the "brittle" nature of the diabetes. *The distinction from classic diabetes mellitus (type 1) is important as chronic pancreatitis damages not only the β-insulin-producing islet cells but also the α cells, δ cells, and F or D1 cells that secrete the counter-regulatory hormones, glucagon, somatostatin, and pancreatic polypeptide.*

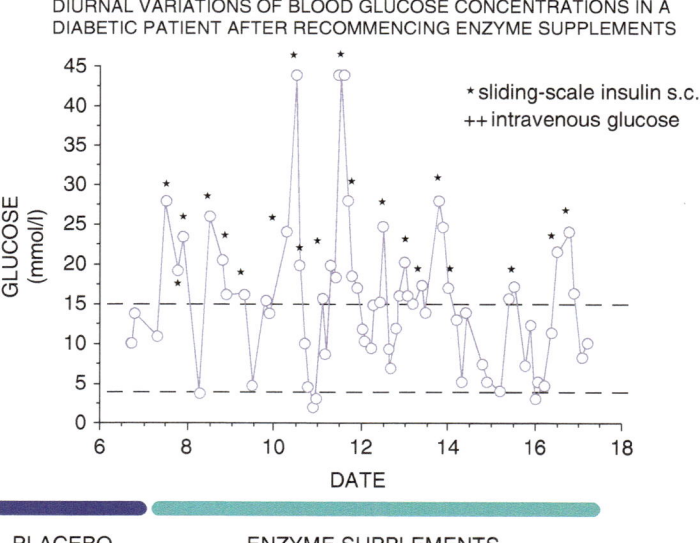

Fig. 13.9 "Brittle diabetes." Diurnal variations in blood glucose concentrations in a diabetic patient after recommencing enzyme supplements. *Asterisk* indicates sliding-scale insulin subcutaneously; ++, intravenous glucose

For this reason, the condition has been termed pancreatogenic diabetes, or type 3c diabetes, which can be diagnosed by an absent pancreatic polypeptide (or absent glucagon) response to mixed-nutrient ingestion or hypoglycemia. It is because of the lack of both regulatory and counter-regulatory hormones that hypoglycemia is particularly dangerous in pancreatic patients with diabetes and accounts for more deaths than does hyperglycemia. For example, the "usual" dose of insulin may precipitate profound unopposed hypoglycemia and life-threatening neuroglycopenia, if the rate of absorption of glucose drops because of a missed meal or forgotten enzyme supplementation. The risk is further increased in malnourished patients who have depleted glycogen stores.

The Practice

Nutritional care is commonly overlooked in the management of chronic pancreatitis; most attention is given to imaging the pancreas and the symptoms that patients complain of, namely, chronic abdominal pain and disturbed gut function. However, as discussed above, the pancreas is in essence the heart of digestion, absorption, and metabolism, and closer attention to what the pancreas is supposed to do will, and to what patients eat and how they eat, inevitably lead to improved overall care, health, and quality of life. Progressive weight loss and the development of diabetes are red flags and should direct management to the investigation of food intake and the need for pancreatic enzyme and insulin supplementation. However, it must be remembered that serious nutritional deficiencies can develop without weight loss earlier in the disease as a consequence of mild chronic malabsorption and poor food consumption—particularly in alcoholics. Fat malabsorption coupled to fat-soluble vitamin malabsorption can result in progressive calcium and vitamin D deficiency, leading to fracture risk and associated comorbidities [260].

The two key problems to look out for are the development of pancreatic insufficiency and diabetes. We suggest the following routine investigations in the clinic in anyone with established chronic pancreatitis:

1. Monitor CBC and CMP.

   (a) If hemoglobin is low, measure iron, TIBC, folate, and B12: if low, give oral supplements.
   (b) If glucose is abnormal, measure HbA_{1c}.
   (c) If HbA_{1c} is >6.5, measure 75 g 2-h glucose tolerance. If any value >200 mg/dl or if BMI <18.5, refer to endocrinology for insulin therapy and joint management (see below).

2. Monitor BMI: red flag if BMI <18.5 kg/m^2.

   (a) Ask dietitian to assess dietary intake.
   (b) Measure fecal elastase or endoscopic duodenal enzymes concentrations (see below).

(c) Measure fecal fat: first. see whether there is an "excess" in a fecal sample; if so, measure 72-h fecal fat, making sure the patient is eating normally and consuming at least 80 g of fat per day.

(d) If either (b) or (c) is abnormal, commence a trial of enteric coated pancreatic enzyme supplements, e.g., Creon (Abbott Labs, Chicago, Il) 10,000 capsules, four with meals, two with snacks (see below).

Management of Weight Loss

1. *Check Intake*: First, make sure the weight loss is not due to chronic anorexia and poor dietary intake. Ask your dietitian to measure usual intakes and to recommend dietary changes and the use of nutritional supplements. The supplements should contain a balanced mixture of all essential nutrients, but in complex form, particularly the carbohydrate with low glycemic indices.

2. *Check Fat Absorption*: If dietary intake is adequate and the above measures are ineffective, check a fecal sample for fat excess. If it is possible, collect stools for 72 h when the patient consumes a diet containing at least 80 g of fat per day. If there is more than 10 g of fat/day in stools, the patient has fat malabsorption. Characteristically, the fat malabsorption in CP is much higher (>20 g/day) than in other diseases, such as mucosal diseases, resulting in classical steatorrhea. In severe steatorrhea, the stools are not only pale in color (note all stools are offensive!) but oil droplets may be seen floating in the toilet bowl after defecation. In this situation, no testing is necessary; start enzyme supplements immediately.

3. *Check Pancreatic Enzyme Secretion*: Many of us spent years developing methods to measure pancreatic enzyme function in clinical practice. The conventional method was to place a double-lumen perfusion–aspiration tube across a 20-cm section of the mid-duodenum and stimulate pancreatic secretion with CCK and secretin, CCK-8, or food or a liquid diet infusion and to aspirate samples every 30 min for 2–4 h, using a PEG marker to calculate amylase, trypsin, and lipase secretions. Figure 13.10 shows that there was a relationship between pancreatic structural damage detected by radiology and pancreatic secretion induced by feeding. Consequently, as CT exams are easy to do (and done in nearly every patient with chronic or acute disease!), while the conventional method for the measurement of secretion is technically challenging, secretion is rarely measured outside research studies. This has led to the search for less invasive methods.

   Next, we examined the use of radio-labeled fat (^{14}C-triolein) and later stable isotope-labeled fat (^{13}C-triolein) given as a bolus drink and measured the secretion of the metabolite, $^{14}CO_2$, in the breath as an index of digestion, absorption, and metabolism [259]. As this might also be abnormal in patients with mucosal disease, the test was repeated with pancreatic enzymes, allowing differentiation, as pancreatic malabsorption would have been improved with enzymes.

   Finally, we developed a *simple endoscopic test*, whereby a normal EGD was performed and duodenal juice was aspirated by the endoscope from the area

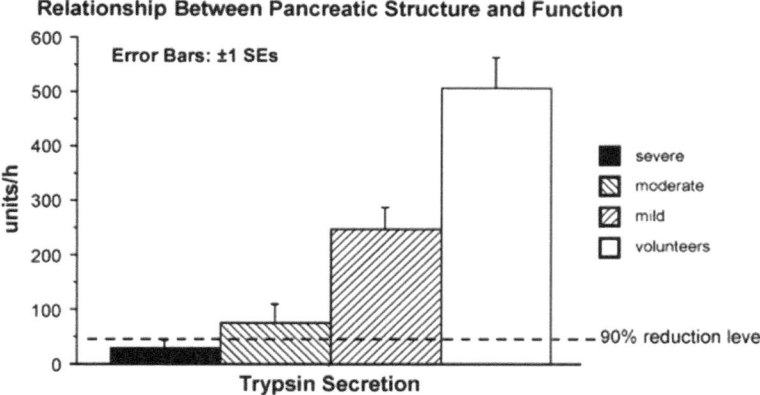

Fig. 13.10 Illustrates the relation between pancreatic structure defined by radiological imaging and pancreatic exocrine function defined by the trypsin secretory response to continuous enteral feeding over a 2-h period. Secretion was significantly reduced in patients with mild ($P=0.001$), moderate ($P=0.0005$), and severe structural disease p<0.0001 (O'Keefe et al. 2007 [262])

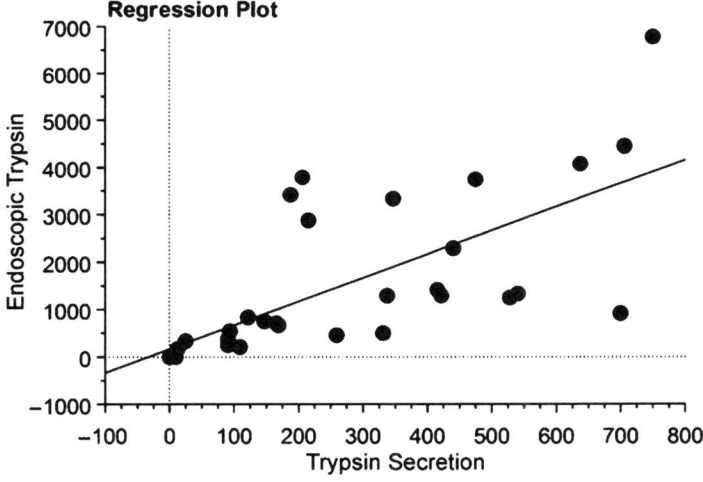

Fig. 13.11 The association between trypsin secretion measured over 2 h in response to feeding and the initial trypsin concentration in duodenal juice aspirated at endoscopy. The correlation was significant ($r^2=0.48$, $P<0.0001$) [260]

adjacent to the ampulla of Vater 5 min after the injection of 20 ml of Ensure into the mid-duodenum. Our results showed that the concentration of enzymes in the aspirated juice correlated well with conventional 2-h secretion studies (Fig. 13.11), allowing the detection of all patients with pancreatic insufficiency [262]. Most hospital labs can do enzyme measurement as an extension of their blood tests for amylase and lipase. The most commonly used test today is the measurement of elastase in fecal samples. Unlike most other secreted pancreatic enzymes that are degraded on their journey down the GI tract, elastase is more resistant, and studies have shown that its concentration in stools is related to pancreatic function—provided the patient does not have diarrhea [263].

4. *Pancreatic Enzyme Supplementation*: Advances in manufacturing have led to the development of high lipase supplements, generally of pig origin, in the form of mini-microspheres contained within gastric acid-resistant capsules, which, when taken with meals, are designed to empty with broken down food particles <2 mm in diameter and be released in the alkaline medium of the duodenum and so get to work digesting. The chief problem is the size and quantity of supplements required, for example, four capsules with meals, two with snacks, or about 500 per month. This exemplifies the remarkably high enzyme synthesis rate of the exocrine pancreas. There is no need for simultaneous acid suppression with PPIs; in fact, this might decrease efficacy by promoting bacterial overgrowth. In patients with malnutrition and diarrhea, it is sometimes more effective to instruct patients to break the capsules and scatter the contents on their meals and to use anti-motility drugs, such as Imodium, to slower the transit in order to give them more time to act.

5. *Treatment of Pancreatic Endocrine Insufficiency*: As discussed above, the onset of diabetes is often insidious and can result in unexpected changes in nutrition. Thus, regular monitoring in the clinic, as outlined above, is essential. Unlike pancreatic exocrine supplementation, endocrine supplementation is only available for insulin, and glucagon, somatostatin, and pancreatic polypeptide replacement is not currently available. This differentiates the management from that of type 1 diabetes, where insulin alone is deficient and where profound hypoglycemia is attenuated by the release of counter-regulatory hormones such as glucagon, which generates gluconeogenesis. Thus, treatment is more complex and difficult, as illustrated by Fig. 13.9, and it is imperative to refer patients to an endocrinologist for commencement and supervision of diabetes. Patient education is critically important with pancreatogenic diabetes, particularly with regard to the prevention and treatment of hypoglycemia:

   (a) Advise patients to *never* inject insulin if unable to eat for any reason.
   (b) Under controlled conditions, allow patients to experience symptoms of early hypoglycemia so that they know urgent action is needed to prevent neuroglycopenia.
   (c) Always carry glucose supplements, or sugar drinks, and take immediately if symptoms occur.

Chapter 14
Liver Disease

Nutritional Immunological Interactions

The liver is often considered the "heart of metabolism", complimenting the functions of the pancreas in digestion, absorption, and assimilation. It tightly regulates the flow of digested and absorbed nutrients throughout the body and maintains their distribution to support vital organ function during fasting and starvation. Consequently, liver dysfunction has a major impact on nutritional requirements and our ability to withstand feast and famine. Furthermore, appetite is often poor in patients with chronic liver disease resulting in chronic malnutrition. The degree of wasting is often masked by fluid retention and edema. In a study of 156 patients admitted to hospital with liver disease, we found that weight/height was within the normal range for all chronic liver disease subgroups, except those with carcinoma [118]. However, triceps skinfold thickness (TSF) was reduced in 49% of patients with cirrhosis and 55% with alcoholic disease. Hypoalbuminemia was common in all groups, with 66% of those with chronic disease having concentrations below 3.5 g/l. As we were concerned that protein deficiency might account for the high rates of spontaneous infections (e.g., peritonitis), in our patients we correlated nutritional parameters with blood lymphocyte counts and reactivity to skin testing with common antigens. Lymphopenia was common with 65% of patients with fulminant hepatic failure (FHF) having counts below 1,000 cells/mm^3. Incidence of total anergy to standard skin tests was 54% overall: 93% in FHF and 60% in cirrhosis and alcoholic disease. There were significant links between reduced TSF and hypoalbuminemia, lymphopenia and anergy, hypoalbuminemia and anergy, and anergy and mortality. Reduced TSF was only associated with anergy in patients with chronic disease. We concluded that the high incidence of immuno-incompetence may underlie the frequent occurrence of spontaneous infections in patients with liver disease and that the association between anergy and malnutrition in patients with chronic liver disease suggested that the anergy may be partly reversible by dietary intervention.

© Springer Science+Business Media New York 2015
S.J.D. O'Keefe, *The Principles and Practice of Nutritional Support*,
DOI 10.1007/978-1-4939-1779-2_14

Table 14.1 Explanations why the liver is essential for nutritional homeostasis. It contains the enzymes essential for the distribution of body fuels during feast and famine

Key enzymes: carbohydrate homeostasis
- *Hepatic hexokinase*: inducable to hepatic portal glucose concentrations of >70,000 mg/dl
- *Glycogen synthetase*: activated when glucose >150 mg/dl
- *Hepatic glucose-6-phosphatase*: activated when glucose <60 mg/dl - glucose release into the bloodstream

Key enzymes: protein metabolism
- *Aromatic amino acid oxidases* tyrosine, tryptophan and phenylalanine clearance
- *Carbamoyl phosphate synthetase* ammonia clearance and urea synthesis

Key enzymes: fat metabolism
- *Acylase* and keto-adaptation in starvation
- Normal glucose requirement of the brain 100–150 g/day. In starvation relative increase in fat oxidation and ketone production by the liver. Acylase permits liberation of free ketones into the bloodstream which substitute 70% of glucose as fuel source for the brain

Table 14.2 Key features that change nutritional requirements in patients with liver failure

Nutritional problems in liver failure

- Can't fast, nor feast
- Hypoglycemia
- Protein and carbohydrate intolerance
- Fat intolerance

However, remember that metabolism is an integrated process, and defects in one pathway will invariable coexist with defects in others

Nutritional support in liver failure

OBJECTIVE:
- Composition of infused nutrients should be designed to nullify the known metabolic abnormalities and thus maintain homeostasis

- *The Liver is the Heart of Metabolism:* As discussed in Chapter 2, the liver enables us to survive through feast and famine. It does this by regulating the flow of nutrients throughout the body and maintaining carbohydrate, protein, and fat homeostasis (Tables 14.1 and 14.2). First, hepatic hexokinase is inducible to hepatic portal glucose concentrations of >70,000 mg/dl allowing the body to tolerate high rates of carbohydrate feeding. At the same time, glycogen synthetase is induced when portal concentrations exceed 150 mg/dl. On the other hand, during starvation, the liver prevents blood glucose from dropping below 60 mg/dl by the activation of hepatic glucose-6-phosphatase which releases glucose from glycogen into the bloodstream. Thus, in liver failure, enteral feeding will produce uncontrolled increases in system glucose flow and hyperglycemia, while in fasting, blood concentrations will drop precipitously producing neuroglycopenia. With regard to protein metabolism, the liver also prevents excessive swings in plasma amino acid levels through feast and starvation and also prevents the accumulation of toxic protein breakdown products, such as ammonia. The increased flow of amino acids following a meal is accommodated by induction of hepatic amino acid oxidases. This results in increased ammonia production, which in turn induces hepatic carbamoyl phosphatase synthetase, which increases ureagenesis and renal excretion. In liver failure, this control mechanism is lost, and excessive quantities of amino acids flow into the systemic circulation. Muscle contains enzymes that oxidize branched-chain amino acids, but not aromatic amino acids, and so an amino acid imbalance occurs in the plasma [135, 265]. The failing liver cannot also detoxify ammonia into urea synthesis, and so ammonia also accumulates in the bloodstream. Finally, the liver plays an essential role in ketoadaptation to starvation, as it alone contains the enzyme, acylase, responsible for ketogenesis. With fasting beyond 48 h, hepatic glycogen stores are spent, and energy provision transitions from glucose to predominantly fat oxidation. Insulin levels drop, and insulin-sensitive lipase activity increases resulting in higher rates of release of free fatty acids from adipose tissue. Blood levels rise. Increased hepatic fat oxidation results in induction of *acylase*, which permits liberation of free ketones into the bloodstream. Ketones substitute for 70% of glucose demand by the brain, reducing the need for gluconeogenesis from protein catabolism and suppressing ureagenesis. In liver failure, this process is disrupted. The ability to withstand even a short fast is impaired by the failure of the liver to synthesize and store glycogen, coupled to its impaired ability to oxidize amino acids for gluconeogenesis. Secondly, ketogenesis is also impaired. This explains why patients with liver failure can easily drop into coma during short-term fasting with permanent brain damage. The dramatic changes in blood concentrations with depletion in urea, glucose, and glycolysis metabolites and increases in ammonia, glutamine, and aromatic amino acids have been associated with hepatic encephalopathy and have been indicted as an etiological factor via increasing tryptophan transport across the blood–brain barrier and disturbing serotonin synthesis [265–267]. It also explains the results of the studies, which have shown that mental performance is improved in patients with chronic liver dysfunction given a late evening meal.

Principles of Treatment and Management

The role of nutritional support in liver failure is to take over the role of the liver in maintaining a constant flow of nutrients to vital organs (Table 14.2). The composition of infused nutrients should be designed to nullify the known metabolic abnormalities and thus maintain homeostasis. First, it is crucial that patients with liver failure are given constant infusions of feeds, delivering 100–200 g glucose daily. Second, provide moderate quantities of protein and fat, and avoid excessive infusions. Third, renal function is often impaired through the hepatorenal syndrome: restrict salt and water to prevent fluid overload. Third, liver injury and failure is associated with increased loss of vitamin and trace element stores. Monitor blood levels and supplement appropriately. Digestion is usually well maintained, and post-pyloric tube feeding is preferable to IV feeding as it optimizes hepatic regeneration and avoids excessive blood fluctuations, although a 5% dextrose drip is usually given simultaneously, as backup. As discussed in Chapter 5, p. 39, "Why Is Enteral Feeding Superior", there is good evidence for compartmentation within the liver such that IV-delivered nutrients will be less well utilized by the liver than enterally delivered nutrients which enter via the portal bloodstream.

Defining Protein Requirements

As a result of the concern about the association between blood ammonia and encephalopathy, the standard management of liver failure up to the 1980s was dietary protein restriction to approximately 20 g/day. To assess the nutritional wisdom of this practice, we measured protein metabolism in patients with cirrhosis and fulminant hepatic failure, employing amino acid isotope-labeled infusion techniques [132]. The results showed that the increases in plasma aromatic amino acid concentrations was mostly due to large increases in the breakdown of endogenous body proteins (988 g/day in fulminant hepatic failure (FHF), 447 g/day in cirrhosis, compared to normal 276 g/day) and not to dietary intake. In addition, although amino acid oxidation was decreased, it continued, and even patients with fulminant hepatic failure lost the equivalent of 25 g/day, which had to be replaced in order to prevent progressive protein depletion. Our calculations suggested that approximately 40–45 g of high biological value protein would be needed in patients with cirrhosis or liver failure to prevent protein deficiency. In follow-up studies, we showed that the infusion of diets containing 60–80 g/day not only prevented protein loss but also suppressed endogenous protein breakdown [135], laying the foundation for modern nutritional management which advocates the use of nutritional formulae that contain moderate quantities of protein, i.e., 80 g/day, and sufficient glucose (150 g/day) to supple basic energy needs as well as suppressing endogenous protein catabolism and the need for gluconeogenesis. Studies of ours have also shown that hepatic protein synthesis can be increased by correcting the abnormal amino acid pattern with a "liver-specific" dietary formula enriched with branched-chain amino acids and low in aromatic amino acids [134] (Fig. 14.1). This information has supported the design and manufacture of "specialized" enteral and parenteral diets for patients with liver failure, e.g., IV Branchamin, Baxter-Travenol, Deerfield Ill, or enteral Hepatonutril, Oxford Nutritionals, UK. There has been much discussion on their efficacy in clinical practice. An early meta-analysis by Naylor et al. concluded that the most conservative interpretation of the published data yielded a significant reduction in mortality ($p=0.023$) [267]. However, given the uncertainty about effects on mortality and short follow-up times in all studies, a confirmatory randomized controlled trial with longer follow-up periods was warranted. Since that time, three further meta-analyses have been published chiefly focusing on their beneficial effects on hepatic encephalopathy, which has led ESPEN to give them a Grade A recommendation for the treatment of hepatic encephalopathy [268].

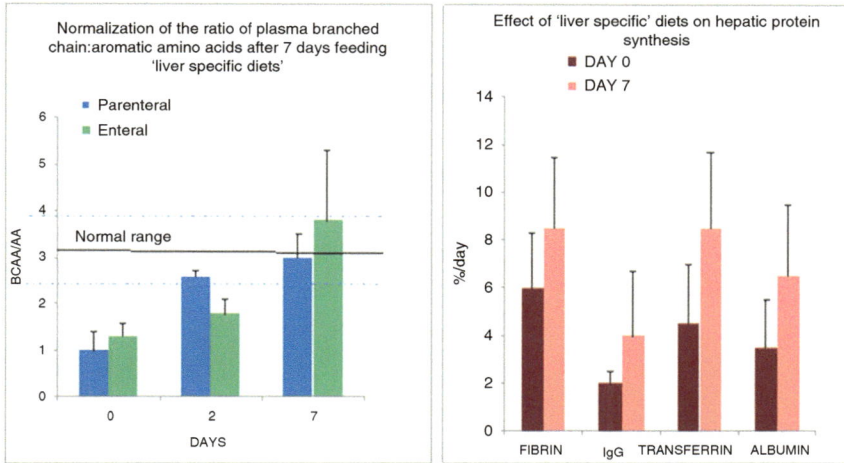

Fig. 14.1 Illustration of the characteristic plasma amino acid imbalance between branched-chain and aromatic amino acids seen in patients with liver failure and their response to enteral and parenteral feeding "liver-specific" formulae designed to nullify the derangement. This was associated with significant increases in hepatic protein synthesis measured by IV infusions of isotope-labeled amino acids (O'Keefe et al. [134])

Practice

Non-encephalopathic Patients

Most of the nutritional problems in patients with chronic liver disease are due to insufficient dietary intake and due to anorexia that accompanies the disease. So, first, assess dietary intake, and consult your dietitian to provide advice on increasing normal feeding or provide nutritionally balanced supplements, such as "Boost," "Ensure," or "Carnation Instant Breakfast." This is particularly important in patients awaiting liver transplantation. In tube-fed patients, use a standard polymeric diet at a rate to provide 1.0 g protein/kg ideal body weight/day. Fluid and salt restriction is mandatory in patients with ascites, accompanied with the use of potassium-retaining diuretics if resistant. There is good evidence that the retention of both water- and fat-soluble vitamins is reduced in patients with chronic liver disease, so all patients should be given daily oral supplements.

Liver Failure or Encephalopathic Patients

1. Avoid periods of fasting: Provide a constant infusion of a standard polymeric diet delivering at least 150–200 g of carbohydrate and 60 g of protein per day preferably by duodenal feeding tube, but don't waste time and use IV infusions if a tube is difficult to place initially.

2. Monitor BUN, plasma ammonia and glucose, and INR: They are all indicators of liver function in these patients. Failure of BUN to rise and a low glucose concentration during the above feeding indicate severe liver failure, as does an increasing blood ammonia and prothrombin time, and likely need for urgent liver transplantation. This would be the indication to switch to a "liver-specific" formula enriched with BCAA, low in AA, high in glucose-maltodextrin, low in sodium, and low in volume.

Chapter 15
Renal Disease

The Principles

The kidney is also a key metabolic organ. Consequently, renal failure affects not only the quantity but also the composition of nutritional requirements. The kidney's most critical functions include the control of fluid and electrolyte balance and the excretion of potentially toxic metabolites. For example, the kidney is responsible for the excretion of water, electrolytes, and nitrogenous breakdown products, including urea, creatinine, and ammonia. As diet and body stores influence the production rate of all these substances, it was not surprising that early management principles advised the restriction of their intake, particularly with regard to protein, which is the precursor for urea and ammonia. However, as with liver failure, the restriction of protein intake was eventually shown to worsen survival as no or low protein diets accelerate the catabolism of body proteins, and patients became progressively malnourished. Infusions of glucose or high-carbohydrate diets were shown to reduce the rate of catabolism as outlined in Chapter 4: "Protein Catabolism" but couldn't prevent the progressive depletion of body protein. Hypothesizing that metabolic balance would best be achieved if only essential amino acids (EAA) were given for the protein component of nutritional support allowing the liver to reincorporate nitrogen oxidative products into the synthesis of nonessential amino acids (NEAA), while simultaneously infusing glucose to prevent protein catabolism, Abel et al performed a prospective double-blind study in patients with acute renal failure (ARF) [269]. Results were encouraging, demonstrating the apparent ability of infusions of EAA and dextrose to improve survival. However, a later study showed that a balanced amino acid mixture was equally effective in maintaining nitrogen balance and suppressing blood urea nitrogen (BUN) concentrations, with no difference in survival [270, 271]. Further concern about the use of EAA was raised by the observation of mental status changes associated with metabolic side effects in children and adults with ARF treated with EAA. Investigation revealed hyperammonemia and hyperchloremic metabolic

© Springer Science+Business Media New York 2015
S.J.D. O'Keefe, *The Principles and Practice of Nutritional Support*,
DOI 10.1007/978-1-4939-1779-2_15

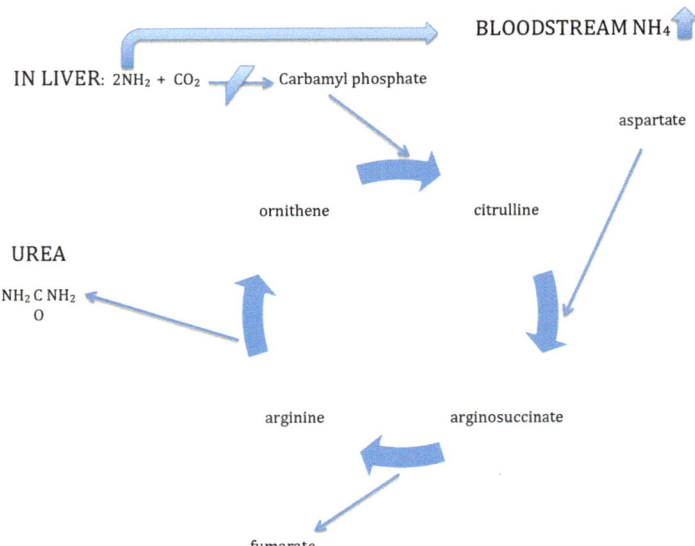

Fig. 15.1 Explanation for the metabolic complications caused by giving essential amino acids alone as a protein source in patients with acute renal failure. Insufficient dietary inessential amino acids result in depletion of citrulline, ornithine, and arginine which are essential for function of the urea cycle. Failure of the urea cycle to incorporate ammonia derived from protein catabolism results in hyperammonemia and mental status changes

acidosis, elevated plasma methionine and ammonia, and depressed plasma citrulline, ornithine, arginine, and histidine levels [272, 273]. The explanation for this appeared to be impairment of the capacity of key urea cycle intermediates (ornithine and citrulline) to accept ammonia from carbamoyl phosphate (Fig. 15.1). In general, controlled clinical trials of the use of specialized nutritional formula for ARF have yielded variable and disappointing results. For example, a recent Cochrane Database meta-analysis examined 8 eligible studies (257 participants) but were unable to perform a pooled analysis because different interventions and different outcomes were employed [274].

The Practice

Appreciation of the results of the above studies has led to the recommendations that, despite the ability of protein restriction to suppress BUN increases, protein restrictions below 0.5 g/kg/day should be avoided. The use of EAA alone should be avoided, but proteins of high biological value (i.e., high EAA:NEAA) should be provided with adequate quantities of energy, chiefly in the form of carbohydrate (4 g/kg/day). As with every other clinical condition, nutritional support should be given by enteral route. Anorexia and delayed gastric emptying are common in chronic renal failure, and supplemental tube feeding may be necessary. In acute renal failure, protein restriction must be avoided as patients are catabolic: increases in BUN, phosphate, and potassium should be treated with timely dialysis. Once established on dialysis, nutritional requirements return to those used in any form of critical illness, namely, protein (or balanced amino acid formulae in PN-fed patients) infusion rates of 1.5 g/kg ideal body weight/day, energy 25 kcal/kg/day. Additional protein supplements of up to 20 g of amino acids may be necessary to cover amino acid loses during dialysis. "Specialized" formula diets ("Nepro," Abbott Nutrition, Columbus, OH) are designed to counteract the metabolic (high biological value protein, complex carbohydrates), electrolyte (low sodium, potassium, and phosphate), and fluid (concentrated) defects and so have theoretical advantages, but whether these translate into better survival compared to standard formula plus dialysis remains to be shown.

Chapter 16
Nutrition Support in the Obese

Principles

The obesity epidemic in westernized populations is reflected by an increasing number of obese hospitalized patients. In the early years of nutritional support, the focus was on the remarkably high incidence of depleted or malnourished patients in hospital, as exemplified by Bistrian and Blackburn's landmark study in 1974, which showed that approximately 50% of surgical patients in an urban hospital had protein-calorie malnutrition [275]. Not surprisingly, we found even higher rates in hospitalized patients in South Africa [276, 277]. In their recent review, Blackburn and colleagues highlighted the facts that over the last 30 years there have been radical changes in the levels of severe obesity, metabolic syndrome, and weight loss surgery in the USA [278]. The prevalence of class III (BMI >40 kg/m^2) obesity has increased nearly tenfold since the late 1960s and doubled since the early 1990s. As of 2002, an estimated 22% of US adults had metabolic syndrome. Between 1996 and 2002, population-adjusted rates of weight loss surgery increased more than sevenfold, with an estimated 220,000 Americans undergoing weight loss procedures in 2008. In our own recent survey of hospitalized patients in Pittsburgh, we noted that the prevalence of obesity and overweight, defined as BMI > or =25, was 43.3%, the prevalence of obesity as defined by BMI > or = 30 was 20.8%, while the prevalence of malnutrition as defined by BMI < or = 18.5 was only 3.9%.

Recognition that many obese patients have the metabolic syndrome and hyperglycemia would lead one to suspect that they would have an increased risk of metabolic complications which, from what we have discussed earlier (Chapter 4: "The Metabolic Response to Acute Illness"), would impair outcome from the underlying disease for which they were admitted. This is certainly true for the obese with acute pancreatitis [279], and studies have reported that mortality is increased in the non-ICU populations. However, remarkably, several good-sized (>600 patients) studies on ICU patients have found that obesity was associated with a *lower* mortality, suggesting that the increased nutrient stores associated with obesity may have survival value. This subject has been well reviewed recently by Choban et al. for the American Society of Enteral and Parenteral Nutrition and summarized in Table 16.1 [280].

© Springer Science+Business Media New York 2015 199
S.J.D. O'Keefe, *The Principles and Practice of Nutritional Support*,
DOI 10.1007/978-1-4939-1779-2_16

Table 16.1 ICU mortality and complications in obese patients compared to non-obese

GRADE table question 1: Do clinical outcomes vary across levels of obesity in critically ill or hospitalized non-ICU patients?

Comparison	Outcome	Quantity, type of evidence	Findings (for individual reference numbers see Choban et al. [278])	Grade for outcome	Overall evidence GRADE
ICU patients					
Obese versus optimal BMI	Mortality (large studies)	8 OBS	1 Increased [21]	Low	Low
			5 Decreased [23, 35, 41, 43, 44]		
			2 No difference [32, 45]		
	Hospital LOS (large studies)	4 OBS	3 Increased [22, 29, 44]	Low	
			1 No difference [45]		
	Complications	6 OBS	5 Increased [25, 36, 44–46]	Low	
			1 No difference [32]		
BMI ≥40 kg/m² versus optimal BMI	Mortality (large studies)	4 OBS	1 Decreased [43]	Low	
			3 No difference [22, 23, 44]		
	Hospital LOS (large studies)	4 OBS	2 Increased [22, 29]	Low	
			2 No difference [44, 45]		
Non-ICU patients					
Obese versus optimal BMI	Mortality	2 OBS	1 Increased [47]	Low	
			1 No difference [3]		

ICU intensive care unit, *LOS* length of stay, *OBS* observational study

Journal of Parenteral and Enteral Nutrition 37(6):724 [280]

The explanation is clearly complex and needs further investigation before we advocate obesity to protect you should you become critically ill!

Nutritional Assessment

Clearly we cannot use the BMI on its own in the assessment of the obese patient with feeding problems as it is going to remain high even with starvation while fluid and electrolytes, protein, vitamins, minerals, and trace elements will be wasting away. Therefore we recommend:

- Ask about recent weight loss: perform a subjective global assessment (Chapter 7: "Nutritional Assessment").
- Measure blood levels: BUN drops in protein starvation; creatinine increases with fluid depletion, potassium, magnesium, and zinc; and iron levels drop in starvation. Water-soluble vitamins such as folate, vitamin C, thiamin, and nicotinamide drop rapidly (within weeks), while fat-soluble vitamins such as vitamins A, E, and D, and trace elements, drop more slowly (within months).

Nutritional Requirements

A major concern, as expressed earlier on in this book, is what are the nutritional requirements of the obese critically ill? As outlined in Chapter 2: "Physiology of Human Nutrition: Starvation and Obesity", overfeeding leads to the retention and accumulation within the body of not only fat, but also many other nutrients, including protein. Consequently, the obese should be able to survive without nutritional support for longer periods than the non-obese. However, the proportionally largest nutrient stores in obesity are undeniably fat in adipose tissue, and so an argument can be made for (a) starting nutritional support later in the obese, and (b) when starting use hypocaloric formulations. The situation is further complicated by the difficulty in defining what is hypocaloric in the obese, in the absence of indirect calorimetry. Clearly the usual figure of 25 kcal/kg/day cannot be used as this would amount to 7,500 kcal per day for a 300 kg person! Some have suggested that the value 12.5 kcal/actual body weight can be used alternatively for calculating energy requirements in the obese. However, while this works well in moderate obesity, it vastly overestimates requirements in the morbidly obese as illustrated in (Fig. 16.1) from the recent review of the subject by McClave et al. [281]. Figure 16.1 shows that in comparison to the energy infusion of 65% of expenditure measured by indirect calorimetry for the obese currently—the level recommended by Guidelines for Nutrition Therapy of the Adult Critically Ill Patient (American Society for Parenteral and Enteral Nutrition (A.S.P.E.N.) and the Society for Critical Care Medicine (SCCM)

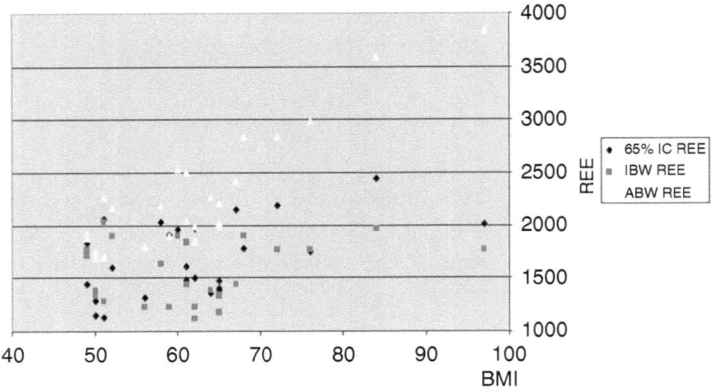

Fig. 16.1 Illustration of the difficulties in estimating energy requirements for obese patients see text for explanation. Data from ref McClave et al. [281]

[108, 130])—the use of 12.5 kcal/kg/day actual body weight would indicate that the super-obese would require up to 4,000 kcal/day! On the other hand, the use of ideal body weight-based calculations produced much more reasonable estimates.

Practice

If an obese patient is admitted unable to eat, the first priority is to perform the assessment as above and, while waiting for the results of blood tests to return, resuscitate the patient with fluid, electrolytes, and multivitamins. Next assess oral intake and correct specific deficiencies when specialized blood tests return. To calculate nutritional requirements, we recommend the use of *ideal body weight* for calculating both energy and protein requirements for the reasons discussed above. In more stable patients, it is reasonable to reduce caloric infusions to 100 g glucose/dextrose per day to help mobilize their own fat stores and initiate weight loss, which *must* be the long-term therapeutic goal. Blood testing for electrolytes and micronutrients must be monitored during refeeding and levels corrected by adjusting levels of supplementation. Thereafter, standard additions of daily vitamins and minerals must be included.

Nutritional Problems Post Bariatric Surgery

Principles

The most popular technique today is the Roux-en-Y gastric bypass procedure, which results in an average weight loss of approximately 95 lbs per year or a 2/3 loss of the excess weight in 2 years [282, 283] (http://win.niddk.nih.gov/

Table 16.2 Summary and meta-analysis of four suitable RCTs showing the superiority of bariatric surgery to nonsurgical approaches to weight loss. For individual references, see Colquitt et al. [283]

Surgery vs Medical Treatment of Obesity

Review: Surgery for weight loss in adults
Comparison: I Surgery versus non-surgery
Outcome: 5 Mean weight at study end

Study or subgroup	Surgery N	Mean(SD)[kg]	No surgery N	Mean(SD)[kg]	Mean Difference IV,Random,95% CI	Mean Difference IV,Random,95% CI
Dixon 2012 (1)	30	107 (22.8)	30	121.8 (21.4)		-14.80 [-25.99, -3.61]
Ikramuddin 2013 (2)	60	73 (13.6)	60	90.1 (17)		-17.10 [-22.61, -11.59]
O'Brien 2006 (3)	40	74.5 (6.7)	40	89.5 (4.8)		-15.00 [-17.55, -12.45]
Schauer 2012 (4)	99	76.4 (12.9)	41	99 (16.4)		-22.60 [-28.23, -16.97]

-20   -10   0   10   20
Favours surgery   Favours no surgery

publications/gastric.htm#reading). The most recent Cochran Review found seven satisfactory RCTs of surgery vs. no surgery to evaluate which are summarized on Table 16.2. All showed significantly higher weight losses with surgery, and some improvements in quality of life and diabetes [283]. Three RCTs compared laparoscopic RYGB to laparoscopic banding, showing higher rates of weight loss with the former at −5.2 kg/m², but higher late complications. Furthermore, more complex surgery in two RCTs found that biliopancreatic diversion with duodenal switch (BDDS) resulted in greater weight loss (−7.3 kg/m²) than RYGB in morbidly obese patients, but that need for reoperations was higher in the BDDS group (16.1–27.6%) compared to the RYGB group (4.3–8.3%). Thus, in general, the more complex the surgery, the better the weight loss, but the higher the complication rates. The authors concluded that across all studies adverse event rates and reoperation rates were generally poorly reported. They also expressed concern that most trials followed participants for only 1 or 2 years, and therefore the long-term effects of surgery remain unclear (Table 16.2).

In RYGB, the most commonly used procedure, weight loss occurs for two major reasons: first the volume of the stomach is reduced, and second, the duodenum and first part of the jejunum are bypassed resulting in malabsorption. However, alteration in GI anatomy results in a wide spectrum of changes in digestive and metabolic physiology, many of which can contribute to weight loss as recently reviewed by Madsbad et al. [284] and summarized in Fig. 16.2.

In our experience, most patients tolerate the procedure remarkably well with a leveling off of weight loss close to the ideal, about 5–10% over-swing and continue to lose weight, become progressively more malnourished, and need for nutritional support or reversal of the surgery. In some, surgical reversal is impossible because of previous surgical complications, and some end up with short bowel-intestinal failure due to loss of small intestine due to ischemia from acute volvulus, and can only be kept alive by home TPN as illustrated in Fig. 16.3.

One such patient recently received a successful small bowel transplant in our institution, and now is again obese! In this group of patients with "gastric bypass

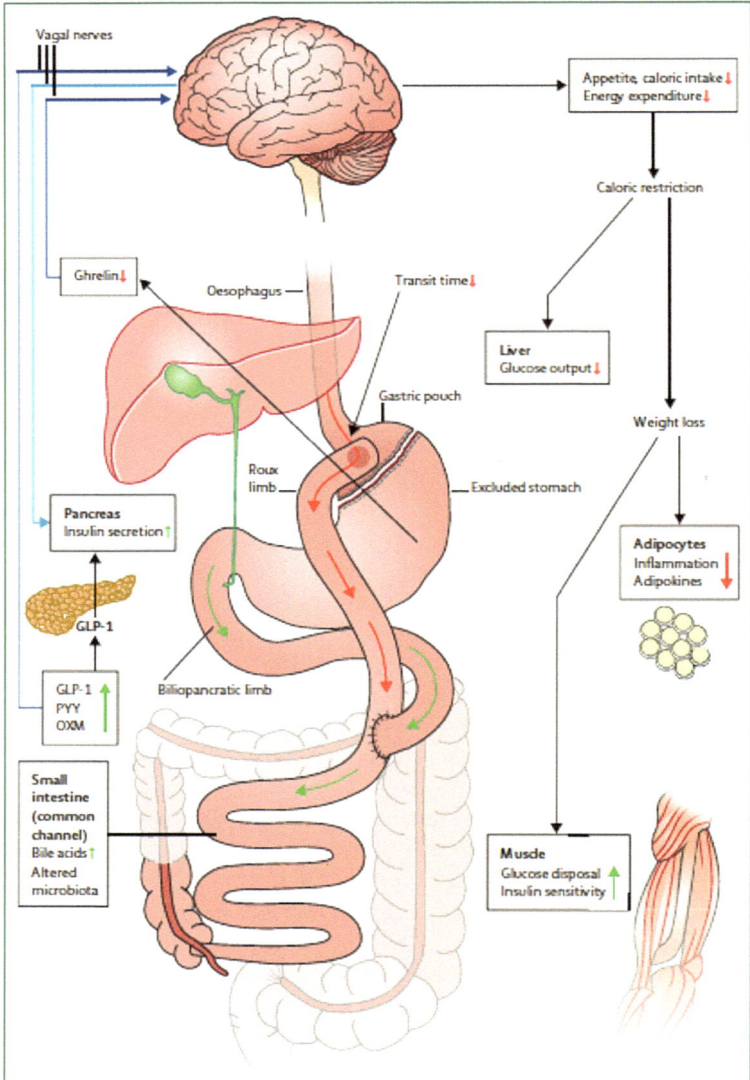

Fig. 16.2 Mechanisms of RYGB important for weight loss and improved glycemic control: Review by Sten Madsbad, Carsten Dirksen, Jens J Holst (2014) [284]. Early effects of Roux-en-Y gastric bypass are induction of postprandial increases in glucagon-like peptide 1 (GLP-1), peptide YY (PYY), and oxyntomodulin (OXM) because of the fast entry of food into the small intestine (alimentary [Roux] limb and common channel), while ghrelin secretion is reduced. Together, these changes are probably the main causes of reduced appetite and food intake. The exaggerated GLP-1 response also accounts for the increase in insulin secretion seen in patients with type 2 diabetes after RYGB. Reduced perioperative caloric intake increases hepatic insulin sensitivity within a few days after surgery. Later effects (i.e., after major weight loss occurs) include improvements in skeletal-muscle insulin sensitivity. Bypass surgery also results in increased concentrations of bile acids in the blood and changes in intestinal microbiota which might also contribute to weight change

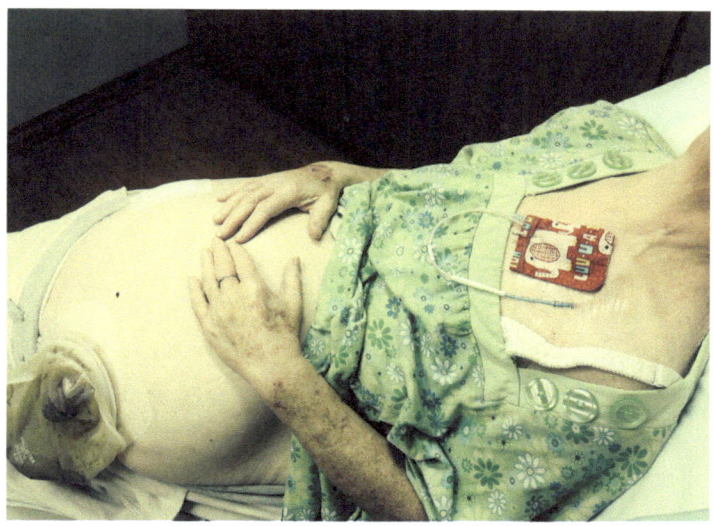

Fig. 16.3 Illustration of a patient s/p gastric bypass for morbid obesity who developed the complication of small intestinal volvulus resulting in massive intestinal loss and the need for home TPN. Her recovery was complicated by anastomosis breakdown and abdominal sepsis, but once stabilized, she was given hypocaloric feeding until her BMI was normal allowing reconstructive surgery with jejunocolic anastomosis and repair of abdominal hernia 2 years later. She is now independent of PN

gone wrong (GBGW)," we recently investigated the effect of bypass on pancreatic secretion due to concern that a state of permanent ileal brake stimulation will exist because of the increased delivery of undigested food into the distal small intestine. Our results confirmed decreased pancreatic enzyme stimulation in response to feeding together with increased ileal brake peptide (GLP-1, peptide YY) release, and showed that absorption could be increased by exogenous pancreatic enzyme supplementation (Fig. 16.4).

Because the surgery is so common, reportedly the most common elective procedure in the USA today, we, as gastroenterologists, are seeing patients referrals for nutritional complications more frequently. Micronutrient deficiencies are particularly common, including *deficiencies in iron, copper, zinc, selenium, thiamine, folate, and vitamins B12 and D* [280]. More serious complications are metabolic acidosis, hepatic steatosis, and liver failure. While gastric bypass surgery in undoubtedly the most effective way of treating morbid obesity today, it modifies natural anatomy and physiology we discussed in Chapter 3: "Physiology of Digestion and Absorption" and in the manner illustrated in Fig. 16.2 to the extent that it destroys the fine orchestration of the digestive process, culminating in malabsorption, dysregulation of gut peptide and neuroendocrine regulation, disturbed bile acid pooling, and changes in the colonic and small bowel microbiome and metabolome, with consequent severe

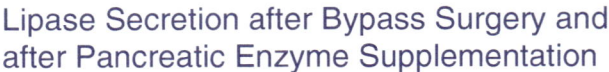

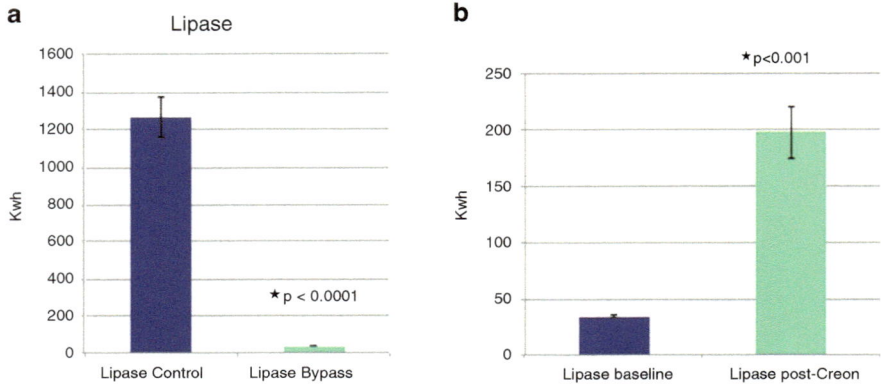

Fig. 16.4 Measurements of pancreatic lipase secretion in response to feeding in RYGB patients show-ing suppression of enzyme secretion in 11 patients compared to 10 healthy volunteers (*left panel*), and a significant increase in 4 patients restudied 3 months after pancreatic enzyme supplementation

malnutrition in those who fail to adapt. Recent studies suggest that changes in the gut microbiome after RYGB contribute to weight loss through reduced microbial short-chain fatty acid (SCFA) production and thus malabsorbed carbohydrate salvage [285]. Patients are also at greater risk of developing NAFLD possibly mediated by the dysbiosis and their potential to stimulate the inflammasome and to produce toxic metabolites, such as ethanol [286–288].

Consequently, gastric bypass surgery cannot be considered the final solution to the treatment of obesity, but may point to new avenues of treatment independent of surgery, for example the therapeutic use of gut peptides or manipulation of the colonic microbiota composition [289].

Practice

The malnourished postgastric bypass patient is one of the most difficult to manage. First, oral intake is usually very low for a variety of reasons including the reduced stomach, chronic stimulation of the ileal brake, and anorexia associated with the need for chronic narcotic pain medications. Secondly, malabsorption is present due to the bypass of the small intestine that is chiefly responsible for digestion and absorption. Third, maldigestion occurs due to improper mixing of food with diges-tive enzymes and insufficient enzyme secretion as described above. Despite the fact that enteral feeding should be able to replete these patients, it is usually better to replete all the micronutrient deficiencies by initial IV infusions while placing an enteral feeding tube to sustain responses. Because digestion and absorption is likely to be impaired, we recommend the use of semi-elemental formulae. In the patient who is able to eat meals, we recommend a trial of pancreatic enzyme supplements taken with meals (e.g., Creon 10,000 three capsules) and snacks (two capsules). It is critical to understand that decompromise in these patients is never due to the deficiency of a single nutrient; the deficiency in one micronutrient is invariable accompanied by the deficiency of others, which may be less apparent or more difficult to measure and monitor. Figure 16.5 illustrates one such patient who was admitted with weight loss, mental confusion, and a desquamated skin rash covering most of the whole body, particularly the limbs. Blood tests revealed a wide range of vitamin and mineral deficiencies, including potassium, magnesium, zinc, iron, thiamine, nicotinamide, ascorbic acid, folate, B12, and vitamin D. Management, as above, resulted in rapid improvements in mental status and healing of the skin rash, in concert with normalization of blood levels. Short-term TPN can be used, but risk of refeeding syndrome is great, so it has to be started at 25% of macronutrient goals and only advanced once the clinical condition improves, usually after 3–5 days. Long-term management is particularly problematic, as the dramatic recovery in hospital will be followed by rapid decline after discharge home on a recommended normal diet because the underlying cause has not been reversed. As food intake is

Fig. 16.5 Skin rash in association with multiple micronutrient deficiencies in a patient following gastric bypass surgery

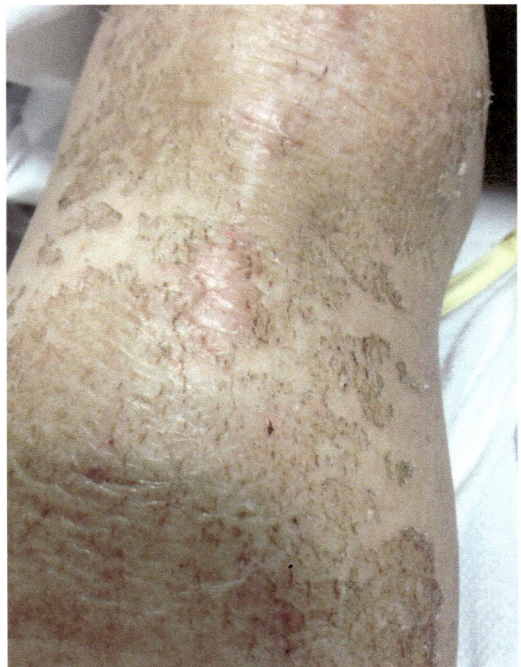

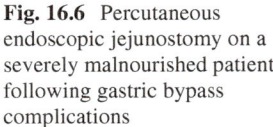

Fig. 16.6 Percutaneous endoscopic jejunostomy on a severely malnourished patient following gastric bypass complications

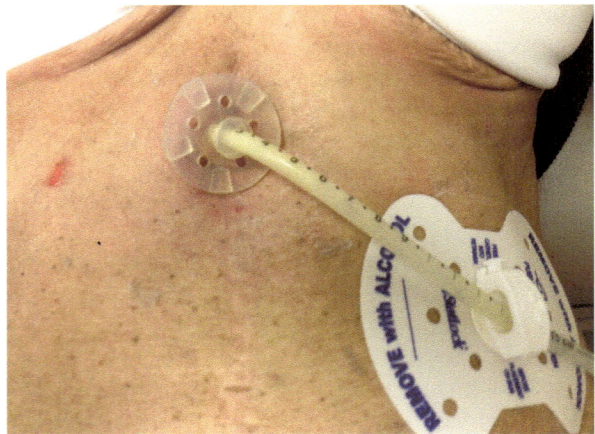

usually the chief problem, placement of a direct percutaneous endoscopic enterostomy (PEJ) as shown in Fig. 16.6 (rather than a PEG, which is difficult because of the diminished stomach size) is often the only solution other than performing a surgical reversal—which is often technically difficult.

Chapter 17
Nutritional Support in the Elderly

Principles

People in developed countries tend to gain weight until about 60 years of age, stay stable for a while, and then lose weight. Women 85 years of age or older were found to have a BMI of 1.8 kg/m² lower than that of women 55–64 years, and men 85 years or older had a BMI of 2.6 kg/m² lower than men of 45–64 years [290]. Community-dwelling men over the age of 65 years were shown to lose about 0.5% of their body weight/year [291].

Weight loss in the elderly is associated with poor outcomes including reduced life expectancy, increased number of hospital admissions, prolonged hospital stay, frailty, functional impairment, pressure ulcers, increased fracture risk, cognitive impairment, and poor QoL among others. Liu et al. showed that mortality in elderly persons a year after hospital discharge was doubled in those with a low BMI [292] (Fig. 17.1).

Body composition changes with age. Fat stores increase and lean body mass decreases due to loss of skeletal muscle. This loss of muscle mass is often referred to as sarcopenia.

Changes in appetite take place with aging. Older persons are often less hungry before meals, consume smaller meals, eat fewer snacks between meals, feel more satiated after a standard meal, and eat a more monotonous diet. The average daily energy intake has been shown to decrease by <30% between 20 and 80 years of age.

When healthy, this age-related decrease in intake is compensated for by a decline in energy expenditure. However, if decrease in intake outpaces the decline in energy expenditure, then weight is lost. This puts elderly persons at increased risk of malnutrition when they are acutely ill or otherwise unable to eat. Chronic disease, lifestyle, and social and environmental factors may further affect nutritional status. Indeed, many studies have now shown that there are significant benefits to being overweight (BMI 25–30) as you age and no disadvantage in being obese over the age of 70 [293–295] (Fig. 17.2).

"Anorexia of aging" occurs as the result of multiple physiological changes that occur with age. These include changes in taste and smell, decreased adaptive

© Springer Science+Business Media New York 2015
S.J.D. O'Keefe, *The Principles and Practice of Nutritional Support*,
DOI 10.1007/978-1-4939-1779-2_17

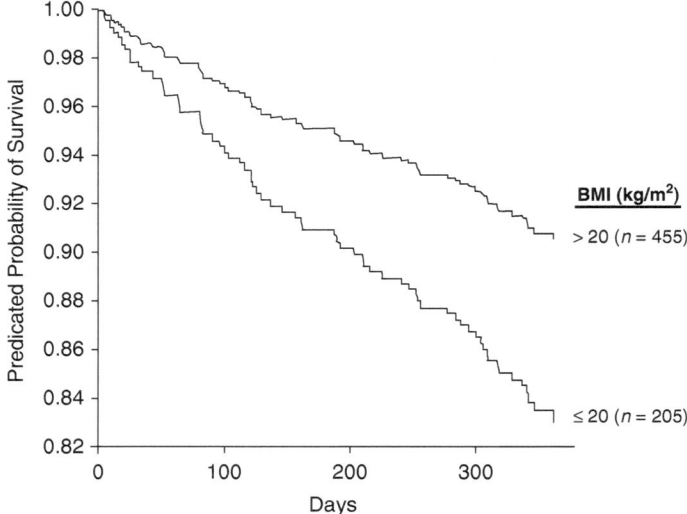

Fig. 17.1 Malnutrition in the elderly is associated with reduced life expectancy 1 year after hospital discharge

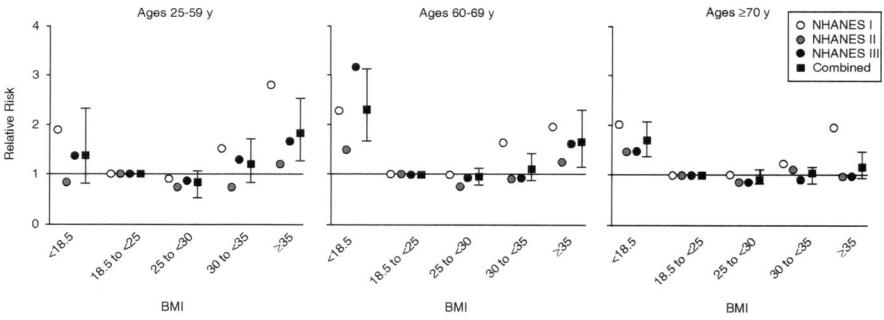

Fig. 17.2 Relative risks of mortality by BMI category, survey, and age [294]

relaxation of the fundus of the stomach, delayed gastric emptying after large meals, changes in orexigenic and anorexic hormones, elevation in pro-inflammatory cytokine levels, and, probably, changes in the central regulation of appetite. It appears to be more pronounced in men than women.

There is a small increase in taste threshold with advancing age, especially in those who smoke or take medications. Older persons are also more likely to be unable to smell the odors associated with food.

Nitric oxide is responsible for the adaptive smooth muscle relaxation in the gastric fundus that occurs with a meal. In the elderly, nitric oxide production in response to food is decreased causing the fundus to be less compliant [296, 297]. The resultant rapid antral filling signals satiety. The delayed gastric emptying seen after large meals in older persons also contributes to increased satiation [298].

Leptin, a hormone released from adipocytes, decreases food intake and increases metabolic rate promoting weight loss. Fasting levels of leptin are elevated in older compared with younger persons [299]. Testosterone suppresses leptin secretion, and hence, lower testosterone levels in older men may partly explain why men are more prone to age-related weight loss.

Ghrelin is released from the fundus of the stomach. It stimulates the release of growth hormone from the pituitary and acts on the hypothalamus to increase appetite. Studies suggest a small decrease in ghrelin levels and a shift towards the inactive deacetylated form in older persons [300–302].

Cholecystokinin (CCK) is released in response to fat and signals satiety. Higher basal levels have been found in the elderly together with a greater release in response to fat [303, 304]. CCK infusion has a greater satiating effect in older than in younger persons [302]. A fatty meal has also been shown to increase levels of glucagon-like peptide-1 (GLP-1), a potent anorexic hormone that slows gastric emptying [305].

The relative increase in adipose tissue usually seen with aging is associated with an increase in TNF-α and other pro-inflammatory cytokines that cause anorexia. IL-6 increases as a function of normal aging, and the level correlates inversely with functional status. The chronic disease present in many elderly will compound this baseline elevation in cytokine levels and push them towards cachexia (Fig. 17.3).

Factors that may compound "physiological" anorexia and result in pathological weight loss include comorbid disease, medications, individual factors, and institutional factors.

Chronic diseases of particular concern in the elderly include:

1. Dementia: Weight loss is almost inevitable in the advanced stages. Affected individuals may appear to become unaware of hunger or fail to respond to it, refuse to open their mouths or spit food out, chew repetitively and pocket food, fail to initiate the swallowing reflex or swallow ineffectively, and aspirate.
2. Dysphagia which is usually secondary to cerebrovascular disease or esophageal dysmotility (presbyesophagus).
3. Chronic constipation is prevalent among the institutionalized elderly and may be associated with abdominal discomfort and bloating that has a negative impact on appetite.
4. Depression is common, especially in long-term care settings, and may be associated with poor appetite and decreased food and fluid intake.

Older persons are likely to be taking more medications, both prescription and over the counter. Anorexia may be a side effect of individual medications and/or related to high pill burden. Common culprits include acetylcholinesterase inhibitors, iron, potassium, digoxin, diuretics, metformin, amiodarone, and narcotics.

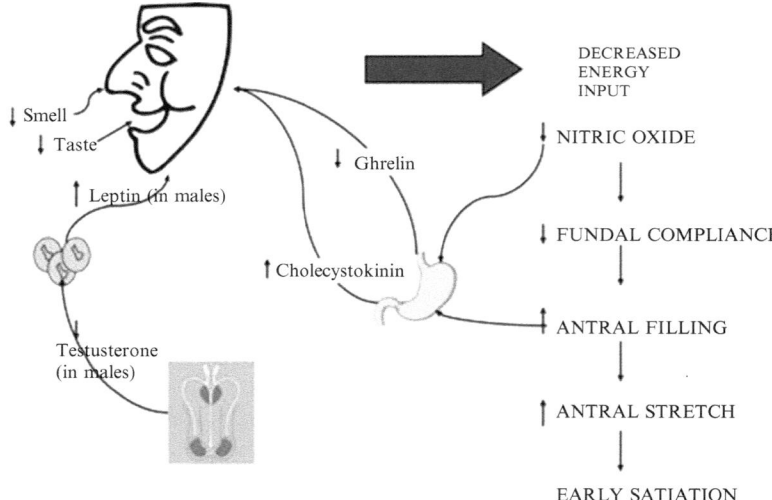

Fig. 17.3 Summary of the multiple factors involved in the pathogenesis of physiological anorexia of aging and energy expenditure [306]

Other factors that may contribute to inadequate intake in older persons include:

1. Poor vision
2. Poor dentition
3. Poor posture
4. Poor manual dexterity
5. Dependence on others/inadequate assistance with eating
6. Unappetizing diet
7. Being left in bed all day
8. Social factors including abuse

Practice

Screening

Several screening tools have been developed to identify older adults at risk of malnutrition. The 2 with the highest quartile for sensitivity (>83%) and specificity (>90%) are the Mini Nutritional Assessment Short Form and the Malnutrition Screening Tool [307, 308]. However, it is safe to assume that all hospitalized and institutionalized elderly persons are at risk of malnutrition, and careful monitoring of food intake should be undertaken.

General Measures

A multidisciplinary approach is mandatory with input from nursing, dietary, speech therapy, pharmacy, and social work, in addition to the physician.

This should include counseling the patient and/or family members about the natural history of their disease and, if appropriate, a discussion of end-of-life goals of care. It is normal to decrease food and fluid intake towards the end of life, and a point will be reached where it is unrealistic to expect improvement in nutritional status.

It is important to address dietary preferences, food texture, and oral factors such as poor dentition. Dietary restrictions have been shown to be associated with weight loss and should be lifted whenever possible. Most long-term care facilities serve "heart-healthy" diets and do not further restrict carbohydrate or salt. Social issues that prevent access to adequate food need to be identified; these include inability to shop or prepare meals, dependence on being fed, and lack of money to buy food.

If there is a problem with swallowing, speech therapy should be consulted to optimize food and liquid consistency and the therapist should work with the patient, if they are able, to find techniques, e.g., chin tuck, that help them swallow without aspirating.

Medical and psychiatric illnesses should be optimally controlled and medication burden reduced with particular attention being paid to the medications discussed above.

Dietary Supplements

Dietary supplements are of questionable benefit. A meta-analysis which evaluated 55 randomized (or quasi-randomized) controlled trials of nutritional supplements in 9,187 participants in the hospital, nursing home, and community suggested a reduction in mortality, but the findings were not significant [309]. The relative risk for mortality was 0.88 (0.74–1.04), 0.65 (0.41–1.02), and 1.05 (0.57–1.95) in elderly subjects in the hospital, nursing home, and community, respectively. However, when they looked at subsets of data, the mortality rate was reduced in hospitalized, undernourished patients over the age of 75 years who received at least 400 kcal/day of supplement.

A study looking at nutritional supplementation in long-term care showed that supplements were not given as often as prescribed, that staff spent minimal time assisting residents in consuming them, and that they provided minimal additional calories (average of 144 kcal/day if given between meals and 230 kcal/day when given with meals) [310].

Appetite Stimulants

Appetite stimulants have not been shown to be of benefit in the majority of elderly persons. There is one randomized placebo-controlled trial of megestrol acetate that was conducted in 69 VA nursing home patients with weight loss >5% in the preceding 3 months or who were 20% or more below ideal body weight. Megestrol acetate 800 mg daily was compared with placebo for 12 weeks. At 12 weeks, there was improvement in appetite, well-being, and enjoyment of life but no weight gain in the treatment group. At week 20 (i.e., 8 weeks post-intervention), weight gains of 2.45 and 0.4 kg were seen in the treatment and placebo groups, respectively. However, megestrol acetate failed to increase weight in a frail subset and it has side effects, including fluid retention and venous thromboembolism (4.9–32% in nursing home residents) that make us anxious about using it in the elderly [311].

Dronabinol, a synthetic cannabis derivative, has been shown to improve appetite in AIDS patients but has not been well studied in older adults. A limited nonrandomized trial showed possible benefit in patients with advanced Alzheimer's disease who were refusing food. However, it is difficult and expensive to obtain and we do not use it in practice.

Mirtazapine, an antidepressant medication that is not related to serotonin reuptake inhibitors, tricyclic antidepressants, or monoamine oxidase inhibitors, has potent histamine (H1) blocking effects that tend to increase appetite and cause weight gain. A retrospective cohort study did not find statistically significant differences in weight change at 3 or 6 months between mirtazapine and other antidepressants. However, in practice, mirtazapine can promote weight gain and is a good choice for treating depression in an elderly person with weight loss [312].

Tube Feeding

Tube feeding is not a viable option to address weight loss in most elderly persons. It can be appropriate to treat dysphagia after CVA or in association with trauma or surgery where a reasonable degree of recovery is expected. In advanced dementia, feeding tubes do not improve survival, prevent malnutrition, decrease aspiration risk, heal pressure ulcers, or improve comfort or QoL. In a review of the evidence for and against tube feeding in persons with dementia, Finucaine stated that "The widespread practice of tube feeding should be carefully reconsidered, and we believe that for severely demented patients the practice should be discouraged on clinical grounds" [164].

A prospective cohort study of 36,492 nursing home residents with advanced dementia and new eating problems looked at survival after the development of the need for eating assistance with, and without, placement of a percutaneous endoscopic gastrostomy (PEG) and, whether timing of feeding tube insertion (<1 month vs. >4 months) affected survival. They showed that neither insertion of PEG tubes nor timing of insertion affected survival [313] (Fig. 17.4).

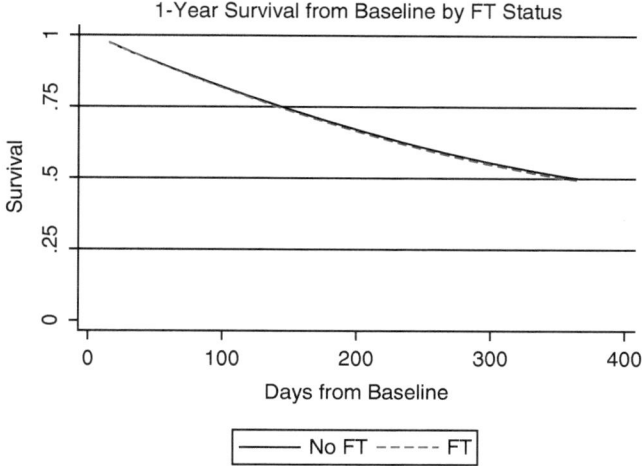

Fig. 17.4 Survival curve comparing 1-year survival from the Minimum Data Set that noted need for assistance with eating in residents with and without a PEG after Teno et al [313]

Acute Care

A duotube may be considered in the acute care setting for temporary nutritional support when recovery is expected. However, older persons are at increased risk of developing delirium, and if they are confused, it may be necessary to use restraints to prevent them from pulling the tube out. Restraints are unpleasant for the patient, have well-documented adverse effects, and may prolong the course of delirium. In my experience it may be better to accept that they are unable to eat for a day or two and resume oral feeding with the safest consistency (usually pureed diet and thickened liquids) and strict aspiration precautions as soon as they are alert enough to be able to cooperate.

Speech therapy can be very helpful, but therapists are often reluctant to recommend resuming oral intake until the patient is not at risk of aspiration. Sometimes this is not practical as the patient, even if at high risk of aspiration, would not want a feeding tube. In this situation it is the responsibility of the physician to have a discussion with the patient and/or their family members about the risks and benefits of resuming oral intake. *It is not uncommon for frail elderly persons to aspirate chronically, but only a proportion of them ever develop aspiration pneumonia.*

As discussed in Chapter 2 (p. 15) and Chapter 7 "The Problem of the Sick, Malnourished, Patient with "Failure to Thrive"", refeeding syndrome (RFS) is caused by severe electrolyte and water imbalance following reintroduction of food after a period of fasting and can lead to CHF, respiratory failure, seizures, and sudden death. Elderly persons are at increased risk of RFS and it may often go unrecognized. In contrast to the young or middle aged, the elderly handle starvation poorly presumably because the rate of mobilization, and depth, of body stores is lower. For this reason it is recommended that vulnerable elderly patients should not only be initially fed at slow rates to avoid RFS, but more care should be taken to commence early enteral feeding if they are unable to eat as they are less tolerant of starvation. Clinicians need to be aware of RFS as a potentially reversible cause of clinical deterioration in frail elderly. After starvation or relative starvation, start feeding with 10 kcal/kg ideal body weight/day and increase slowly over 5–7 days. Excess intravenous fluids, especially normal saline, should be avoided as elderly patients may handle excess salt and water badly.

Micronutrient Deficiencies

B12 deficiency is present in 10–20% of older adults. It may be associated with cognitive impairment and depression in the elderly but rarely causes anemia. B12 absorption from protein requires gastric acid as well as intrinsic factor. About 15% of persons over 60 years of age poorly absorb protein-bound B12 as a result of gastric achlorhydria. New onset of pernicious anemia is relatively uncommon at this age. Consequently, the majority of older persons with B12 deficiency can be treated with crystalline B12 supplements by mouth as these do not require the presence of acid for absorption.

Vitamin D deficiency is particularly common in older adults. Contributing factors include lack of sun exposure, impaired skin synthesis of pre-vitamin D, decreased hydroxylation in the kidney, and poor dietary intake. 25-Hydroxyvitamin D level should be used as a screening test. Levels <30 ng/ml are considered inadequate and should be replaced with high-dose vitamin D2 50,000 U/week for 12 weeks. All elderly persons should be encouraged to supplement with at least 800 U of vitamin D daily, combined with a calcium supplement.

The recommended intake of calcium in elderly persons is 1,200 mg daily as they absorb calcium less efficiently from the gastrointestinal tract. As much of this as possible should come from dietary sources as calcium supplements have adverse side effects such as constipation, nephrolithiasis, and possibly, increased risk of heart disease. Pill burden, with the associated risk of noncompliance with essential medications, is a real issue in elderly patients so it is sometimes wise to forego calcium supplementation if dairy intake is good.

Multivitamins (MVI): There is no clear evidence that MVI supplementation is of benefit either in decreasing incidence of infections or mortality. Older persons often have many prescription medications to take, and it is prudent not to increase their pill burden without a good reason. Therefore, supplementation with MVI should only be considered in persons with poor intake who may not be meeting their micronutrient needs. As a general principle, isolated vitamin or mineral deficiencies do not occur, and if there is concern about nutritional status or intake, whole foods (solid or liquid) should be given, when possible.

End-of-Life Issues

Family members often find it hard to accept that a patient is not able to eat or drink and are concerned about him/her suffering from hunger and thirst. It is important to explain to them that death from any chronic illness involves a gradual decrease in nutritional intake. Studies in cancer patients and Irish Republican Army hunger strikers have documented that discomfort as a result of hunger and thirst is not felt as death approaches. Indeed, providing intravenous fluids may have adverse effects in the terminally ill, e.g., edema and increased skin breakdown as a result of incontinence. Consequently, patients should be kept as comfortable as possible and interventions should be avoided. When still alert, pleasure foods should be offered. Excellent mouth care is important to keep the mouth moist and clear of secretions.

ERRATUM TO

Nutritional Support in the Elderly

© Springer Science+Business Media New York 2015
S.J.D. O'Keefe, *The Principles and Practice of Nutritional Support*,
DOI 10.1007/978-1-4939-1779-2_17

DOI 10.1007/978-1-4939-1779-2_18

Chapter 17: "Nutritional Support in the Elderly" was written by Elizabeth A. O'Keefe. The publisher regrets that her name was not included on the opening page of her chapter and in the table of contents.

The online version of the original chapter can be found at
http://dx.doi.org/10.1007/978-1-4939-1779-2_17

References

1. Alberts B. Cell biology: the endless frontier. Mol Biol Cell. 2010;21(22):3785.
2. Molecular Biology of the Cell. Ed Alberts B et al. 5th edition. Garland Science, Taylor and Francis Group, LLC 2008, New York.
3. Greer JB, O'Keefe SJ. Microbial induction of immunity, inflammation and cancer. Front Physiol. 2011;1:168.
4. Cahill Jr GF. Starvation in man. N Engl J Med. 1970;282(12):668–75.
5. Keys A. Experimental studies of starvation on men. Bull Chic Med Soc. 1946;49:42–6.
6. Monro HN. Mammalian protein metabolism. Chapter 10: regulation of protein metabolism. In: Munro, editor. vol. 1. New York, NY: Academic; 1964. p 382–468
7. Marik P, Varon J. The obese patient in the ICU. Chest. 1998;113(2):492–8.
8. Prentice AM et al. Energy expenditure in overweight and obese adults in affluent societies: an analysis of 319 doubly-labelled water measurements. Eur J Clin Nutr. 1996;50(2):93–7.
9. McLaren DS. The great protein fiasco. Lancet. 1974;2(7872):93–6.
10. Bartholomew M. James Lind's Treatise of the Scurvy (1753). Postgrad Med J. 2002;78(925):695–6.
11. Lowe H et al. Vitamin D toxicity due to a commonly available "over the counter" remedy from the Dominican Republic. J Clin Endocrinol Metab. 2011;96(2):291–5.
12. Russell RM. The vitamin A spectrum: from deficiency to toxicity. Am J Clin Nutr. 2000;71(4):878–84.
13. Mason JB. Unraveling the complex relationship between folate and cancer risk. Biofactors. 2011;37(4):253–60.
14. Wang YC et al. Health and economic burden of the projected obesity trends in the USA and the UK. Lancet. 2011;378(9793):815–25.
15. Tsai AG, Williamson DF, Glick HA. Direct medical cost of overweight and obesity in the USA: a quantitative systematic review. Obes Rev. 2011;12(1):50–61.
16. Gamble JL, Physiological Information from Studies on the Life Raft Ration. The Harvey Lectures, ser. 42, 1946–1947, p. 247.
17. O'Keeffe T. Suicide and self-starvation. Philosophy. 1984;59(229):349–63.
18. Finch CE. Evolution in health and medicine Sackler colloquium: evolution of the human lifespan and diseases of aging: roles of infection, inflammation, and nutrition. Proc Natl Acad Sci U S A. 2010;107 Suppl 1:1718–24.
19. Voit C. Handbuch der Physiologie. Herman L, editors. vol. IV. Leipzig: Vogel; 1881. p. 3.
20. McGilvery RW. Biochemistry: a functional approach. Philadelphia, PA: WB Saunders; 1979.

© Springer Science+Business Media New York 2015
S.J.D. O'Keefe, *The Principles and Practice of Nutritional Support*,
DOI 10.1007/978-1-4939-1779-2

21. Voit C Protein Metabolism. In Handbuch der Physiologie. Editor L Herman: 1881; vol IV, p3, Vogel publishers, Leipzig, Germany.
22. Addis T, Lew W. J Biol Chem. 1936;116:343
23. Prentice AM. Starvation in humans: evolutionary background and contemporary implications. Mech Ageing Dev. 2005;126(9):976–81
24. Burkhalter TM, Hillman CH. A narrative review of physical activity, nutrition, and obesity to cognition and scholastic performance across the human lifespan. Adv Nutr. 2011;2(2):201S–6.
25. Wang C, Hegsted DM, Lapi A, et al. J Lab Clin Med. 1949;34:953.
26. Miller LL, W.G., Am J Med Sci. 1940;199:204.
27. Sitzmann JV et al. Total parenteral nutrition and alternate energy substrates in treatment of severe acute pancreatitis. Surg Gynecol Obstet. 1989;168(4):311–7.
28. Winter TA et al. The effect of severe undernutrition, and subsequent refeeding on digestive function in human patients. Eur J Gastroenterol Hepatol. 2000;12(2):191–6.
29. O'Keefe SJ et al. Severe malnutrition associated with alpha-heavy chain disease: response to tetracycline and intensive nutritional support. Am J Gastroenterol. 1988;83(9):995–1001.
30. O'Keefe SJ et al. Physiological effects of enteral and parenteral feeding on pancreaticobiliary secretion in humans. Am J Physiol Gastrointest Liver Physiol. 2003;284(1):G27–36.
31. O'Keefe SJ et al. Trypsin and splanchnic protein turnover during feeding and fasting in human subjects. Am J Physiol Gastrointest Liver Physiol. 2006;290(2):G213–21.
32. Fukatsu K, Kudsk KA. Nutrition and gut immunity. Surg Clin North Am. 2011;91(4):755–70. vii.
33. O'Keefe SJ. Nutrition and colonic health: the critical role of the microbiota. Curr Opin Gastroenterol. 2008;24(1):51–8.
34. O'Keefe SJ et al. Effect of fiber supplementation on the microbiota in critically ill patients. World J Gastrointest Pathophysiol. 2011;2(6):138–45.
35. Windmueller HG, Spaeth AE. The journal of biological chemistry, volume 249, 1974: uptake and metabolism of plasma glutamine by the small intestine. Nutr Rev. 1990;48(8):310–2.
36. Stoll B et al. Enteral nutrient intake level determines intestinal protein synthesis and accretion rates in neonatal pigs. Am J Physiol Gastrointest Liver Physiol. 2000;279(2):G288–94.
37. Burrin DG et al. Minimal enteral nutrient requirements for intestinal growth in neonatal piglets: how much is enough? Am J Clin Nutr. 2000;71(6):1603–10.
38. Castillo L et al. Splanchnic metabolism of dietary arginine in relation to nitric oxide synthesis in normal adult man. Proc Natl Acad Sci U S A. 1993;90(1):193–7.
39. Tsujinaka T et al. Effect of parenteral and enteral nutrition on hepatic albumin synthesis in rats. Nutrition. 1999;15(1):18–22.
40. Bollhalder L et al. A systematic literature review and meta-analysis of randomized clinical trials of parenteral glutamine supplementation. Clin Nutr. 2013;32(2):213–23.
41. Li N et al. Effects of protein deprivation on growth and small intestine morphology are not improved by glutamine or glutamate in gastrostomy-fed rat pups. J Pediatr Gastroenterol Nutr. 2004;39(1):28–33.
42. DiMagno EP, Go VL, Summerskill WH. Relations between pancreatic enzyme ouputs and malabsorption in severe pancreatic insufficiency. N Engl J Med. 1973;288(16):813–5.
43. Leach SD et al. Intracellular activation of digestive zymogens in rat pancreatic acini. Stimulation by high doses of cholecystokinin. J Clin Invest. 1991;87(1):362–6.
44. Vipperla K, O'Keefe SJ. The microbiota and its metabolites in colonic mucosal health and cancer risk. Nutr Clin Pract. 2012;27(5):624–35.
45. Sellon RK et al. Resident enteric bacteria are necessary for development of spontaneous colitis and immune system activation in interleukin-10-deficient mice. Infect Immun. 1998;66(11):5224–31.
46. O'Keefe SJ et al. Products of the colonic microbiota mediate the effects of diet on colon cancer risk. J Nutr. 2009;139(11):2044–8.
47. O'Keefe SJD LJ, Lahti L et al. Fat, Fiber and Cancer Risk in African Americans and Rural Africans *Nature communications. March* 2015.

48. Greiner T, Bäckhed F. Effects of the gut microbiota on obesity and glucose homeostasis. Trends Endocrinol Metab. 2011;22(4):117–23.
49. Hinton P, Allison SP, Littlejohn S, Lloyd J. Insulin and glucose to reduce catabolic response to injury in burned patients. Lancet. 1971;1:767–9.
50. O'Keefe SJ, Moldawer LL, Young VR, Blackburn GL. The influence of intravenous nutrition on protein dynamics following surgery. Metabolism. 1981;30:1150–8.
51. Cuthbertson DP. The distribution of nitrogen and sulphur in the urine during conditions of increased catabolism. Biochem J. 1931;25:236–44.
52. O'Keefe SJ, Sender PM, James WP. "Catabolic" loss of body nitrogen in response to surgery. Lancet. 1974;2:1035–8.
53. O'Keefe SJ, Wesley A, Jialal I, Epstein S. The metabolic response and problems with nutritional support in acute tetanus. Metabolism. 1984;33:482–7.
54. Munro HN, Chalmers MI. Fracture metabolism at different levels of protein intakes. Br J Expt Path. 1945;XXVI:396–403.
55. Van den Berghe G. How does blood glucose control with insulin save lives in intensive care? J Clin Invest. 2004;114:1187–95. doi:10.1172/jci23506.
56. Wolfe RR. Sepsis as a modulator of adaptation to low and high carbohydrate and low and high fat intakes. Eur J Clin Nutr. 1999;53 Suppl 1:S136–42.
57. Gamble JL, Physiological Information from Studies on the Life Raft Ration. The Harvey Lectures, ser. 42,1946-1947, p. 247.
58. Abou-Assi SG, Craig K, Mihas A, O'Keefe S. The nutritional management of acute pancreatitis: a prospective randomized study of jejunal versus intravenous feeding. Am J Clin Nutr. 2002;75:P284.
59. Van den Berghe G et al. Intensive insulin therapy in the medical ICU. N Engl J Med. 2006;354:449–61. doi:10.1056/NEJMoa052521.
60. Dudrick SJ et al. Long-term total parenteral nutrition with growth, development, and positive nitrogen balance. Surgery. 1968;64(1):134–42.
61. Sax HC et al. Early total parenteral nutrition in acute pancreatitis: lack of beneficial effects. Am J Surg. 1987;153(1):117–24.
62. Abou-Assi S, Craig K, O'Keefe SJD. Hypocaloric jejunal feeding is better than total parenteral nutrition in acute pancreatitis: results of a randomized comparative study. Am J Gastroenterol. 2002;97(9):2255–62.
63. O'Keefe SJ. A guide to enteral access procedures and enteral nutrition. Nat Rev Gastroenterol Hepatol. 2009;6(4):207–15.
64. Perioperative total parenteral nutrition in surgical patients. The Veterans Affairs Total Parenteral Nutrition Cooperative Study Group. N Engl J Med. 1991;325(8):525–32.
65. Moore EE, Moore FA. Immediate enteral nutrition following multisystem trauma: a decade perspective. J Am Coll Nutr. 1991;10(6):633–48.
66. Kudsk KA et al. Enteral versus parenteral feeding. Effects on septic morbidity after blunt and penetrating abdominal trauma. Ann Surg. 1992;215(5):503–11. discussion 511–3.
67. Braunschweig CL et al. Enteral compared with parenteral nutrition: a meta-analysis. Am J Clin Nutr. 2001;74(4):534–42.
68. Harvey SE et al., Trial of the route of early nutritional support in critically ill adults. N Engl J Med, 2014;371(18):1673–84.
69. Kelly DA. Intestinal failure-associated liver disease: what do we know today? Gastroenterology. 2006;130(2 Suppl 1):S70–7.
70. Carter BA, Shulman RJ. Mechanisms of disease: update on the molecular etiology and fundamentals of parenteral nutrition associated cholestasis. Nat Clin Pract Gastroenterol Hepatol. 2007;4(5):277–87.
71. Chan S et al. Incidence, prognosis, and etiology of end-stage liver disease in patients receiving home total parenteral nutrition. Surgery. 1999;126(1):28–34.
72. Craig RM et al. Severe hepatocellular reaction resembling alcoholic hepatitis with cirrhosis after massive small bowel resection and prolonged total parenteral nutrition. Gastroenterology. 1980;79(1):131–7.

73. Mullady DK, O'Keefe SJ. Treatment of intestinal failure: home parenteral nutrition. Nat Clin Pract Gastroenterol Hepatol. 2006;3(9):492–504.
74. Jain AK et al. Enteral bile acid treatment improves parenteral nutrition-related liver disease and intestinal mucosal atrophy in neonatal pigs. Am J Physiol Gastrointest Liver Physiol. 2012;302(2):G218–24.
75. Ammori BJ et al. Early increase in intestinal permeability in patients with severe acute pancreatitis: correlation with endotoxemia, organ failure, and mortality. J Gastrointest Surg. 1999;3(3):252–62.
76. Fukatsu K et al. Lack of enteral feeding increases expression of E-selectin after LPS challenge. J Surg Res. 2001;97(1):41–8.
77. Gray KD et al. Endotoxin potentiates lung injury in cerulein-induced pancreatitis. Am J Surg. 2003;186(5):526–30.
78. Fong YM et al. Total parenteral nutrition and bowel rest modify the metabolic response to endotoxin in humans. Ann Surg. 1989;210(4):449–56. discussion 456–7.
79. Kotani J et al. Enteral nutrition prevents bacterial translocation but does not improve survival during acute pancreatitis. Arch Surg. 1999;134(3):287–92.
80. Beger HG et al. Bacterial contamination of pancreatic necrosis. A prospective clinical study. Gastroenterology. 1986;91(2):433–8.
81. Marshall JC et al. Multiple organ dysfunction score: a reliable descriptor of a complex clinical outcome. Crit Care Med. 1995;23(10):1638–52.
82. Buijs N, et al., Novel nutritional substrates in surgery. Proc Nutr Soc. 2013:1–11.
83. Krishnan JA et al. Caloric intake in medical ICU patients: consistency of care with guidelines and relationship to clinical outcomes. Chest. 2003;124(1):297–305.
84. Rolandelli RH et al. The effect of enteral feedings supplemented with pectin on the healing of colonic anastomoses in the rat. Surgery. 1986;99(6):703–7.
85. Yuan Y et al. Early enteral nutrition improves outcomes of open abdomen in gastrointestinal fistula patients complicated with severe sepsis. Nutr Clin Pract. 2011;26(6):688–94.
86. Dahly EM et al. Role of luminal nutrients and endogenous GLP-2 in intestinal adaptation to mid-small bowel resection. Am J Physiol Gastrointest Liver Physiol. 2003;284(4):G670–82.
87. Drucker DJ. Biological actions and therapeutic potential of the glucagon-like peptides. Gastroenterology. 2002;122(2):531–44.
88. Liu X et al. Synergistic effect of supplemental enteral nutrients and exogenous glucagon-like peptide 2 on intestinal adaptation in a rat model of short bowel syndrome. Am J Clin Nutr. 2006;84(5):1142–50.
89. Rahman SH et al. Intestinal hypoperfusion contributes to gut barrier failure in severe acute pancreatitis. J Gastrointest Surg. 2003;7(1):26–35. discussion 35–6.
90. Murphy MS. Growth factors and the gastrointestinal tract. Nutrition. 1998;14(10):771–4.
91. Kudsk KA et al. Visceral protein response to enteral versus parenteral nutrition and sepsis in patients with trauma. Surgery. 1994;116(3):516–23.
92. Ley R, Peterson D, Gordon J. Ecological and evolutionary forces shaping microbial diversity in the human intestine. Cell. 2006;124:837–48.
93. Nicholson JK. Global systems biology, personalized medicine and molecular epidemiology. Mol Syst Biol. 2006;2:52.
94. Roediger WE. Utilization of nutrients by isolated epithelial cells of the rat colon. Gastroenterology. 1982;83(2):424–9.
95. Harig JM et al. Treatment of diversion colitis with short-chain-fatty acid irrigation. N Engl J Med. 1989;320(1):23–8.
96. Goodlad RA et al. Effects of an elemental diet, inert bulk and different types of dietary fibre on the response of the intestinal epithelium to refeeding in the rat and relationship to plasma gastrin, enteroglucagon, and PYY concentrations. Gut. 1987;28(2):171–80.
97. O'Keefe SJ. Tube feeding, the microbiota, and Clostridium difficile infection. World J Gastroenterol. 2010;16(2):139–42.
98. McDonald LC et al. An epidemic, toxin gene-variant strain of Clostridium difficile. N Engl J Med. 2005;353(23):2433–41.

99. Hell M et al. Probiotics in Clostridium difficile infection: reviewing the need for a multistrain probiotic. Benef Microbes. 2013;4(1):39–51.
100. van Nood E et al. Duodenal infusion of donor feces for recurrent Clostridium difficile. N Engl J Med. 2013;368(5):407–15.
101. Pickard, J.M., et al., *Rapid fucosylation of intestinal epithelium sustains host-commensal symbiosis in sickness.* Nature, 2014;514(7524):638–41.
102. Rice TW et al. Initial trophic vs full enteral feeding in patients with acute lung injury: the EDEN randomized trial. JAMA. 2012;307(8):795–803.
103. Shaw JH, Wolfe RR. Glucose, fatty acid, and urea kinetics in patients with severe pancreatitis. The response to substrate infusion and total parenteral nutrition. Ann Surg. 1986;204(6):665–72.
104. Dvir D, Cohen J, Singer P. Computerized energy balance and complications in critically ill patients: an observational study. Clin Nutr. 2006;25(1):37–44.
105. Bartlett RH et al. Measurement of metabolism in multiple organ failure. Surgery. 1982;92(4):771–9.
106. Casaer MP et al. Early versus late parenteral nutrition in critically ill adults. N Engl J Med. 2011;365(6):506–17.
107. Singer P et al. ESPEN guidelines on parenteral nutrition: intensive care. Clin Nutr. 2009;28(4):387–400.
108. Martindale RG et al. Guidelines for the provision and assessment of nutrition support therapy in the adult critically ill patient: Society of Critical Care Medicine and American Society for Parenteral and Enteral Nutrition: Executive Summary. Crit Care Med. 2009;37(5):1757–61.
109. Heyland DK et al. Canadian clinical practice guidelines for nutrition support in mechanically ventilated, critically ill adult patients. J Parenter Enteral Nutr. 2003;27(5):355–73.
110. Rice TW et al. Enteral omega-3 fatty acid, gamma-linolenic acid, and antioxidant supplementation in acute lung injury. JAMA. 2011;306(14):1574–81.
111. Nehme AE. Nutritional support of the hospitalized patient. The team concept. JAMA. 1980;243(19):1906–8.
112. O'Keefe SJ, Haffejee AA. Nutritional support of the hospitalized patient. Part I. Background, methodology and techniques. S Afr Med J. 1983;63(16):610–5.
113. Apovian CM et al. Board certification and credentialing in nutrition. J Parenter Enteral Nutr. 2010;34 Suppl 6:78S–85S.
114. Marik PE, Pinsky M. Death by parenteral nutrition. Intensive Care Med. 2003;29(6):867–9.
115. O'Keefe S, Foody W, Gill S. Transnasal endoscopic placement of feeding tubes in the intensive care unit. J Parenter Enteral Nutr. 2003;27(5):349–54.
116. O'Keefe S et al. Enteral feeding patients with gastric outlet obstruction. Nutr Clin Pract. 2012;27(1):76–81.
117. O'Keefe SJ, Dicker J. Is plasma albumin concentration useful in the assessment of nutritional status of hospital patients? Eur J Clin Nutr. 1988;42:41–5.
118. O'Keefe SJ, El-Zayadi AR, Carraher TE, Davis M, Williams R. Malnutrition and immuno-incompetence in patients with liver disease. Lancet. 1980;2:615–7.
119. Buzby GP, Mullen JL, Matthews DC, Hobbs CL, Rosato EF. Prognostic nutritional index in gastrointestinal surgery. Am J Surg. 1980;139:160–7.
120. Detsky AS et al. What is subjective global assessment of nutritional status? J Parenter Enteral Nutr. 1987;11:8–13.
121. Baker JP et al. Nutritional assessment. New Engl J Med. 1982;306:969–72. doi:10.1056/NEJM198204223061606.
122. Detsky AS et al. Evaluating the accuracy of nutritional assessment techniques applied to hospitalized patients: methodology and comparisons. J Parenter Enteral Nutr. 1984;8:153–9.
123. Waterlow JC. Classification and definition of protein-calorie malnutrition. Br Med J. 1972;3:566–9.
124. Waterlow JC. Classification and definition of protein-energy malnutrition. Monogr Ser World Health Organ. 1976:530–555.
125. Hill GL, Church J. Energy and protein requirements of general surgical patients requiring intravenous nutrition. Br J Surg. 1984;71:1–9.

126. Elwyn DH, Gump FE, Munro HN, Iles M, Kinney JM. Changes in nitrogen balance of depleted patients with increasing infusions of glucose. Am J Clin Nutr. 1979;32:1597–611.

127. Baker JP et al. Randomized trial of total parenteral nutrition in critically ill patients: metabolic effects of varying glucose-lipid ratios as the energy source. Gastroenterology. 1984;87:53–9.

128. O'Keefe SJ et al. Trypsin secretion and turnover in patients with acute pancreatitis. Am J Physiol Gastrointest Liver Physiol. 2005;289:G181–7. doi:10.1152/ajpgi.00297.2004.

129. Hoffer LJ, Bistrian BR. Appropriate protein provision in critical illness: a systematic and narrative review. Am J Clin Nutr. 2012;96:591–600. doi:10.3945/ajcn.111.032078.

130. McClave SA et al. Guidelines for the provision and assessment of nutrition support therapy in the adult critically ill patient: Society of Critical Care Medicine (SCCM) and American Society for Parenteral and Enteral Nutrition (A.S.P.E.N.). J Parenter Enteral Nutr. 2009;33:277–316. doi:10.1177/0148607109335234.

131. Blackburn GL, O'Keefe SJ. Nutrition in liver failure. Gastroenterology. 1989;97:1049–51.

132. O'Keefe SJ et al. Increased plasma tyrosine concentrations in patients with cirrhosis and fulminant hepatic failure associated with increased plasma tyrosine flux and reduced hepatic oxidation capacity. Gastroenterology. 1981;81:1017–24.

133. O'Keefe SJ, Abraham RR, Davis M, Williams R. Protein turnover in acute and chronic liver disease. Acta Chir Scand Suppl. 1981;507:91–101.

134. O'Keefe SJ, Ogden J, Dicker J. Enteral and parenteral branched chain amino acid-supplemented nutritional support in patients with encephalopathy due to alcoholic liver disease. J Parenter Enteral Nutr. 1987;11:447–53.

135. O'Keefe SJ, Ogden J, Ramjee G, Moldawer LL. Short-term effects of an intravenous infusion of a nutrient solution containing amino acids, glucose and insulin on leucine turnover and amino acid metabolism in patients with liver failure. J Hepatol. 1988;6:101–8.

136. Labadarios D et al. Plasma vitamin levels in patients on prolonged total parenteral nutrition. J Parenter Enteral Nutr. 1988;12:205–11.

137. From the Centers for Disease Control and Prevention. Lactic acidosis traced to thiamine deficiency related to nationwide shortage of multivitamins for total parenteral nutrition – United States, 1997. JAMA. 1997;278:109, 111.

138. Lactic acidosis traced to thiamine deficiency related to nationwide shortage of multivitamins for total parenteral nutrition – United States, 1997. Morb Mortal Wkly Rep. 1997;46:523–8.

139. Deaths associated with thiamine-deficient total parenteral nutrition. Morb Mortal Wkly Rep. 1989;38:43–6.

140. Silk DB, Perrett D, Clark M. Absorption of amino acids and peptides in man. Gut. 1972;13:854–5.

141. Heyland DK et al. Should immunonutrition become routine in critically ill patients? A systematic review of the evidence. JAMA. 2001;286:944–53.

142. Marik PE, Zaloga GP. Immunonutrition in critically ill patients: a systematic review and analysis of the literature. Intensive Care Med. 2008;34:1980–90. doi:10.1007/s00134-008-1213-6.

143. Heyland DK, Samis A. Does immunonutrition in patients with sepsis do more harm than good? Intensive Care Med. 2003;29:669–71. doi:10.1007/s00134-003-1710-6.

144. Esparza J, Boivin MA, Hartshorne MF, Levy H. Equal aspiration rates in gastrically and transpylorically fed critically ill patients. Intensive Care Med. 2001;27:660–4.

145. Heyland DK, Drover JW, MacDonald S, Novak F, Lam M. Effect of postpyloric feeding on gastroesophageal regurgitation and pulmonary microaspiration: results of a randomized controlled trial. Crit Care Med. 2001;29:1495–501.

146. Davies AR et al. Randomized comparison of nasojejunal and nasogastric feeding in critically ill patients. Crit Care Med. 2002;30:586–90.

147. Montejo JC et al. Multicenter, prospective, randomized, single-blind study comparing the efficacy and gastrointestinal complications of early jejunal feeding with early gastric feeding in critically ill patients. Crit Care Med. 2002;30:796–800.

148. Marik PE, Zaloga GP. Early enteral nutrition in acutely ill patients: a systematic review. Crit Care Med. 2001;29:2264–70.

149. Marik PE, Zaloga GP. Gastric versus post-pyloric feeding: a systematic review. Crit Care. 2003;7:R46–51. doi:10.1186/cc2190.
150. Reignier J et al. Early enteral nutrition in mechanically ventilated patients in the prone position. Crit Care Med. 2004;32:94–9. doi:10.1097/01.ccm.0000104208.23542.a8.
151. van der Voort PH, Zandstra DF. Enteral feeding in the critically ill: comparison between the supine and prone positions: a prospective crossover study in mechanically ventilated patients. Crit Care. 2001;5:216–20.
152. Staudinger T et al. Continuous lateral rotation therapy to prevent ventilator-associated pneumonia. Crit Care Med. 2010;38:486–90. doi:10.1097/CCM.0b013e3181bc8218.
153. Montejo JC et al. Gastric residual volume during enteral nutrition in ICU patients: the REGANE study. Intensive Care Med. 2010;36:1386–93. doi:10.1007/s00134-010-1856-y.
154. McClave SA et al. Poor validity of residual volumes as a marker for risk of aspiration in critically ill patients. Crit Care Med. 2005;33:324–30.
155. Jiyong J, Tiancha H, Huiqin W, Jingfen J. Effect of gastric versus post-pyloric feeding on the incidence of pneumonia in critically ill patients: observations from traditional and Bayesian random-effects meta-analysis. Clinical Nutr. 2013;32:8–15. doi:10.1016/j.clnu.2012.07.002.
156. Ho KM, Dobb GJ, Webb SA. A comparison of early gastric and post-pyloric feeding in critically ill patients: a meta-analysis. Intensive Care Med. 2006;32:639–49. doi:10.1007/s00134-006-0128-3.
157. Nguyen NQ et al. Feed intolerance in critical illness is associated with increased basal and nutrient-stimulated plasma cholecystokinin concentrations. Crit Care Med. 2007;35:82–8. doi:10.1097/01.ccm.0000250317.10791.6c.
158. MacLaren R et al. Sequential single doses of cisapride, erythromycin, and metoclopramide in critically ill patients intolerant to enteral nutrition: a randomized, placebo-controlled, crossover study. Crit Care Med. 2000;28:438–44.
159. Kaushik N, Pietraszewski M, Holst JJ, O'Keefe SJD. Enteral feeding without pancreatic stimulation. Pancreas. 2005;31:353–9.
160. O'Keefe SJ, McClave SA. Feeding the injured pancreas. Gastroenterology. 2005;129:1129–30. doi:10.1053/j.gastro.2005.06.077.
161. O'Keefe SJ, Sharma S. Nutrition support in severe acute pancreatitis. Gastroenterol Clin North Am. 2007;36:297–312. doi:10.1016/j.gtc.2007.03.009. viii.
162. O'Keefe S, Foody W, Gill S. Transnasal endoscopic placement of feeding tubes in the intensive care unit. J Parenter Enteral Nutr. 2003;27:349–54. doi:10.1177/0148607103027005349.
163. DeLegge MH et al. Ethical and medicolegal aspects of PEG-tube placement and provision of artificial nutritional therapy. Gastrointest Endosc. 2005;62:952–9. doi:10.1016/j.gie.2005.08.024.
164. Finucane TE, Christmas C, Travis K. Tube feeding in patients with advanced dementia: a review of the evidence. JAMA. 1999;282:1365–70.
165. Lipp A, Lusardi G. Systemic antimicrobial prophylaxis for percutaneous endoscopic gastrostomy. Cochrane Database Syst Rev (online) 2006;CD005571. doi:10.1002/14651858.CD005571.pub2
166. Shike M, Latkany L. Direct percutaneous endoscopic jejunostomy. Gastrointest Endosc Clin N Am. 1998;8:569–80.
167. Waldhausen JH, Shaffrey ME, Skenderis 2nd BS, Jones RS, Schirmer BD. Gastrointestinal myoelectric and clinical patterns of recovery after laparotomy. Ann Surg. 1990;211:777–84. discussion 785.
168. Warren J, Bhalla V, Cresci G. Postoperative diet advancement: surgical dogma vs evidence-based medicine. Nutr Clin Pract. 2011;26:115–25. doi:10.1177/0884533611400231.
169. Pearl ML, Valea FA, Fischer M, Mahler L, Chalas E. A randomized controlled trial of early postoperative feeding in gynecologic oncology patients undergoing intra-abdominal surgery. Obstet Gynecol. 1998;92:94–7.
170. Andersen HK, Lewis SJ, Thomas S. Early enteral nutrition within 24h of colorectal surgery versus later commencement of feeding for postoperative complications. Cochrane Database Syst Rev (online) 2006;CD004080. doi:10.1002/14651858.CD004080.pub2

171. Caddell KA, Martindale R, McClave SA, Miller K. Can the intestinal dysmotility of critical illness be differentiated from postoperative ileus? Curr Gastroenterol Rep. 2011;13:358–67. doi:10.1007/s11894-011-0206-8.

172. Lewis SJ, Franco S, Young G, O'Keefe SJ. Altered bowel function and duodenal bacterial overgrowth in patients treated with omeprazole. Aliment Pharmacol Ther. 1996;10:557–61.

173. O'Keefe SJ et al. Short bowel syndrome and intestinal failure: consensus definitions and overview. Clin Gastroenterol Hepatol. 2006;4(1):6–10.

174. Koretz RL. What supports nutritional support? Dig Dis Sci. 1984;29(6):577–88.

175. Koretz RL. My grandmother's intravenous chicken soup. Gastroenterology. 1993;105(1):299–300.

176. Rhee, P., et al., What happened to total parenteral nutrition? The disappearance of its use in a trauma intensive care unit. J Trauma, 2007. 63(6): p. 1215–22.

177. Wischmeyer PE, Heyland DK. The future of critical care nutrition therapy. Crit Care Clin. 2010;26(3):433–41. vii.

178. Lidder P et al. Combining enteral with parenteral nutrition to improve postoperative glucose control. Br J Nutr. 2010;103(11):1635–41.

179. Denny Jr DF. Placement and management of long-term central venous access catheters and ports. Am J Roentgenol. 1993;161(2):385–93.

180. Maisonneuve N et al. Parenteral nutrition practices in hospital pharmacies in Switzerland, France, and Belgium. Nutrition. 2004;20(6):528–35.

181. Solomons NW. Trace elements. In: Rombeau JL, editor. Clinical nutrition parenteral nutrition. 2nd ed. Philadelphia, USA: WB Saunders; 1993. p. 150–83. Chapter 8.

182. Fahy BG, Sheehy AM, Coursin DB. Glucose control in the intensive care unit. Crit Care Med. 2009;37(5):1769–76.

183. Burnes JU, O'Keefe SJ, Fleming CR, Devine RM, Berkner S, Herrick L. Home parenteral nutrition–a 3-year analysis of clinical and laboratory monitoring. J Parenter Enteral Nutr. 1992;16(4):327–32.

184. Howard L, Heaphey L, Fleming CR, Lininger L, Steiger E. Four years of North American registry home parenteral nutrition outcome data and their implications for patient management. J Parenter Enteral Nutr. 1991;15(4):384–93.

185. Howard L, Ament M, Fleming CR, Shike M, Steiger E. Current use and clinical outcome of home parenteral and enteral nutrition therapies in the United States. Gastroenterology. 1995;109(2):355–65.

186. Denny Jr DF. Placement and management of long-term central venous access catheters and ports. AJR Am J Roentgenol. 1993;161(2):385–93.

187. Nordgaard I, Hansen BS, Mortensen PB. Importance of colonic support for energy absorption as small-bowel failure proceeds. Am J Clin Nutr. 1996;64(2):222–31.

188. Matarese LE, Jeppesen PB, O'Keefe SJ. Short bowel syndrome in adults: the need for an interdisciplinary approach and coordinated care. J Parenter Enteral Nutr. 2014;38:60S–4S.

189. O'Keefe SJ, Burnes JU, Thompson RL. Recurrent sepsis in home parenteral nutrition patients: an analysis of risk factors. J Parenter Enteral Nutr. 1994;18(3):256–63.

190. John BK, Khan MA, Speerhas R, et al. Ethanol lock therapy in reducing catheter-related bloodstream infections in adult home parenteral nutrition patients: results of a retrospective study. J Parenter Enteral Nutr. 2012;36(5):603–10.

191. Bern MM, Lokich JJ, Wallach SR, et al. Very low doses of warfarin can prevent thrombosis in central venous catheters. A randomized prospective trial. Ann Intern Med. 1990;112(6):423–8.

192. O'Keefe SJ, Emerling M, Koritsky D, et al. Nutrition and quality of life following small intestinal transplantation. Am J Gastroenterol. 2007;102(5):1093–100.

193. Robinovitch AE. Home total parenteral nutrition: a psycho-social viewpoint. J Parenter Enteral Nutr. 1981;5(6):522–5.

194. Jeppesen PB, Langholz E, Mortensen PB. Quality of life in patients receiving home parenteral nutrition. Gut. 1999;44(6):844–52.

195. Bern MM, Bothe Jr A, Bistrian B, Champagne CD, Keane MS, Blackburn GL. Prophylaxis against central vein thrombosis with low-dose warfarin. Surgery. 1986;99(2):216–21.

196. Cavicchi M, Beau P, Crenn P, Degott C, Messing B. Prevalence of liver disease and contributing factors in patients receiving home parenteral nutrition for permanent intestinal failure. Ann Intern Med. 2000;132(7):525–32.

197. Kelly DA. Preventing parenteral nutrition liver disease. Early Hum Dev. 2010;86(11):683–7.

198. Puder M, Valim C, Meisel JA, et al. Parenteral fish oil improves outcomes in patients with parenteral nutrition-associated liver injury. Ann Surg. 2009;250(3):395–402.

199. Le HD, de Meijer VE, Robinson EM, et al. Parenteral fish-oil-based lipid emulsion improves fatty acid profiles and lipids in parenteral nutrition-dependent children. Am J Clin Nutr. 2011;94(3):749–58.

200. Mennigen R, Bruewer M. Effect of probiotics on intestinal barrier function. Ann N Y Acad Sci. 2009;1165:183–9.

201. White JS, Hoper M, Parks RW, Clements WD, Diamond T, Bengmark S. The probiotic bacterium Lactobacillus plantarum species 299 reduces intestinal permeability in experimental biliary obstruction. Lett Appl Microbiol. 2006;42(1):19–23.

202. Raphael BP, Duggan C. Prevention and treatment of intestinal failure-associated liver disease in children. Semin Liver Dis. 2012;32(4):341–7.

203. Beau P, Labat-Labourdette J, Ingrand P, Beauchant M. Is ursodeoxycholic acid an effective therapy for total parenteral nutrition-related liver disease? J Hepatol. 1994;20(2):240–4.

204. Anderson CM. Long-term survival with six inches of small intestine. Br Med J. 1965;1(5432):419–22.

205. Buchman AL. The medical and surgical management of short bowel syndrome. MedGenMed: Medscape general medicine. 2004;6(2):12.

206. Carbonnel F, Cosnes J, Chevret S, et al. The role of anatomic factors in nutritional autonomy after extensive small bowel resection. JPEN. Journal of parenteral and enteral nutrition. Jul-Aug 1996;20(4):275–280.

207. O'Keefe SJ et al. Long-acting somatostatin analogue therapy and protein metabolism in patients with jejunostomies. Gastroenterology. 1994;107(2):379–88.

208. Vipperla K, O'Keefe SJ. Teduglutide for the treatment of short bowel syndrome. Expert Rev Gastroenterol Hepatol. 2011;5(6):665–78.

209. O'Keefe SJ, Peterson ME, Fleming CR. Octreotide as an adjunct to home parenteral nutrition in the management of permanent end-jejunostomy syndrome. J Parenter Enteral Nutr. 1994;18(1):26–34.

210. McIntyre PB, Fitchew M, Lennard-Jones JE. Patients with a high jejunostomy do not need a special diet. Gastroenterology. 1986;91(1):25–33.

211. Woolf GM et al. Diet for patients with a short bowel: high fat or high carbohydrate? Gastroenterology. 1983;84(4):823–8.

212. Simko V et al. High-fat diet in a short bowel syndrome. Intestinal absorption and gastroenteropancreatic hormone responses. Dig Dis Sci. 1980;25(5):333–9.

213. DiCecco S et al. Nutritional intake of gut failure patients on home parenteral nutrition. J Parenter Enteral Nutr. 1987;11(6):529–32.

214. Lennard-Jones JE. Oral rehydration solutions in short bowel syndrome. Clin Ther. 1990;12(Suppl A):129–37. discussion 138.

215. Williamson RC. Intestinal adaptation (second of two parts). Mechanisms of control. N Engl J Med. 1978;298(26):1444–50.

216. Williamson RC. Intestinal adaptation (first of two parts). Structural, functional and cytokinetic changes. N Engl J Med. 1978;298(25):1393–402.

217. Byrne TA et al. Growth hormone, glutamine, and a modified diet enhance nutrient absorption in patients with severe short bowel syndrome. J Parenter Enteral Nutr. 1995;19(4):296–302.

218. Wales PW et al. Human growth hormone and glutamine for patients with short bowel syndrome. Cochrane Database Syst Rev. 2010;6, CD006321.

219. Gleeson MH et al. Endocrine tumour in kidney affecting small bowel structure, motility, and absorptive function. Gut. 1971;12(10):773–82.

220. Drucker DJ et al. Induction of intestinal epithelial proliferation by glucagon-like peptide 2. Proc Natl Acad Sci U S A. 1996;93(15):7911–6.

221. Martin GR, Beck PL, Sigalet DL. Gut hormones, and short bowel syndrome: the enigmatic role of glucagon-like peptide-2 in the regulation of intestinal adaptation. World J Gastroenterol. 2006;12(26):4117–29.

222. Jeppesen PB et al. Randomised placebo-controlled trial of teduglutide in reducing parenteral nutrition and/or intravenous fluid requirements in patients with short bowel syndrome. Gut. 2011;60(7):902–14.

223. O'Keefe SJ et al. Safety and efficacy of teduglutide after 52 weeks of treatment in patients with short bowel intestinal failure. Clin Gastroenterol Hepatol. 2013;11(7):815–23.e1-3.

224. Jeppesen PB et al. Teduglutide reduces need for parenteral support among patients with short bowel syndrome with intestinal failure. Gastroenterology. 2012;143(6):1473–81.e3.

225. Kunkel D et al. Efficacy of the glucagon-like peptide-1 agonist exenatide in the treatment of short bowel syndrome. Neurogastroenterol Motil. 2011;23(8):739–e328.

226. Seguy D et al. Low-dose growth hormone in adult home parenteral nutrition-dependent short bowel syndrome patients: a positive study. Gastroenterology. 2003;124(2):293–302.

227. O'Keefe SJ. Candidacy for intestinal transplantation. Am J Gastroenterol. 2006;101(7): 1644–6.

228. Grant D et al. 2003 Report of the intestine transplant registry: a new era has dawned. Ann Surg. 2005;241(4):607–13.

229. O'Keefe SJ et al. Endoscopic evaluation of small intestine transplant grafts. Transplantation. 2012;94(7):757–62.

230. Pironi L et al. Candidates for intestinal transplantation: a multicenter survey in Europe. Am J Gastroenterol. 2006;101(7):1633–43. quiz 1679.

231. O'Keefe SJ et al. Nutrition in the management of necrotizing pancreatitis. Clin Gastroenterol Hepatol. 2003;1(4):315–21.

232. Makhija R, Kingsnorth AN. Cytokine storm in acute pancreatitis. J Hepatobiliary Pancreat Surg. 2002;9(4):401–10.

233. Giakoustidis A, Mudan SS, Giakoustidis D. Dissecting the stress activating signaling pathways in acute pancreatitis. Hepatogastroenterology. 2010;57(99–100):653–6.

234. Shi C et al. Role of nuclear factor-kappaB, reactive oxygen species and cellular signaling in the early phase of acute pancreatitis. Scand J Gastroenterol. 2005;40(1):103–8.

235. Steer ML. Frank Brooks memorial lecture: the early intraacinar cell events which occur during acute pancreatitis. Pancreas. 1998;17(1):31–7.

236. Liu HS et al. Effect of NF-kappaB and p38 MAPK in activated monocytes/macrophages on pro-inflammatory cytokines of rats with acute pancreatitis. World J Gastroenterol. 2003;9(11):2513–8.

237. Vaquero E et al. Localized pancreatic NF-kappaB activation and inflammatory response in taurocholate-induced pancreatitis. Am J Physiol Gastrointest Liver Physiol. 2001;280(6):G197–208.

238. Leindler L et al. Importance of cytokines, nitric oxide, and apoptosis in the pathological process of necrotizing pancreatitis in rats. Pancreas. 2004;29(2):157–61.

239. Inoue K et al. Further evidence for endothelin as an important mediator of pancreatic and intestinal ischemia in severe acute pancreatitis. Pancreas. 2003;26(3):218–23.

240. Fong YM et al. The acute splanchnic and peripheral tissue metabolic response to endotoxin in humans. J Clin Invest. 1990;85(6):1896–904.

241. Ammori BJ. Role of the gut in the course of severe acute pancreatitis. Pancreas. 2003;26(2):122–9.

242. Johnson CD et al. Double blind, randomised, placebo controlled study of a platelet activating factor antagonist, lexipafant, in the treatment and prevention of organ failure in predicted severe acute pancreatitis. Gut. 2001;48(1):62–9.

243. O'Keefe SJ, Lee R, Abou-Assi S. The effect of acute pancreatitis on the synthesis and turnover of trypsin in humans. Gastroenterology. 2002;122(4):439.

244. Keller J, Holst JJ, Layer P. Inhibition of human pancreatic and biliary output but not intestinal motility by physiological intraileal lipid loads. Am J Physiol Gastrointest Liver Physiol. 2006;290(4):G704–9.

245. Vu MK et al. Does jejunal feeding activate exocrine pancreatic secretion? Eur J Clin Invest. 1999;29(12):1053–9.

246. Hegazi R et al. Early jejunal feeding initiation and clinical outcomes in patients with severe acute pancreatitis. JPEN J Parenter Enteral Nutr. 2011;35(1):91–6.

247. Bakker OJ et al. Early versus on-demand nasoenteric tube feeding in acute pancreatitis. New Engl J Med. 2014:372;21.

248. Ranson JH et al. Prognostic signs and the role of operative management in acute pancreatitis. Surg Gynecol Obstet. 1974;139(1):69–81.

249. Knaus WA et al. APACHE II: a severity of disease classification system. Crit Care Med. 1985;13(10):818–29.

250. Mofidi R et al. Association between early systemic inflammatory response, severity of multiorgan dysfunction and death in acute pancreatitis. Br J Surg. 2006;93(6):738–44.

251. Simchuk EJ et al. Computed tomography severity index is a predictor of outcomes for severe pancreatitis. Am J Surg. 2000;179(5):352–5.

252. Papachristou GI, Whitcomb DC. Inflammatory markers of disease severity in acute pancreatitis. Clin Lab Med. 2005;25(1):17–37.

253. Besselink MG et al. Probiotic prophylaxis in predicted severe acute pancreatitis: a randomised, double-blind, placebo-controlled trial. Lancet. 2008;371(9613):651–9.

254. Villatoro E, Mulla M, Larvin M. Antibiotic therapy for prophylaxis against infection of pancreatic necrosis in acute pancreatitis. Cochrane Database Syst Rev. 2010;5, CD002941.

255. Bai Y et al. Prophylactic antibiotics cannot reduce infected pancreatic necrosis and mortality in acute necrotizing pancreatitis: evidence from a meta-analysis of randomized controlled trials. Am J Gastroenterol. 2008;103(1):104–10.

256. Bradley 3rd EL, Dexter ND. Management of severe acute pancreatitis: a surgical odyssey. Ann Surg. 2010;251(1):6–17.

257. Marotta F et al. Pancreatic enzyme replacement therapy. Importance of gastric acid secretion, H2-antagonists, and enteric coating. Dig Dis Sci. 1989;34(3):456–61.

258. O'Keefe SJD. Physiological response of the human pancreas to enteral and parenteral feeding. Curr Opin Clin Nutr Metab Care. 2006;9(5):622–8.

259. O'Keefe SJD, Cariem AK, Levy M. The exacerbation of pancreatic endocrine dysfunction by potent pancreatic exocrine supplements in patients with chronic pancreatitis. J Clin Gastroenterol. 2001;32(4):319–23.

260. Duggan SN et al. High prevalence of osteoporosis in patients with chronic pancreatitis: a systematic review and meta-analysis. Clin Gastroenterol Hepatol. 2013;12:219–28.

261. O'Keefe SJ, Adam J. Assessment of adequacy of pancreatic enzyme replacement with the multiple-phase carbon-14-triolein test. S Afr Med J. 1984;66(20):763–5.

262. O'Keefe SJD et al. Physiological evaluation of the severity of pancreatic exocrine dysfunction during endoscopy. Pancreas. 2007;35(1):30–6.

263. Ayling RM. New faecal tests in gastroenterology. Ann Clin Biochem. 2012;49(Pt 1):44–54.

264. Plauth M, Schutz T. Branched-chain amino acids in liver disease: new aspects of long known phenomena. Curr Opin Clin Nutr Metab Care. 2011;14(1):61–6.

265. Munro HN, Fernstrom JD, Wurtman RJ. Insulin, plasma aminoacid imbalance, and hepatic coma. Lancet. 1975;1(7909):722–4.

266. James JH et al. Hyperammonaemia, plasma aminoacid imbalance, and blood-brain aminoacid transport: a unified theory of portal-systemic encephalopathy. Lancet. 1979;2(8146):772–5.

267. Naylor CD et al. Parenteral nutrition with branched-chain amino acids in hepatic encephalopathy. A meta-analysis. Gastroenterology. 1989;97(4):1033–42.

268. Plauth M et al. ESPEN guidelines on enteral nutrition: liver disease. Clin Nutr. 2006;25(2):285–94.

269. Abel RM et al. Improved survival from acute renal failure after treatment with intravenous essential L-amino acids and glucose. Results of a prospective, double-blind study. N Engl J Med. 1973;288(14):695–9.

270. Feinstein EI et al. Total parenteral nutrition with high or low nitrogen intakes in patients with acute renal failure. Kidney Int Suppl. 1983;16:S319–23.
271. Mirtallo JM, Kudsk KA, Ebbert ML. Nutritional support of patients with renal disease. Clin Pharm. 1984;3(3):253–63.
272. Nakasaki H et al. Complication of parenteral nutrition composed of essential amino acids and histidine in adults with renal failure. J Parenter Enteral Nutr. 1993;17(1):86–90.
273. Motil KJ, Harmon WE, Grupe WE. Complications of essential amino acid hyperalimentation in children with acute renal failure. J Parenter Enteral Nutr. 1980;4(1):32–5.
274. Li Y et al. Nutritional support for acute kidney injury. Cochrane Database Syst Rev. 2012;8, CD005426.
275. Bistrian BR, Blackburn GL, Hallowell E, Heddle R. Protein status of general surgical patients. JAMA. 1974;230:858–60.
276. O'Keefe SJ, Dicker J, Delport I. Incidence of malnutrition in adult patients at Groote Schuur Hospital, 1984. S Afr Med J. 1986;70:16–20.
277. O'Keefe SJ. Malnutrition among adult hospitalized patients in Zululand during the drought of 1983. S Afr Med J. 1983;64:628–9.
278. Blackburn GL, Wollner S, Bistrian BR. Nutrition support in the intensive care unit: an evolving science. Arch Surg. 2010;145:533–8. doi:10.1001/archsurg.2010.97.
279. Hegazi R et al. Early jejunal feeding initiation and clinical outcomes in patients with severe acute pancreatitis. J Parenter Enteral Nutr. 2011;35:91–6. doi:10.1177/0148607110376196.
280. Choban P, Dickerson R, Malone A, Worthington P, Compher C. A.S.P.E.N. Clinical guidelines: nutrition support of hospitalized adult patients with obesity. J Parenter Enteral Nutr. 2013;37:714–44. doi:10.1177/0148607113499374.
281. McClave SA, Martindale RG, Kiraly L. The use of indirect calorimetry in the intensive care unit. Curr Opin Clin Nutr Metab Care. 2013;16:202–8. doi:10.1097/MCO.0b013e32835dbc54.
282. National Institutes of Health. Clinical guidelines on the identification, evaluation, and treatment of overweight and obesity in adults – the evidence report. Obes Res. 1998;6 Suppl 2:51S–209S.
283. Colquitt JL, Pickett K, Loveman E, Frampton GK. Surgery for weight loss in adults. Cochrane Database Syst Rev. 2014;8, CD003641. doi:10.1002/14651858.CD003641.pub4.
284. Madsbad S, Dirksen C, Holst JJ. Mechanisms of changes in glucose metabolism and body-weight after bariatric surgery. Lancet Diabetes Endocrinol. 2014;2:152–64. doi:10.1016/s2213-8587(13)70218-3.
285. Liou AP et al. Conserved shifts in the gut microbiota due to gastric bypass reduce host weight and adiposity. Sci Transl Med. 2013;5:178ra141. doi:10.1126/scitranslmed.3005687.
286. Wong VW et al. Molecular characterization of the fecal microbiota in patients with nonalcoholic steatohepatitis – a longitudinal study. PLoS One. 2013;8:e62885. doi:10.1371/journal.pone.0062885.
287. Zhu L et al. Characterization of gut microbiomes in nonalcoholic steatohepatitis (NASH) patients: a connection between endogenous alcohol and NASH. Hepatology. 2013;57:601–9. doi:10.1002/hep.26093.
288. Henao-Mejia J et al. Inflammasome-mediated dysbiosis regulates progression of NAFLD and obesity. Nature. 2012;482:179–85. doi:10.1038/nature10809.
289. Li JV et al. Metabolic surgery profoundly influences gut microbial-host metabolic cross-talk. Gut. 2011;60:1214–23. doi:10.1136/gut.2010.234708.
290. Stevens J et al. The effect of age on the association between body-mass index and mortality. N Engl J Med. 1998;338(1):1–7.
291. Wallace JI et al. Involuntary weight loss in older outpatients: incidence and clinical significance. J Am Geriatr Soc. 1995;43(4):329–37.
292. Liu L et al. Undernutrition and risk of mortality in elderly patients within 1 year of hospital discharge. J Gerontol A Biol Sci Med Sci. 2002;57(11):M741–6.
293. Grabowski DC, Ellis JE. High body mass index does not predict mortality in older people: analysis of the longitudinal study of aging. J Am Geriatr Soc. 2001;49(7):968–79.
294. Flegal KM et al. Excess deaths associated with underweight, overweight, and obesity. JAMA. 2005;293(15):1861–7.

295. Wassertheil-Smoller S et al. Relation of low body mass to death and stroke in the systolic hypertension in the elderly program. The SHEP Cooperative Research Group. Arch Intern Med. 2000;160(4):494–500.

296. Smits GJ, Lefebvre RA. Influence of age on the signal transduction pathway of non-adrenergic non-cholinergic neurotransmitters in the rat gastric fundus. Br J Pharmacol. 1995;114(3):640–7.

297. Sturm K et al. Energy intake and appetite are related to antral area in healthy young and older subjects. Am J Clin Nutr. 2004;80(3):656–67.

298. Brogna A et al. Radioisotopic assessment of gastric emptying of solids in elderly subjects. Aging Clin Exp Res. 2006;18(6):493–6.

299. Di Francesco V et al. Unbalanced serum leptin and ghrelin dynamics prolong postprandial satiety and inhibit hunger in healthy elderly: another reason for the "anorexia of aging". Am J Clin Nutr. 2006;83(5):1149–52.

300. Schneider SM et al. Effects of age, malnutrition and refeeding on the expression and secretion of ghrelin. Clin Nutr. 2008;27(5):724–31.

301. Serra-Prat M et al. The role of ghrelin in the energy homeostasis of elderly people: a population-based study. J Endocrinol Invest. 2007;30(6):484–90.

302. Rigamonti AE et al. Plasma ghrelin concentrations in elderly subjects: comparison with anorexic and obese patients. J Endocrinol. 2002;175(1):R1–5.

303. Tai K et al. Effects of nutritional supplementation on the appetite and energy intake responses to IV cholecystokinin in older adults. Appetite. 2010;55(3):473–7.

304. Sturm K et al. Appetite, food intake, and plasma concentrations of cholecystokinin, ghrelin, and other gastrointestinal hormones in undernourished older women and well-nourished young and older women. J Clin Endocrinol Metab. 2003;88(8):3747–55.

305. Di Francesco V et al. The quantity of meal fat influences the profile of postprandial hormones as well as hunger sensation in healthy elderly people. J Am Med Dir Assoc. 2010;11(3):188–93.

306. Wilson MM, Morley JE. Invited review: aging and energy balance. J Appl Physiol (1985). 2003;95(4):1728–36.

307. Kaiser MJ et al. Validation of the mini nutritional assessment short-form (MNA-SF): a practical tool for identification of nutritional status. J Nutr Health Aging. 2009;13(9):782–8.

308. Ferguson M et al. Development of a valid and reliable malnutrition screening tool for adult acute hospital patients. Nutrition. 1999;15(6):458–64.

309. Milne AC, Avenell A, Potter J. Meta-analysis: protein and energy supplementation in older people. Ann Intern Med. 2006;144(1):37–48.

310. Simmons SF, Patel AV. Nursing home staff delivery of oral liquid nutritional supplements to residents at risk for unintentional weight loss. J Am Geriatr Soc. 2006;54(9):1372–6.

311. Yeh SS et al. Improvement in quality-of-life measures and stimulation of weight gain after treatment with megestrol acetate oral suspension in geriatric cachexia: results of a double-blind, placebo-controlled study. J Am Geriatr Soc. 2000;48(5):485–92.

312. Mihara IQ, McCombs JS, Williams BR. The impact of mirtazapine compared with non-TCA antidepressants on weight change in nursing facility residents. Consult Pharm. 2005;20(3):217–23.

313. Teno JM et al. Does feeding tube insertion and its timing improve survival? J Am Geriatr Soc. 2012;60(10):1918–21.

Further Reading

Molecular biology of the cell. Alberts B, et al., editors. 5th ed. Garland Science. New York, NY: Taylor and Francis Group, LLC; 2008.

Index

© Springer Science+Business Media New York 2015
S.J.D. O'Keefe, *The Principles and Practice of Nutritional Support*,
DOI 10.1007/978-1-4939-1779-2